Find What You Need in This Book

Index: Look up your health issues in the index at the back.

Symptom Guides: Look for your symptoms in the easy-to-use charts starting on **page 59**.

Table of Contents: Check the table of contents on **pages vi** to **ix**. It lists all the topics in the book. Each colored section has its own table of contents on the first page.

Color Bars: Use the color bars on the edge of the pages to browse for topics that interest you:

Green	Saving money and getting better care
Red	First aid and emergency topics, A to Z
Orange	Common health problems, A to Z
Blue	Major chronic diseases, A to Z
Purple	Healthy habits, preventive care, and safety tips
Gold	Aging issues, caregiving tips, and end-of-life planning

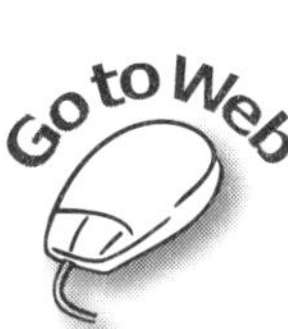

Find Even More

Get more of what you're looking for!

When you see this icon in the book, go to the Healthwise® Knowledgebase at **gotoweb.healthwise.net/life**. Just enter the code in the Web site's search box to reach decision-focused, action-oriented tools related to the information in this book.

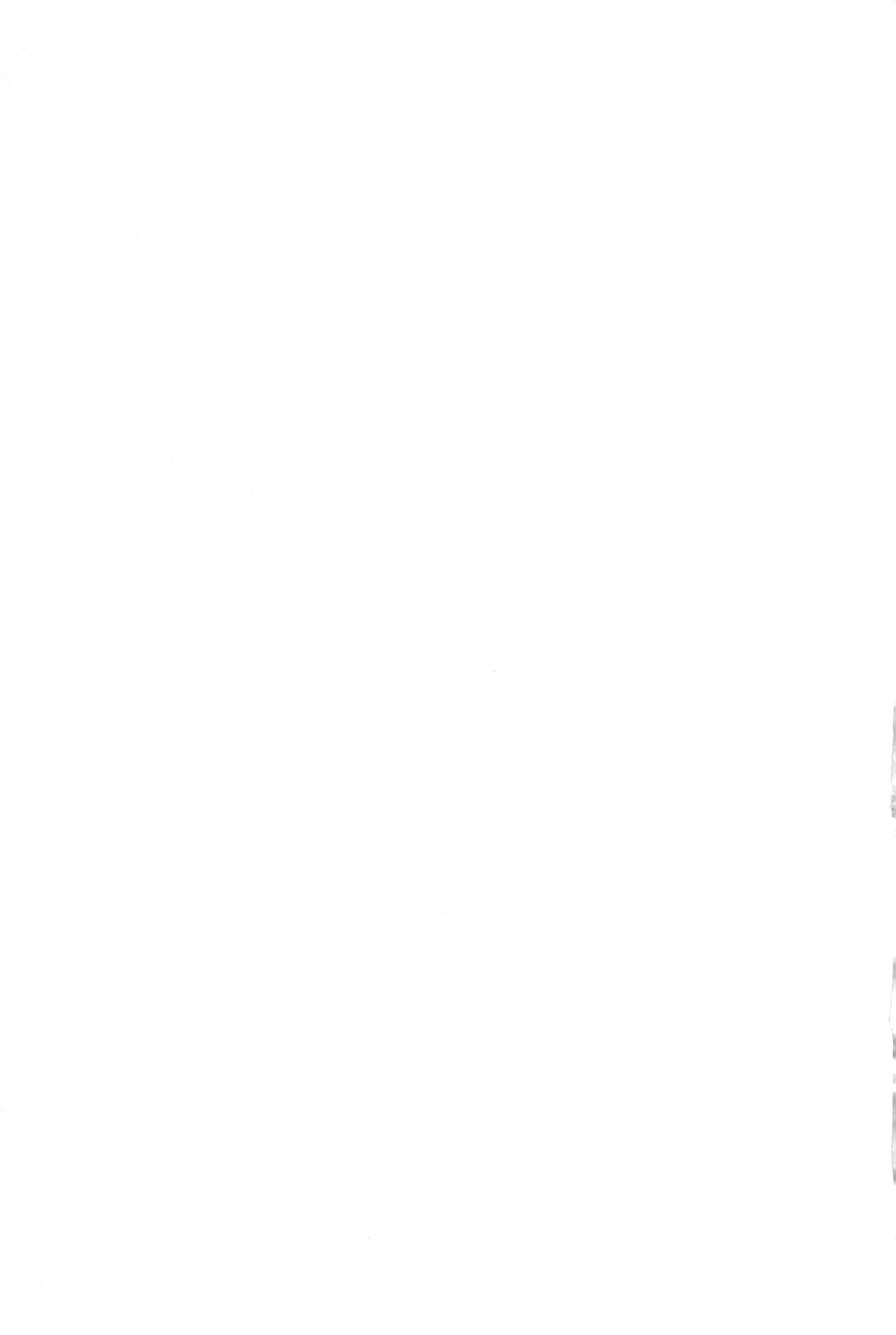

Healthwise® for Life

A Self-Care Guide for People Age 50 and Better

Better Care, Lower Costs

First Aid and Emergencies

Common Health Problems

Living Better With Chronic Disease

Staying Healthy

Growing Older: Myths, Gifts, and Realities

7th Edition

Molly Mettler and Donald W. Kemper

Katy E. Magee, Editor
Steven L. Schneider, MD, Medical Editor
A. Patrice Burgess, MD, Medical Editor

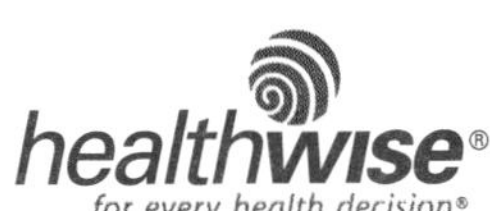

Healthwise
P.O. Box 1989
Boise, Idaho 83701

This information is not intended to replace the advice of a doctor. Healthwise disclaims any liability for your use of this information.

First edition 1992
Seventh edition 2007

7hwfl/1st/5-07
ISBN 1-932921-31-1

Printed in the United States of America

Printed on recycled paper

About Healthwise

Healthwise is a nonprofit organization. Our mission is to help people make better health decisions. People use our handbooks, online content, and nurse call center resources nearly 90 million times a year for help with their health decisions. To learn more about us, please visit www.healthwise.org.

About This Book

No book can replace the need for doctors. And no doctor can replace the need for people to care for themselves. This new edition of *Healthwise® for Life* will help people over age 50 deal with common health problems and chronic diseases, stay healthy as they grow older, work well with their doctors, and avoid unnecessary care and costs. We trust that you will find the book easy to use and easy to understand.

If you have access to the Internet, you can get much more in-depth information about your health questions. Each time you see the "Go to Web" icon, you will find instructions on how to reach information in the Healthwise® Knowledgebase that can help you make a decision, master a skill, or learn more about your health.

If your doctor gives you advice that conflicts with this book, follow your doctor's advice. Because your doctor knows your specific history and needs, his or her advice may be the best for you. Likewise, if you follow the book's self-care tips but do not get positive results, be sure to talk with your doctor.

This book is only a guide. We cannot guarantee that it will work for you in every case. Nor will Healthwise accept responsibility for any problems that may occur from following its guidelines. Remember to use your common sense and good judgment.

We wish you the best of health!

Molly Mettler and Donald W. Kemper

Table of Contents

About Healthwise v
Acknowledgements x

Better Care, Lower Costs

Better Care at Lower Costs 2
Work Closely With Your Doctor 2
Smart Money Tips for Medicines . . . 3
Save the Emergency Room for Emergencies. 6
Smart Money Tips for Medical Tests . 7
Smart Decisions: Know Your Treatment Options . . . 8
Medicare: The Basics 9

First Aid and Emergencies

Bites—Animals and Humans 12
Bites and Stings—Insects, Spiders, and Ticks. 13
Bleeding Emergencies 17
Blood Under a Nail 18
Breathing Emergencies and CPR. . 19
Bruises. 22
Burns. 23
Chemical Burns 25
Choking 26
Cuts and Punctures 27
Dehydration 29
Eye (Object in) 31
Fainting and Unconsciousness . . . 33
Falls 34
Frostbite 35
Head Injury 36
Heart Attack 38
Heat Sickness 39
Hypothermia. 41
Nosebleeds 43
Scrapes 44
Seizures 45
Shock 47
Splinters 49
Strains, Sprains, and Broken Bones 49
Stroke 54
Suicide. 55
Sunburn 56

Common Health Problems

Symptom Guides 59
Chest, Heart, and Lung Problems 59
Digestive Problems 60
Skin Problems 61
Eye and Vision Problems 62
Ear and Hearing Problems 63
Nose and Throat Problems 63
Headaches. 64
Urinary Problems 65
Abdominal Pain 66
Abuse and Violence 68
Alcohol and Drugs. 70
Allergies 73

Anger and Hostility 76
Anxiety and Panic 77
Back Pain 79
Bladder and Kidney Infections . . . 90
Bladder Control 92
Blisters. 95
Blood Clots in the Leg. 96
Boils 98
Breast Problems. 99
Breathing Problems 101
Bronchitis 102
Bunions and Hammer Toes. . . . 103
Bursitis and Tendinosis 105
Calluses and Corns 109
Canker Sores 109
Carpal Tunnel Syndrome 110
Cataracts 113
Chest Pain 114
Cold Hands and Feet 117
Cold Sores 118
Colds 119
Colorectal Cancer 121
Confusion and Memory Loss . . . 122
Constipation 124
Cough 126
Diarrhea 127
Diverticular Disease. 129
Dizziness and Vertigo 130
Dry Mouth 133
Dry Skin 134
Ear Infections 135
Earwax 137
Erection Problems. 138
Eye Problems 140
Pinkeye. 140
Dry Eyes 143
Blood in the Eye 143
Eyelid Problems 144
Fatigue and Weakness 145
Female Pelvic Problems. 148
Fever 150
Fibromyalgia 152
Flu 153
Food Poisoning 155
Fungal Infections 157
Gallstones 159
Gas. 161
Glaucoma 162
Gout 163
Gum Disease 164
Hair Loss. 165
Headaches. 166
Hearing Problems 170
Hearing Loss. 171
Ringing in the Ears 173
Heartbeat Changes 174
Heartburn 176
Heel Pain and Plantar Fasciitis . . 178
Hemorrhoids and Rectal Problems 180
Hernia 182
High Blood Pressure 183
High Cholesterol. 186
Hives 188

Ingrown Toenail 189
Irritable Bowel Syndrome 190
Jaw Pain and Temporomandibular Disorder. . 192
Kidney Stones 193
Knee Problems 194
Laryngitis 196
Leg Pain and Muscle Cramps. . . 197
Lung Cancer 200
Menopause 201
Neck Pain 204
Osteoporosis. 207
Peripheral Artery Disease. 208
Pneumonia 210
Polymyalgia Rheumatica 212
Pressure Sores 213
Prostate Cancer 214
Prostate Enlargement. 215
Prostatitis 217
Rashes. 218
Rosacea 221
Sexually Transmitted Diseases (STDs) 222
Shingles 225
Sinusitis 227
Skin Cancer 230
Skin Growths and Spots 231
Sleep Problems 232
Sore Throat 235
Swollen Lymph Nodes. 236
Thyroid, Low (Hypothyroidism) . . 238
Toothache 240
Tooth Injury 241
Tremor (Shaking) 241
Ulcers 243
Vaginitis 245
Varicose Veins 247
Vision Changes 248
Vomiting 253
Warts. 254

Living Better With Chronic Disease

Mastering Chronic Disease: The Basics 258
Living Better With Alzheimer's Disease. 261
Living Better With Arthritis 266
Living Better With Asthma 271
Living Better With Cancer. 276
Living Better With COPD 282
Living Better With Coronary Artery Disease 287
Living Better With Depression . . 292
Living Better With Diabetes. . . . 296
Living Better With Heart Failure . 303
Living Better With Chronic Kidney Disease. 308
Living Better After a Stroke 314

Staying Healthy

Get Immunized 320
Wellness Exams and Screening Tests 321
Reaching a Healthy Weight 326
Healthy Eating. 333
Exercise for Health 340

Quitting Smoking 351
Take Care of Your Teeth. 354
Managing Stress 356
Keep Your Brain Healthy 359
Sex and Aging 361
Safe Sex 363
Preventing Falls 364
Driving: Are You Safe?. 365
Master Your Medicines 367

Growing Older: Myths, Gifts, and Realities

Myths of Aging. 372
Gifts of Aging 374
The Biggest Challenge of Aging: Loss and Life Change 376
A Caregiver's Guide 378
Planning for the Future 382
Dying Well 387
Index. 389

Acknowledgements

To make a book "easy to use and easy to understand" is not an easy task; it takes skill and dedication. We are especially grateful to our editor, Katy Magee, whose patient good humor and persistent quest for excellence made this edition of *Healthwise® for Life* possible. Big thanks also go to the ever-hardworking book production team: Terrie Britton and John Kubisiak, for their layout, design, and typesetting expertise; Jo-Ann Kachigian, whose careful proofreading made the book better; Kourtney Funke, for her work in creating the new cover; and Andrea Blum, who kept it all together. Lila Havens helped readable content emerge from the myriad comments of our medical reviewers and wrote some of the new material. And both she and Michele Cronen found elegant ways to improve on what was already there.

Patrice Burgess, MD, and Steve Schneider, MD, provided thoughtful guidance and ensured the medical accuracy of every topic. We also thank the following health professionals for the clinical wisdom and experience they shared in reviewing the book:

Heather O. Chambliss, PhD
Arden G. Christen, DDS
Alan C. Dalkin, MD
Jeffrey Ginsberg, MD
William M. Green, MD
Carla Herman, MD
Barrie G. Hurwitz, MD
Adam Husney, MD
Carol L. Karp, MD
Robert B. Keller, MD
Robert A. Kloner, MD
Steven Kmucha, MD
Karin Lindholm, DO
Patrick McMahon, MD
Joy Melnikow, MD
David Mendelssohn, MD
Alexander Murray, MD
Joseph F. O'Donnell, MD
Theresa O'Young, PharmD
Anne Poinier, MD
Caroline S. Rhoads, MD
Ruth Schneider, RD
Avery L. Seifert, MD
Peter Shalit, MD
Brent T. Shoji, MD
R. Steven Tharratt, MD
Arvydas D. Vanagunas, MD
Lisa Weinstock, MD
Richard D. Zorowitz, MD

Special acknowledgement goes to Michael Linkinhoker, MA, CMI, at Link Studio, for creating the book's illustrations.

This seventh edition of *Healthwise for Life* stands on the shoulders of the six that came before it—and the hundreds of health professionals, educators, writers, editors, and readers who have ensured that Healthwise content keeps improving. Your work has given millions of people a better chance at better health. This book is dedicated to you.

Better Care, Lower Costs

Better Care at Lower Costs 2

Work Closely With Your Doctor 2

Smart Money Tips for Medicines 3

Save the Emergency Room for Emergencies. 6

Smart Money Tips for Medical Tests . . . 7

Smart Decisions: Know Your Treatment Options 8

Medicare: The Basics 9

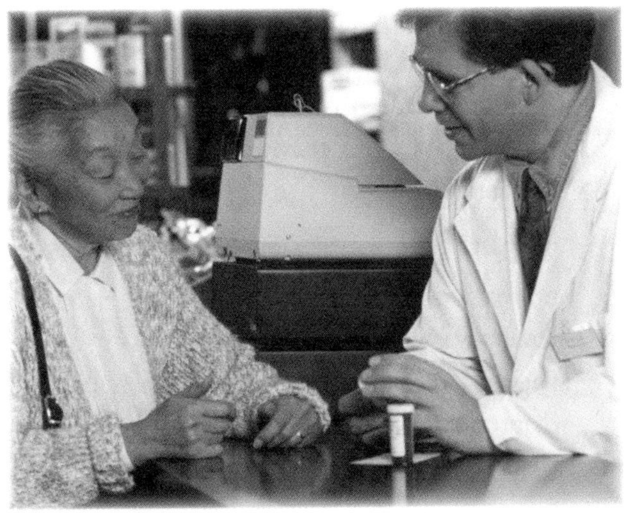

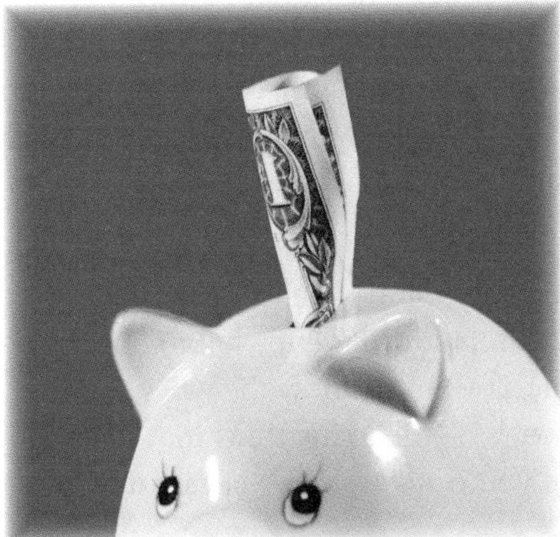

Better Care at Lower Costs

Good health care doesn't just happen. You have to do your part.

This chapter will help you take an active role in getting the care you need—no more and certainly no less. And it may also help you get that care for the best price. It has practical tips in five areas where you can affect both the cost and quality of your care:

- Working closely with your doctor
- Being smart about medicines
- Saving the emergency room for emergencies
- Using medical tests wisely
- Considering your options before you decide on treatment

You also may want to read Medicare: The Basics on page 9.

Wellness: The Best Way to Save

The best way to reduce health care costs is to stay healthy. Everything you do to eat right and stay fit will help you avoid medical costs later. So will getting the right screening tests and immunizations, not smoking, and avoiding accidents.

To learn how to start living healthier today, see page 319.

Work Closely With Your Doctor

A strong partnership between you and your main doctor is key to getting great care and reducing costs. A doctor who not only knows your medical history but understands what's important to you may be the resource you need most when you face a major health care decision. Pick your doctor wisely, and then stick with him or her.

1. Use your doctor as a teacher and coach. Some patients just want their doctors to tell them what to do. They don't want to know the whys and the hows. Some of the time, that's fine. But if you really want to get care that best meets your needs, learn as much as you can from your doctor.

- Don't just ask your doctor what you should do. Ask why. The more you understand, the better choices you can make.
- Ask if you have options. Often, your doctor can't tell which is best for you without your help. Together you can make the right choice.
- Benefit from your doctor's experience with other patients. Every person's situation is a little different, but your doctor has probably helped other patients work through the same issues that you are facing.

2. Tell your doctor that you care about cost. He or she may suggest safe, lower-cost options first before trying more costly tests or treatments. Your doctor can also give you an idea of how the cost of one choice compares to another.

3. Prepare for every doctor visit.

- Bring a list of your main symptoms. Have notes on when they started or changed and what you have done to treat them so far.
- Bring a list with the three questions that you most want to have answered. There may not be time for lots of questions, so focus on the ones that matter most.
- Bring a list of all medicines, vitamins, and herbal supplements that you are taking.
- Bring copies of any recent test results that your doctor may not have.
- Bring a friend or family member who can take notes during the visit.

4. Take an active role in every visit or call. Pay attention. Ask questions if you don't understand something. Write down the diagnosis, the treatment plan, and any guidelines for self-care and follow-up visits or calls. Be honest and direct about what you do or do not plan to do.

Smart Money Tips for Medicines

If you and your doctor have decided that you need prescription medicine, these three tips can help you get it at a lower cost:

- Ask for a generic medicine instead of a brand name.
- If there is no generic option, know whether your health plan or prescription plan makes you pay more for one brand name than another.
- Compare prices and shop smart. Prices for the same drug vary a lot. And they change often, so check them regularly.

Generics and Brand Names

All drugs have a generic name, also known as the scientific name. Many also have one or more brand names. For example, the diabetes medicine Glucophage is a brand name for the generic drug metformin.

Three Simple Rules to Reduce Costs

1. Do as much for yourself as you can do well. Good self-care can reduce your need for care.
2. Find out the care guidelines for your health problem. There are treatment guidelines for most common conditions, but doctors don't always follow them. Asking about the guidelines may improve your care.
3. Learn to say no to care that you don't think will help. Often doctors offer treatment options because they think that's what you want them to do. Always ask how a treatment will help you. If you are fully informed and do not think you need the care, you can feel good about saying no. Keep your options open in case things change.

For years after a new drug is created, patent laws prevent other companies from making the same drug. But after the patent expires, other drug companies can make and sell the drug. They just can't sell it by its brand name. So they use the generic name.

A generic drug has the same active ingredients as its brand-name versions and almost always costs less. In many cases, generics are less than half the cost of the brands.

Are generics really as good as brand-name drugs?

- Yes. Generics are very carefully tested to make sure they have the same ingredients, same effects, and same safety profile as the brands. The medicines may look or taste slightly different.
- For a few medicines, the body does not respond to the generic drug in quite the same way as it does the brand-name drug. The U.S. Food and Drug Administration (FDA) gives these generics a "B" rating. This does not mean that the generic is not as good or that you can't use it. It does mean that you should talk to your doctor or pharmacist before you switch from the brand to the generic (or vice versa). A pharmacist can tell you whether a drug is rated "B."

That's it. The safety and quality of FDA-approved generics are the same as brands. Generics just cost less. If you want to save money, always ask your doctor or pharmacist, "Is there a generic I can take?"

Medicines and Your Health Plan

Most health plans use a **drug formulary** to help control costs. A formulary is simply a list of preferred prescription medicines. The plan will pay more of the cost of drugs on the list than it will for other drugs that treat the same health problem.

The formulary may put drugs into three groups, or "tiers," based on how much your plan will pay and how much you have to pay.

- **Group 1: Generic drugs.** These are usually drugs that have been in use for a long time, have proven benefits, and cost less to make and sell. You pay the least for drugs in this group.
- **Group 2: Brand-name drugs that are on the formulary.** For the same health problem, there often are competing drugs from different companies. Your plan may put one drug on the formulary instead of the others if the drug company agrees to reduce the price. You still pay more for the "formulary" brand-name drug than for the generic, but it costs less than brand-name drugs that are not on the formulary.
- **Group 3: Brand-name drugs that are not on the formulary.** These drugs cost more because your health plan does not have an agreement with the drug company to reduce the price. When the plan pays more, so do you. Your other choice is to switch to a generic or a brand-name drug that is on the formulary.

The difference in cost to you among these three groups can be huge. If your doctor prescribes a medicine, make sure you know whether a different choice would save you money without giving up quality.

Sometimes there are good reasons to use a brand-name drug that's not on the formulary instead of one that is. The drug may have a dosing schedule that works better for you. Or it may have fewer or different side effects. You can still get the drug, but you'll have to pay more for it than for the one that's on the formulary.

But in most cases, there probably is a medicine on the list that will work just as well. Keeping medicine costs low is partly up to you.

- Know how your plan pays for medicines.
- If your doctor prescribes a medicine that is not on your plan's preferred list, ask if there is a medicine on the list that will cost you less and work just as well.
- If a drug you need is not on the list, call your plan and ask about it. This is your right as a consumer and a member of that plan.

Smart Shopping for Medicines

If you pay for medicines out of your own pocket or through a health savings account (HSA), you have even more to gain from careful spending.

1. Compare prices. The speed and convenience of a local pharmacy helps in emergencies or if you're in a rush. But for medicines you take on a regular basis, mail-order or online pharmacies may be cheaper. They may be more convenient too, sending the medicines right to your mailbox.

If you order online, look for Web sites that have the VIPPS (Verified Internet Pharmacy Practice Sites) seal from the National Association of Boards of Pharmacy. This means the site has met state and federal requirements.

2. Ask your doctor for free samples if you are trying a new medicine. This can let you try out the medicine for a couple of weeks without buying a full prescription.

But beware—often the samples doctors get are for newer, more expensive drugs. If you don't switch to a cheaper drug later, you may be paying more than you need to.

3. Buy in bulk. When you know you will be using a medicine for a long time, you can often save money and time by ordering a large supply (90 days' worth, for example). Ask your doctor to write a prescription that covers a few months.

4. Ask your doctor about pill splitting. You can buy some pills at twice the dose you need (100 mg instead of 50 mg, for instance) for nearly the same cost as the lower dose. By splitting the larger dose, you can get two doses for the price of one. To split the dose, you cut the pill in half. It is best to use a pill splitter for this, which is a small tool that helps make a clean cut. (You can buy one at most drugstores.)

It is not safe to split all medicines this way. Capsules and time-release pills should never be split. With many medicines, the dose needs to be extremely precise. So be sure to check with your doctor about whether splitting your pills is safe.

5. Find out about discounts and patient assistance programs. Some drug companies offer free or discounted drugs for people who need help paying for medicine. Your doctor may need to contact them on your behalf. To learn more about these programs, look online at RxAssist (www.rxassist.org) or at the Partnership for Prescription Assistance (www.pparx.org). If you have Medicare, see page 9.

Help may also be available through your state, your community, or the Veterans Administration (for veterans and their families). Some pharmacies and organizations, such as AARP, may offer discounts for older adults.

Save the Emergency Room for Emergencies

Hospital emergency rooms (ERs) are set up to focus on medical emergencies. They are not set up to focus on routine health care. If you go to the ER for a problem that is not an emergency:

- It will cost a lot more than it would at your doctor's office or a "walk-in" clinic.
- It will take a lot longer.
- It will likely be with a doctor who doesn't know you.

Go to the ER if you think you are having a medical emergency. That's what the ER is for. Otherwise, call your doctor's office first, or go to a walk-in clinic.

What's a "Walk-in" Clinic?

Walk-in clinics are often called "minor emergency," "urgent care," or "immediate care" centers. They deal with all kinds of health problems and are often open in the evenings and on weekends. You do not need an appointment.

These types of clinics can be a great option when:

- You can't or don't want to wait for an appointment at your doctor's office.
- You don't need the level of care an ER provides.

Care at a walk-in clinic costs a lot less than care for the same problem at an ER. And if it turns out you are having a true medical emergency, a walk-in clinic will send you to the ER.

Unless you have a walk-in clinic in your neighborhood or already know where one is, it may be hard to find one when you need it. So, at your next doctor visit, ask your doctor to recommend one. Check with your health plan to see if it offers better coverage at some clinics than others.

How do you know when it's an emergency?

There are few clear rules about what is an emergency and what isn't. Most health problems are *not* emergencies, but it's not always easy to tell. Some problems that seem minor can become serious if you ignore them. And it may be even harder to know what to do when a frail older adult is sick.

One good question to ask yourself is, "Am I thinking about going to the ER because it's *convenient* or because it's *necessary*?" If you are choosing the ER because you can get in without an appointment, keep in mind the high price you will pay for that convenience. And you may have other options.

You can always call your doctor's office or a nurse line for help. You can also look for information about your problem in this book or at a Web site you trust.

What if a problem happens on a weekend or at night?

If you think you are having a medical emergency, go to the ER.

If you don't think the problem is an emergency:

- Look up your problem in this book or at a Web site you trust, and look for information about when to call a doctor. See if there is home treatment you can try.
- Call your doctor's office and see if there is a number to call for after-hours service.
- Call a nurse line for advice. The nurse can help you decide whether you need to get help now or whether it is safe to wait.
- Go to a walk-in clinic (if one is open).
- Go to the ER if you feel the problem cannot wait until your doctor's office or a walk-in clinic is open.

Smart Money Tips for Medical Tests

Medical tests are expensive. If you need a test, the tips below can help save you money:

1. Follow instructions about how to prepare. Are you supposed to stop eating the night before? Not drink alcohol? Stop taking medicines, or take a special medicine? Get written instructions from your doctor or nurse, and follow them. This reduces the chance of error and the need to repeat the test.

2. Get a copy of the test results, even if they're normal. This helps in three ways:

- You can compare the results to past or future tests.
- You have a backup record of the test to show to other doctors if needed.
- Having the results helps you better understand what's going on with your health.

3. Don't have tests more often than you need to. If you have a health problem that requires frequent tests and you are worried about the cost, tell your doctor. Maybe you can go a little longer between tests. Maybe you can have a less costly test some of the time and the more expensive one less often.

4. Ask about options, and shop around. The cost of some testing can vary widely without any difference in how reliable the results are. For expensive tests, it may pay to compare the costs of your best options.

Smart Decisions: Know Your Treatment Options

Good health decisions can help you reduce costs and get better care. A good decision takes into account:

- The benefits of each option.
- The risks of each option.
- The costs of each option.
- Your own needs and wants.

1. Always ask why. Too much care can be just as bad as—or worse than—too little. Most medicines can have side effects. Medical tests can give false results that lead to the wrong care. Surgery almost always has risks. And anytime you get care, there is a chance of error.

When your doctor suggests or orders a medicine, surgery, a test, or any other kind of care, ask why you need it and what would happen if you waited. If you don't need it now, you might want to wait.

But also remember that there can be costs to doing nothing. The "wait and see" option is not always the best. If you don't get care when you need it and a health problem gets worse, you may face higher costs than you would have if you had taken care of the problem sooner.

Asking why can help you and your doctor make the decision that's right for you.

2. Know the pros and cons. Every treatment choice has pros and cons. It's up to you to know what they are.

Your doctor can be a big help here. Partner with your doctor to help you understand what a decision might mean for you now and in the long run.

Remember, the goal is to get the care you need, no more and no less, and to get it at the lowest cost you can.

3. Think about your needs and wants. Which option is best often depends on you. People value things differently. When you have a health care decision to make, you have to balance issues like:

- Your desire for better health versus the risks of treatment.
- Your willingness to change your behavior and habits (diet or exercise, for example) versus the risks and costs of medical treatment.
- The certainty of doing something versus the uncertainty of waiting (the known versus the unknown).
- Convenience versus cost.

You are the only person who knows what mix is right for you. You may be willing to pay more if you can get the problem taken care of quickly. You may be willing to go through a very risky surgery if it could cure a serious health problem. Or you may be willing to put

Surgery Decisions

Surgery tends to come with high costs and risks. When the choice to have surgery is not clear, good decisions are especially important.

Before you have surgery for anything other than an urgent, life-threatening problem, make sure you can answer these key questions:

- How might surgery help you?
- What results would you have to get from the surgery for you to consider it a success? How likely are those results?
- What could go wrong if you have surgery?
- How long would it take to recover from surgery? How much time off from work would you have to take? What kind of rehab would you need?
- What happens in the short term if you don't have surgery? What might happen over the long run if you don't have it?
- Are there other treatments you could try first?
- Can the problem come back after surgery? How often does that happen?
- If you need surgery, where should you have it? How can you reduce the chance of an error?

up with some pain if it means you can avoid a treatment with bad side effects or high cost.

For many decisions, these issues are just as important as the medical facts. They are part of what makes a decision right for you.

Medicare: The Basics

Medicare is health insurance that the U.S. government provides for people 65 or older. Your taxes have paid for it.

Medicare is complex, and you will have to make a lot of decisions. Which is the best plan for you? Which drug plan should you choose? Will you need "Medigap" insurance? Start learning about Medicare before you need it. You can get information at www.medicare.gov or by calling the Medicare Helpline at 1-800-633-4227.

Here are the basics. Medicare is divided into Part A, Part B, and Part D.

- Part A helps cover hospital services. Most people get Part A without paying a monthly premium.
- Part B helps cover the cost of doctor and outpatient services. For this coverage, you pay an amount each month that is based on your income.
- Part D covers prescription drugs. You pay for this coverage, and you have a choice of plans.

There are different ways to get the services that Medicare offers.

- Most people choose the Original Medicare Plan, which is managed by the government. Then they join a prescription drug plan. They may also buy a "Medigap" policy to help with costs not covered by the Original Plan.
- Other people choose a Medicare Advantage Plan (sometimes called Part C). This insurance is approved by Medicare but run by private insurance companies. It includes Part A and Part B coverage. Many policies also include a drug plan.

Here are a few things to know about Medicare:

- **Get your "Welcome to Medicare" exam.** You can get a free physical exam within the first 6 months after you sign up for Part B. This includes a review of your health, screening tests and shots, and prevention information.
- **Sign up for Part B soon.** If you don't sign up for Part B as soon as you are eligible for Medicare, the cost may be higher, and you may have to pay this extra amount as long as you have Part B.
- **Sign up for a drug plan soon.** If you don't sign up for a drug plan under Part D as soon as you are eligible, you may have to pay a penalty if you enroll later.
- **Know when to change your coverage.** If you want to change your Medicare coverage, you can do so in the fall of each year.
- **Find out if you can get cheaper drugs.** Medicare gives extra help with prescription drug costs for low-income people. The income limits change each year.
    - You have to apply through the Social Security Administration. Go to www.ssa.gov/prescriptionhelp, or call toll-free at 1-800-772-1213.
    - To find out if you qualify for other low-cost drug programs, go to www.benefitscheckup.org. This is a service run by the National Council on Aging.
- **Don't forget about long-term care.** Medicare does not pay for long-term care. To get this coverage, you will need to buy it from a private insurance company. See page 385 to learn more.

First Aid and Emergencies

Bites—Animals and Humans 12

Bites and Stings—Insects, Spiders, and Ticks. 13

Bleeding Emergencies 17

Blood Under a Nail 18

Breathing Emergencies and CPR. . . 19

Bruises. 22

Burns. 23

Chemical Burns 25

Choking 26

Cuts and Punctures 27

Dehydration 29

Eye (Object in) 31

Fainting and Unconsciousness 33

Falls 34

Frostbite 35

Head Injury 36

Heart Attack 38

Heat Sickness 39

Hypothermia. 41

Nosebleeds 43

Scrapes 44

Seizures 45

Shock 47

Splinters 49

Strains, Sprains, and Broken Bones 49

Stroke 54

Suicide. 55

Sunburn 56

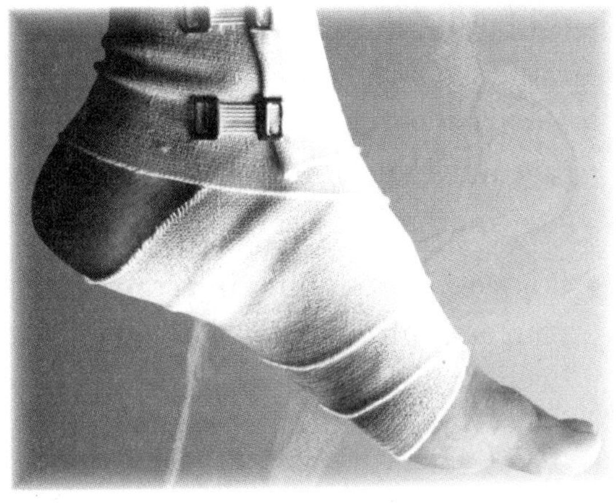

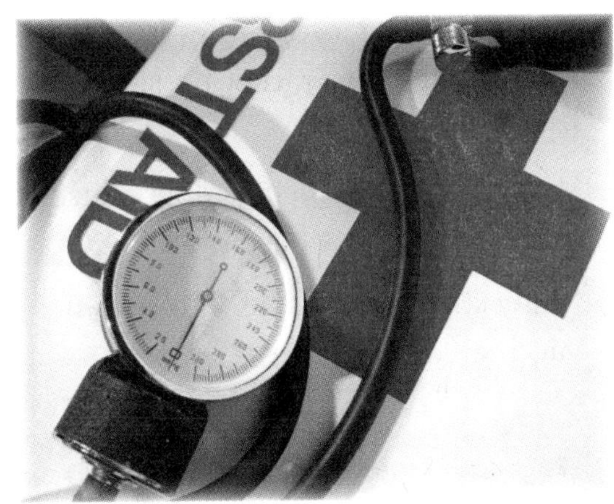

Bites—Animals and Humans

When to Call a Doctor

- The wound is severe and may need stitches, or it is on your face, hand, or foot or over a joint. If the wound needs stitches, be sure to get them within 6 to 8 hours. See page 29.
- The bite or scratch is from a bat or other wild animal.
- The bite is from a human or a cat. These bites get infected easily.
- The bite is from a dog, cat, or ferret that foams at the mouth, acts strangely, or attacked for no clear reason. Also call the local animal control or public health office.
- You can't find the owner of a pet that bit you, or the owner can't confirm that the pet's rabies vaccine is up to date.
- You lose feeling or movement below the wound.
- You have signs of infection. These may include increased pain, swelling, warmth, or redness; red streaks leading from the wound; pus; or fever.
- You have not had a tetanus shot in the past 5 years. If you need a shot, get it within 2 days.

Infection and scarring are the main concerns with bites and scratches that break the skin. You can also get tetanus if your shots are not up to date. See page 320.

After an animal bite, you may want to know if you need a rabies shot. Rabies is quite rare, but it is deadly if you are not vaccinated soon after a bite from an infected animal.

- The main carriers of rabies in North America are bats, raccoons, skunks, foxes, and coyotes.
- Vaccinated pets, such as dogs, cats, and ferrets, rarely have rabies.
- Many stray animals have not been vaccinated.

Home Treatment

- Let the wound bleed freely for up to 5 minutes, unless the bleeding is heavy. If you are bleeding a lot, see Stopping Severe Bleeding on page 17.
- Scrub the wound with soap and water. Do not use alcohol, iodine, or any other cleansers.
- If a pet dog, cat, or ferret bites you, find out if the animal has a current rabies vaccine. A healthy pet without a current vaccine should be confined and watched for up to 10 days by a veterinarian.
- If a wild animal bites or scratches you, ask animal control or the public health office if you need a rabies shot.

Bites and Stings—Insects, Spiders, and Ticks

When to Call a Doctor

Call 911 if:

- You have signs of a severe allergic reaction soon after a bite or sting. These may include:
  - Wheezing or trouble breathing.
  - Swelling around the lips, tongue, or face.
  - Severe swelling around the bite or sting (for example, your entire arm or leg is swollen).
  - Fainting or other signs of shock. See page 47.
- You have just been bitten or stung by something that caused a serious reaction in the past.

Call a doctor if:

- You get a spreading skin rash, itching, a feeling of warmth, or hives.
- You get a blister at the site of a spider bite, or the skin around it changes color.
- A black widow, brown recluse, or hobo spider bites you.
- Your symptoms are not better in 2 to 3 days.
- You have signs of infection. These may include increased pain, swelling, warmth, or redness; red streaks leading from the bite; pus; swollen lymph nodes near the bite; or fever.
- A tick is attached to you and you cannot remove the whole tick.
- You were recently exposed to ticks and have a spreading red rash. The rash may or may not be in the bite area and may or may not occur with flu-like symptoms, such as fever, headache, body aches, and fatigue.
- You want to talk about allergy kits or allergy shots because you have had a serious allergic reaction in the past.

Insects and Spiders

Bites and stings from insects (bees, wasps, yellow jackets) and spiders usually cause pain, swelling, redness, and itching at the site of the sting or bite. In some people, the redness and swelling may last up to a few days.

A few people have severe allergic reactions that affect the whole body. This type of reaction can be deadly. If you have had a severe allergic reaction to a past sting or bite, you may want to keep an allergy kit with an epinephrine syringe (such as EpiPen) with you at all times. Ask your doctor or pharmacist how and when to use it.

Spider bites are rarely serious. But any bite can be serious if it causes an allergic reaction.

More

A single bite from a poisonous spider, such as a black widow, brown recluse, or hobo spider, may cause a severe reaction and needs medical care right away.

- A bite from a female black widow spider may cause chills, fever, nausea, and severe belly cramps.

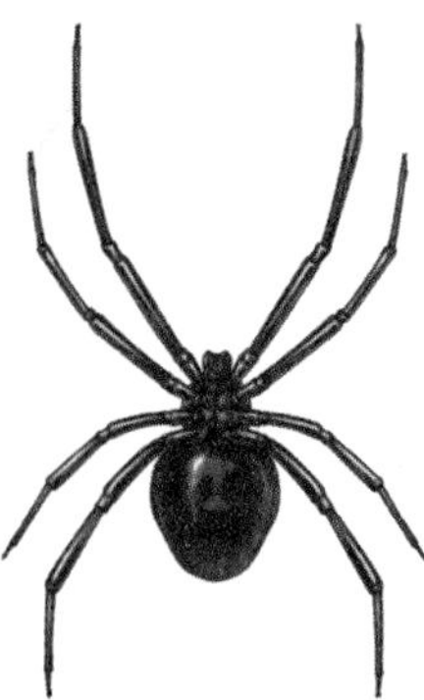

Black widow spiders can be up to 2 inches across and are shiny black with a red or yellow hourglass mark on their undersides.

- A bite from a brown recluse or hobo spider causes intense pain, and you may get a blister that turns into a large, open sore. The bite may also cause nausea, vomiting, headaches, and chills.

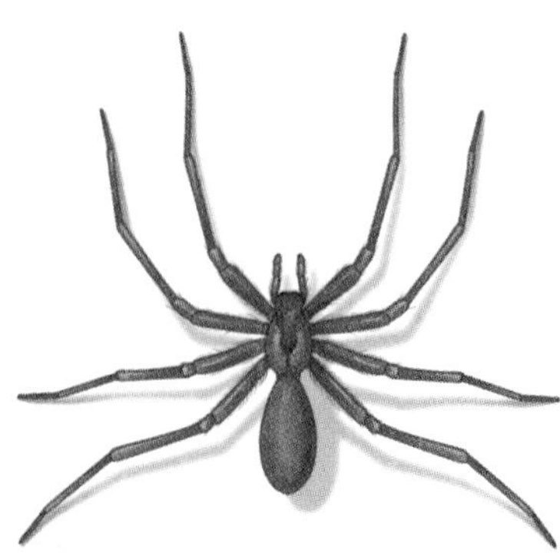

Brown recluse (fiddler) spiders are smaller than black widows and have long legs. They are brown with a violin-shaped mark on their heads.

Ticks

Ticks are small bugs that bite into the skin and feed on blood. They live in bird feathers and animal fur and in wooded or grassy areas. Tick bites occur more often in early spring to late summer.

- Most ticks do not carry diseases, and most tick bites do not cause serious health problems. Still, it is best to remove a tick as soon as you find one.
- Many of the diseases that ticks may pass to humans (such as Lyme disease, Rocky Mountain spotted fever, relapsing fever, and Colorado tick fever) have the same flu-like symptoms: fever, headache, body aches, and fatigue.
- Sometimes a rash or sore may occur with the flu-like symptoms. A red rash that gets bigger is a classic early sign of Lyme disease. It may appear 1 day to 1 month after a tick bite.

Home Treatment

For insect and spider bites and stings:

- Remove a bee stinger by scraping or flicking it out. Do not squeeze it, because you may release more venom into the skin. If you can't see the stinger, assume it's not there.
- If a black widow, brown recluse, or hobo spider bites you, put ice on the bite and call a doctor. Do not use a tourniquet.

- Put ice or a cold pack on the bite or sting. A paste of baking soda or unseasoned meat tenderizer mixed with a little water may help relieve pain and decrease the reaction.
- Take an antihistamine to relieve pain, swelling, and itching. Look for types that won't make you sleepy, such as Claritin or Alavert. Calamine lotion or hydrocortisone cream may also help.
- Wash the area with soap and water.
- Trim your fingernails so you don't scratch too hard.
- Do not break any blisters that form. They could get infected.

For ticks:

- Check your body often for ticks when you are out in the woods. Closely check your clothes, skin, and scalp when you get home. Check your pets for ticks too. The sooner you remove ticks, the less likely they are to spread infection.
- If you find a tick, try to remove it. Use tweezers to gently pull on it as close to the skin (where its mouth is) as you can get. Fine-tipped tweezers may work best. Pull straight out, and try not to crush the tick's body. Do not try to "unscrew" the tick.

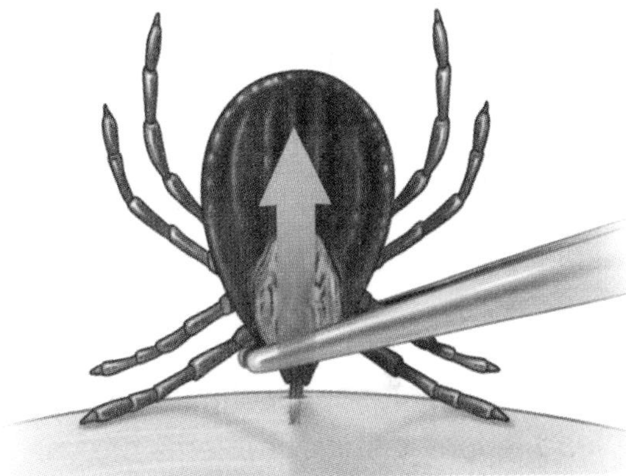

Use tweezers to pull the tick straight out.

- Do not try to burn off the tick or smother it with petroleum jelly, nail polish, gasoline, or rubbing alcohol.
- Save the tick in a jar for tests in case you get flu-like symptoms after the bite.
- Wash the area with soap and water.

More

Mosquitoes and West Nile Virus

West Nile virus is an infection spread to humans by mosquitoes. Most people who get the virus do not get sick.

When symptoms do occur, they appear 3 to 14 days after the bite and include fever, headache, body aches, and sometimes a skin rash. This is called West Nile fever. It is usually a mild illness.

Rarely, West Nile virus may affect the brain, causing serious illness that can lead to long-lasting problems or even death. Older adults and people with weakened immune systems (because of diabetes, cancer, or HIV, for instance) are most likely to have serious illness from the West Nile virus.

When to Call a Doctor

Call a doctor if you were exposed to mosquitoes in the past 2 weeks and have any of these symptoms:

- Fever, headache, stiff neck, and confusion.
- Muscle weakness or loss of movement.
- Mild fever, rash, body aches, or swollen lymph nodes in your neck, armpits, or groin that last more than 2 or 3 days.

How to Avoid West Nile Virus

- Stay indoors at dawn, at dusk, and in the early evening. Mosquitoes are most active at these times.
- Wear long-sleeved shirts and pants made of thick fabric.
- Use an insect repellent that contains DEET, picaridin, or oil of lemon eucalyptus. For the best protection, apply and reapply as the label says.
- Don't keep open containers of water near your home. Mosquitoes can breed in even a small amount of standing water.

Bleeding Emergencies

When to Call a Doctor

Call 911 if:

- You have severe bleeding that you cannot stop.
- You are bleeding and you faint or feel lightheaded.
- You vomit a lot of blood or what looks like coffee grounds.
- You have severe rectal bleeding. Severe means that you are passing a lot of stool that is maroon or mostly blood.
- You have unexpected vaginal bleeding and lower belly pain, and you faint or feel lightheaded.

Stopping Severe Bleeding From a Wound

- Raise the area that is bleeding—higher than the heart, if you can.
- Wash your hands well with soap and water. Put on medical gloves, or place several layers of fabric or plastic bags between your hands and the wound.
- Remove any objects you can see on the surface of the wound. Do not try to clean out the wound.
- Press firmly on the wound with a clean cloth or the cleanest material you can find. If there is an object deep in the wound, put pressure around the object but not directly over it. Do not try to remove the object.
- Apply steady pressure for a full 15 minutes. Do not lift your hands to see if bleeding has stopped before 15 minutes are up. **If bleeding from a large or deep wound has not slowed down or stopped after 15 minutes, call 911** and continue to put pressure on the wound. If blood soaks through the cloth, put another cloth on top of the first one.
- If bleeding slows down after 15 minutes but a little bleeding starts again after you release the pressure, apply pressure for another 15 minutes. For light bleeding, you can apply pressure for up to three 15-minute periods (45 minutes total). If there is any bleeding after 45 minutes of direct pressure, call a doctor.

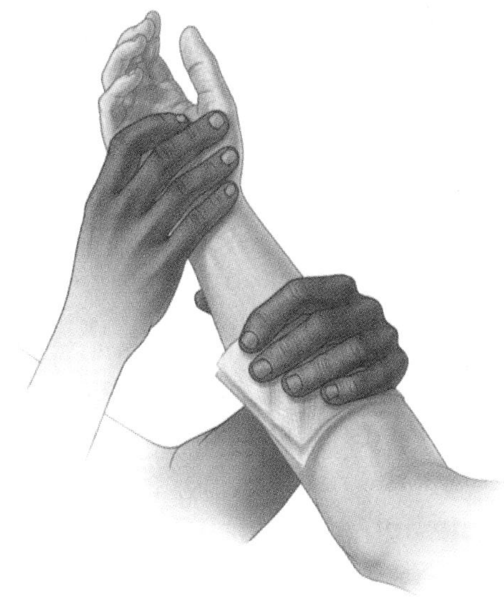

Elevate the area and apply pressure with a clean cloth.

Blood Under a Nail

When to Call a Doctor

- The pain is severe, and you do not want to drain the blood from the nail yourself.
- You drained the blood from under the nail, but your finger or toe still hurts a lot.
- You have diabetes, blood flow problems, or a weak immune system (from HIV, steroid use, cancer treatment, or organ transplant) and need help with blood under a nail.
- You have signs of infection. These may include increased pain, swelling, warmth, or redness; red streaks leading from the nail; pus; or fever.
- You need help removing a nail that has torn or separated from the nail bed.

When a fingernail or toenail gets banged or smashed, blood may build up under the nail. The pressure can hurt a lot. Ice and ibuprofen (Advil, Motrin) or naproxen (Aleve) may help with the pain.

If the pain is severe and throbbing, the only way to relieve it is to make a hole in the nail to drain the blood. Do not try this unless you have severe pain. If you have diabetes, blood flow problems, or a weakened immune system, don't try it at all.

To drain the blood:

- Straighten a paper clip. Then heat the tip in a flame until it is red-hot.
- Place the tip of the paper clip over the area with blood, and let it melt through the nail. Do not push. This should not hurt, because the nail has no nerves. Go slowly, and reheat the clip as needed. A thick nail may take a few tries.
- As soon as there is a hole, blood will drain out and the pain should go away. If the pain does not go away, you may have a more serious injury, such as a broken bone or a deep cut. In this case, see a doctor.
- Soak the finger or toe in warm, soapy water 2 times a day for 10 minutes each time. Apply an antibiotic ointment and a bandage.
- If the pressure builds up again in a few days, repeat the process. Use the same hole.

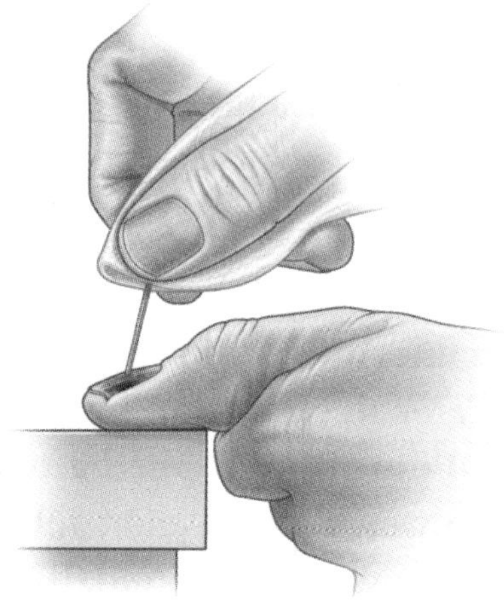

When to Call a Doctor

Call 911 if:

- A person stops breathing for longer than 15 to 20 seconds.
- A person has severe trouble breathing. The person may:
  - Have chest tightness so severe that the person is worried he or she can't keep breathing.
  - Be so short of breath that he or she can't speak.
  - Gasp for breath or have severe wheezing.
  - Feel very anxious, afraid, or restless.
  - Have a gray, blotchy, or blue color to the skin. Look for color changes in the nail beds, lips, and earlobes.
  - Respond slowly or have trouble waking up or staying awake.

For less severe breathing problems, see When to Call a Doctor on page 101.

Rescue Breathing and CPR on Adults

Doing CPR the wrong way or on a person whose heart is still beating can cause serious harm. Do not do CPR unless:

1. The person is not breathing normally (may be gasping for breath) or is not breathing at all.
2. The person does not breathe or move in response to rescue breaths.
3. No one with more training in CPR than you is present. If you are the only one there, do the best you can.

Step 1: Check to see if the person is conscious.

Tap or gently shake the person and shout, "Are you okay?" But do not shake someone who might have a neck or back injury. That could make the injury worse.

If the person does not respond, call 911.

Step 2: Check for breathing for 5 to 10 seconds.

- Kneel next to the person with your head close to his or her head.
- Look to see if the person's chest rises and falls.
- Listen for breathing sounds.
- Put your cheek near the person's mouth and nose to feel whether air is moving out.

More

- If the person is not breathing normally or not breathing at all, roll the person onto his or her back. If you think the person might have a neck or back injury, gently roll the head, neck, and shoulders together as a unit.

Step 3: Start rescue breaths.

- Use your hand to tilt the chin up to keep the airway open. Put your other hand on the person's forehead, and pinch the person's nostrils shut with your thumb and finger. Be very careful if you think the person could have a neck injury.

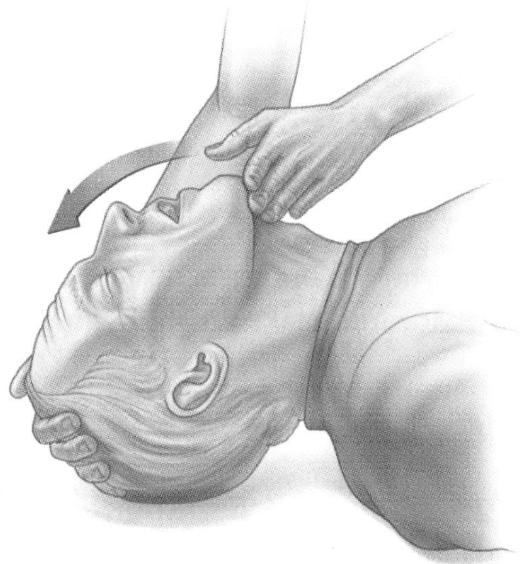

Tilt the chin up to open the airway.

- Take a normal breath (not a deep one), and place your mouth over the person's mouth, making a tight seal. Blow into the person's mouth for 1 second, and watch to see if the person's chest rises.

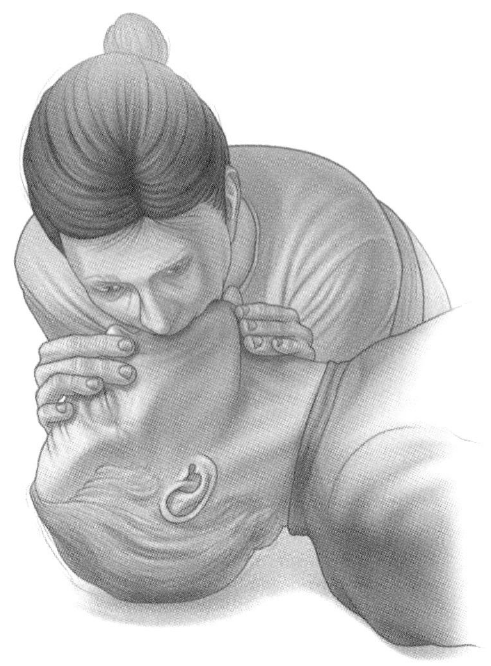

Blow into the person's mouth for 1 second.

- If the chest does not rise, tilt the person's head again, and give another breath.
- Between rescue breaths, remove your mouth from the person's mouth and take a normal breath. Let his or her chest fall, and feel the air escape.
- If the person is still not breathing normally after 2 rescue breaths, start chest compressions.

Step 4: Start chest compressions.

- Kneel next to the person. Use your fingers to find the end of the person's breastbone, where the ribs come together. Place two fingers at the tip of the breastbone.

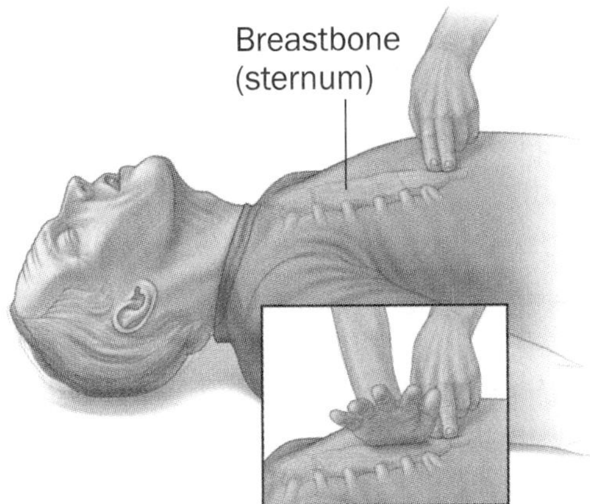

Place two fingers at the tip of the breastbone. Then put the heel of the other hand right above your fingers.

- Place the heel of the other hand right above your fingers (on the side closest to the person's face).
- Use both hands to give compressions. Stack your other hand on top of the one that you just put in position. Lace the fingers of both hands together, and raise your fingers so they do not touch the chest.
- Straighten your arms, lock your elbows, and center your shoulders directly over your hands.
- Press down in a steady rhythm, using your body weight. The force from each thrust should go straight down onto the breastbone, pressing it down 1½ to 2 inches for an adult or from one-third to one-half of the chest's depth for a child.

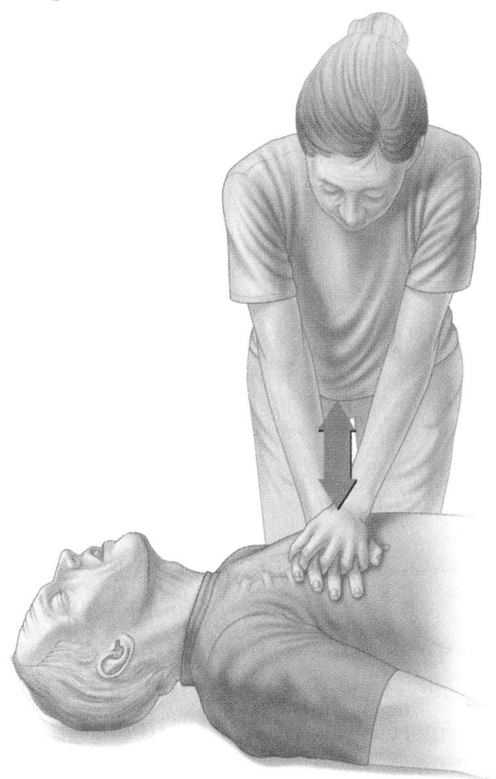

Keep your shoulders directly over your hands with your elbows straight as you push on the chest.

- **Give 30 compressions. Push hard and push fast.** (Do between 1 and 2 compressions each second. It should take a little less than 20 seconds to do 30 compressions.) After 30 compressions, give 2 rescue breaths.
- Keep repeating the cycle of 30 compressions and 2 breaths until help arrives or the person is breathing normally.

Bruises

When to Call a Doctor

- The pain is severe.
- You can't use or move the bruised body part.
- You have signs of infection. These may include increased pain, swelling, warmth, or redness; red streaks leading from the bruise; or fever.
- You suddenly start to bruise easily, or you have lots of bruises for no clear reason.
- Bruises appear while you're sick and you don't know why.
- You take aspirin or a blood thinner such as warfarin (Coumadin) and you are getting lots of bruises.
- After a blow to the eye:
  - You have any blood in the colored part of your eye or a lot of blood in the white part of your eye.
  - You have vision changes.
  - You can't move your eye normally in all directions.
  - You have severe pain.

Bruises occur when small blood vessels under the skin break or tear after a bump or fall. You may bruise easily if you take aspirin or blood thinners like warfarin (Coumadin). As you get older, you may bruise more because the tiny veins in the skin get weaker. Bruises also take longer to heal as we get older.

A **black eye** is a type of bruise. If you get a black eye, use the home treatment for a bruise, and check the eye for blood.

Home Treatment

- Put ice or cold packs on the bruise for 10 minutes several times a day for the first 2 days. The sooner you use ice, the less bleeding and swelling there will be. Always put a thin cloth between the ice and your skin.
- Take acetaminophen (Tylenol), ibuprofen (Advil, Motrin), or naproxen (Aleve) for pain.
- Keep the bruised area above the level of your heart when you can. This helps keep the swelling down. For example, if you bruise your foot, prop it up on a pillow when you are sitting or lying down.
- Rest the area so you don't hurt it more.
- If the area still hurts after 2 days, put a warm towel or heating pad on it.
- If you get a lot of bruises, ask your doctor or pharmacist if bruising could be a side effect of any medicines you take.

Burns

When to Call a Doctor

- You have a third-degree or worse burn. The burned skin may be dry, pale white or charred black, and swollen, or it may have broken open.
- You have severe pain.
- You are not sure how serious the burn is.
- You have a burn worse than a mild sunburn on your face, ears, eyes, hands, feet, genitals, or a joint.
- The burn goes all the way around an arm or leg, or it covers more than 25 percent of any body part.
- Pain from the burn lasts longer than 48 hours.
- You have signs of infection. These may include increased pain, swelling, warmth, or redness; red streaks leading from the burn; pus; or fever.
- A frail older adult or a person with a weak immune system or a chronic health problem (such as cancer, heart disease, or diabetes) is burned.
- There is a chance a person was burned on purpose.

The degree of a burn is based on how deep it is, not on how much pain it causes.

A **first-degree burn** involves only the outer layer of skin. The skin is dry and painful and hurts when you touch it. A mild sunburn is a first-degree burn.

A **second-degree burn** involves several layers of skin. The skin may be swollen, puffy, oozing, or blistered.

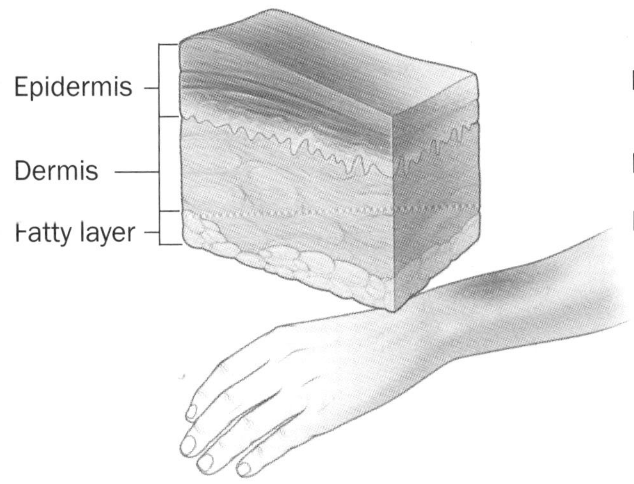

First-degree burn

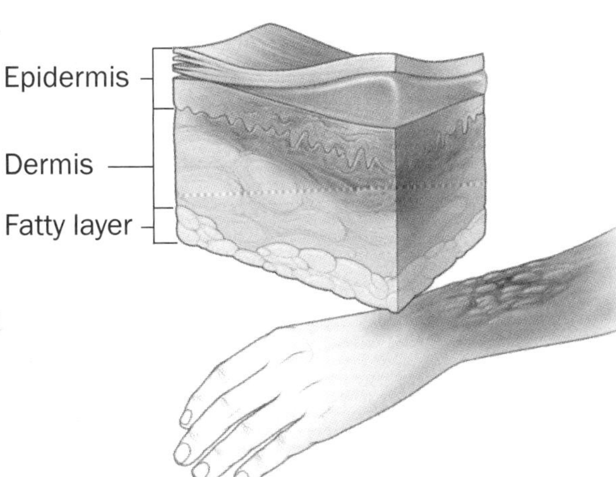

Second-degree burn

More

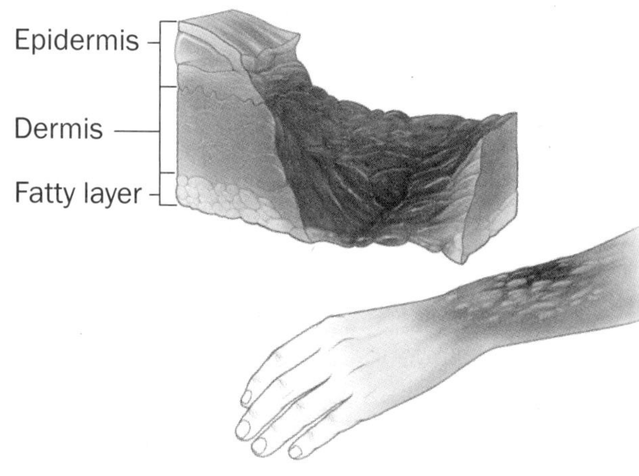

Third-degree burn

- A **third-degree burn** involves all layers of skin and may include tissue beneath the skin. The skin is dry, pale white or charred black, and swollen. It sometimes breaks open. This kind of burn destroys the nerves, so it may not hurt except on the edges.
- A **fourth-degree burn** extends through the skin to muscle and bone.

Home Treatment

For third-degree and fourth-degree burns:

These burns need medical care right away. Call for help, and then:

- Make sure the fire that caused the burn has been put out.
- Have the person lie down to prevent shock. See page 47.
- Cover the burned area with a clean sheet.
- Do not put any ice, salve, or medicine on the burn.

For first- and second-degree burns:

You can treat most of these burns at home.

- Run cool water over the burn until the pain stops (15 to 30 minutes). Do not use ice or ice water, because it may further damage the skin.
- Do not touch the burned area with your hands or any unclean objects. Burns get infected easily.
- Remove rings, jewelry, or clothing from the burned limb. Swelling may make these items hard to remove later. And if they are left on, they may damage nerves or blood vessels.
- Clean the burn with mild soap and water.
- Use an antibiotic ointment such as bacitracin, Polysporin, or Silvadene. Do not use butter, grease, or oil. They increase the risk of infection and do not help the burn heal.
- If the skin breaks open, use a bandage. Otherwise, don't cover the burn unless clothing rubs on it. If you need to cover the burn:
    - Use a nonstick gauze pad. Make sure the tape does not touch the burn.
    - Do not wrap tape all the way around a hand, arm, or leg.
    - Keep the bandage clean and dry. If it gets wet, replace it.
    - Remove the bandage once a day, clean the burn, and put on a new bandage.

- If blisters form, don't break them. If they break on their own, use water and mild soap to clean the area. Don't cut off the flap over a blister. It's a natural bandage. Apply an antibiotic ointment, and cover the burn with a nonstick gauze pad.
- Take acetaminophen (Tylenol), ibuprofen (Advil, Motrin), or naproxen (Aleve) to help relieve pain. Do not take aspirin—it can increase swelling and bleeding.
- After 2 to 3 days, use aloe to soothe the burn.

Chemical Burns

When to Call a Doctor

Call 911 if:

- A strong chemical such as acid or lye splashes into your eye.
- You swallow a chemical that may cause burning or be poisonous.

Call a doctor or Poison Control if:

- A large area of skin (more than 25 percent of any body part) or any part of the face is exposed to a strong acid, such as battery acid, or to a caustic substance, such as lye or Drano.
- A burned eye still hurts after 30 minutes of rinsing with water.
- Your eye is very red; has yellow, green, bloody, or watery discharge; or has a gray or white discolored area.
- You have vision problems that do not clear with blinking.
- Your skin is red, blistered, or blackened.

Burns can occur when a harmful chemical, such as a cleaning product, gasoline, or turpentine, splashes into an eye or onto the skin. Fumes can also burn the eyes, the skin, and the airways and lungs.

A burned eye may be red and watery and may be sensitive to light. If the damage is severe, the eye may look white.

Chemically burned skin may be red, blistered, or blackened. It depends on how strong the chemical was.

Be careful when you work with chemicals. Wear safety glasses, goggles, or a face shield. Follow the product label's advice about wearing gloves. And always know where the nearest sink or shower is.

Home Treatment

- Call Poison Control for specific advice. Have the chemical's container or label nearby.

More

- Right away, flush your eye or skin with a lot of water. Use a cold shower for skin burns. For eye burns, fill a sink or bowl with water, put your face in the water, and open and close your eyelids with your fingers to force the water to all parts of the eye. Or rinse your eye under a faucet or shower. A sink with a sprayer also works well.
- Keep rinsing with water for 30 minutes or until the pain stops, whichever takes longer.

Choking

When to Call a Doctor

Call 911 if a person who is choking faints.

Choking is most often caused by food or an object stuck in the windpipe. A person who is choking cannot talk, cough, or breathe, and may turn gray or blue. The Heimlich maneuver can help get the food or object out.

WARNING: Do not try the Heimlich maneuver unless you are sure the person is choking.

If Someone Is Choking

- Stand behind the person, and wrap your arms around his or her waist. If the person is standing, place one of your feet between his or her legs so you can support the person if he or she faints.
- Make a fist with one hand. Place the thumb side of your fist against the person's belly, just above the belly button but well below the breastbone.
- Grasp your fist with your other hand. Give a quick upward thrust into the belly. This may cause the object to pop out. You may need to use more force for a large person and less for a small one.
- Repeat thrusts until the object pops out or the person faints.

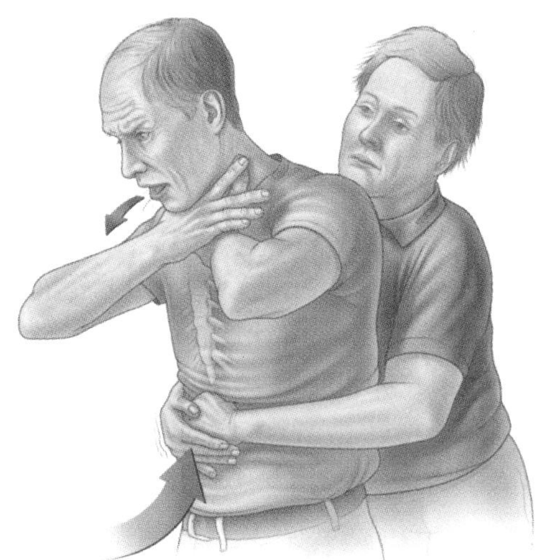

Give quick upward thrusts.

Call 911 if the person faints. Then:

- Start CPR if you know how. See page 19.
- Each time you open the airway during CPR, look for an object in the mouth. If you see an object, remove it.
- Do not do any more Heimlich thrusts.
- Keep doing CPR until the person is breathing on his or her own or until help arrives.

If You Are Choking

If you choke while you are alone, use your fists to do thrusts on yourself. Or lean over the back of a chair and press hard to pop out the object.

Cuts and Punctures

When to Call a Doctor

Call 911 if:

- The person faints or has other signs of shock (see page 47), even if the bleeding has stopped.
- A large or deep cut continues to bleed through bandages after 15 minutes of direct pressure. See page 17.

Call a doctor if:

- The skin near the wound is blue, white, or cold.
- You have numbness, tingling, or loss of feeling or movement below the wound.
- You have a puncture wound to the head, neck, chest, or belly, unless you are sure it is minor.
- You cannot remove an object from the wound, or you think part of the object may still be in the wound.
- A cut has removed all the layers of skin.
- Bleeding is under control but has not stopped after 45 minutes of direct pressure.
- The cut needs stitches. See page 29. Stitches usually need to be done within 6 to 8 hours.
- A deep puncture to the foot occurred through a shoe.
- A cat or human bite punctured the skin.
- You have not had a tetanus shot in the past 5 years. If you need a shot, make sure to get it within 2 days.
- You have signs of infection. These may include increased pain, swelling, warmth, or redness; red streaks leading from the wound; pus; or fever.

More

Cuts

When you get a cut, the first steps are to stop the bleeding and to decide whether to see a doctor. Bleeding from a minor cut will usually stop on its own or after you apply a little pressure.

If the cut is bleeding heavily or spurting blood, you need to stop the bleeding before you do anything else. Raise the area and apply firm pressure with a clean cloth for at least 15 minutes. See Stopping Severe Bleeding on page 17.

Home Treatment

- Wash the cut well with soap and water. Do not use any other cleanser.
- If you think the cut may need stitches, see a doctor right away. If the cut does not need stitches, proceed with home treatment. (See Do You Need Stitches? on page 29.)
- Bandage the cut if it is large or in an area that may get dirty or irritated.
    - Use antibiotic ointment, such as bacitracin or Polysporin, to keep the cut from sticking to the bandage.
    - Use an adhesive strip (such as a Band-Aid) to put pressure on the cut and protect it. Always put the bandage across a cut rather than lengthwise. Butterfly bandages can help hold the edges of the cut together.
    - Replace the bandage once a day and anytime it gets wet or dirty.

Punctures

Punctures are caused by sharp, pointed objects (nails, tacks, knives, needles, teeth) that go through the skin. These wounds get infected easily because they are hard to clean and are a warm, moist place for bacteria to grow.

Home Treatment

- If the object that caused the wound is small, such as a tack or a sewing needle, remove it. Be careful not to break it off in the wound. If the object is large or caused a deep wound, leave it in place and call a doctor right away.
- Let the wound bleed freely for up to 5 minutes to clean itself out, unless you are losing a lot of blood or the blood is squirting out. If bleeding is heavy, raise the area and apply firm pressure for at least 15 minutes. If there is an object in the wound, press around it, not directly on it. See Stopping Severe Bleeding on page 17.
- Clean the wound with soap and water 2 times a day. Do not use any other cleansers.
- Put antibiotic ointment on the wound, and cover it with a nonstick bandage. Replace the bandage when you clean the wound and whenever the bandage gets wet or dirty.
- Watch for signs of infection. If the wound closes, an infection under the skin may be hidden for several days.

Do You Need Stitches?

For best results, cuts that need stitches should get them within 6 to 8 hours. Stitches can help some cuts heal with less scarring. Sometimes stitches are needed to stop the bleeding.

After you have washed the cut and the bleeding has stopped, pinch the sides of the cut together. If it looks better that way, you may want to get stitches. If you think you need stitches, do not use an antibiotic ointment until after a doctor has looked at the cut.

If the cut does not need stitches, you can clean and bandage it at home.

You may need stitches for:

- Deep cuts (more than ¼ inch deep) that have jagged edges or gape open.
- Deep cuts on a joint, such as an elbow, knuckle, or knee.
- Deep cuts on the hands or fingers.
- Cuts on the face, eyelids, or lips.
- Cuts in any area where you are worried about scarring.
- Cuts that go down to the muscle or bone.
- Cuts that keep bleeding after you have applied direct pressure for 15 minutes.

Dehydration

When to Call a Doctor

Call 911 if there are signs of severe dehydration. These include:

- Sunken eyes, no tears, and a dry mouth and tongue.
- Little or no urine for 12 hours.
- Skin that sags when you pinch it.
- Feeling very dizzy when you move from lying down to sitting up.
- Fast breathing and heartbeat.
- Not acting alert, or having trouble waking up.

Call a doctor if:

- You are sick to your stomach and cannot hold down even small sips of fluid.
- Symptoms of mild dehydration (dry mouth, dark urine, not much urine) get worse even with home treatment.

One of these topics may be helpful as well:

- Diarrhea, page 127
- Vomiting, page 253

More

Dehydration means that your body has lost too much fluid. When you stop drinking water or lose a lot of fluids through diarrhea, vomiting, sweating, or exercise, your body's cells take fluid from the blood and other tissues. Severe dehydration can be life-threatening.

Dehydration is harmful for everyone, but it is especially dangerous for older adults. Watch closely for its early signs anytime you have high fever, vomiting, or diarrhea. The early symptoms are:

- A dry, sticky mouth.
- Dark yellow urine, and not much of it.
- Having no energy, or feeling cranky or restless.

Home Treatment

- To stop vomiting or diarrhea, do not eat any solid foods for several hours or until you feel better. During the first 24 hours, take frequent, small sips of water or a rehydration drink.
- As soon as the vomiting or diarrhea is controlled, drink water, weak broth, or sports drinks a sip at a time until your stomach can handle larger amounts. Drinking too much fluid too soon can make you vomit again.
- If vomiting or diarrhea lasts longer than 24 hours, sip a rehydration drink to replace lost fluids and minerals. See Rehydration Drinks on this page.

Rehydration Drinks

Diarrhea, vomiting, and sweating can cause you to lose large amounts of water and important minerals called electrolytes. If you are too sick to eat for a few days, you also lose nutrients.

Plain water replaces fluids only and has no nutrition. If you have diarrhea, your body may not absorb the water anyway.

A better choice is a rehydration drink or sports drinks (like Gatorade or Powerade). These replace fluids and electrolytes in amounts your body can use. These drinks won't make diarrhea or vomiting go away faster, but they will help prevent serious dehydration.

You can make a cheap drink at home. Measure everything exactly. Small changes can make the drink less effective or even harmful. Mix:

- 1 quart water
- ½ teaspoon baking soda
- ½ teaspoon table salt *or* ¼ teaspoon salt substitute
- 3 to 4 tablespoons sugar

If You Exercise or Work in the Heat

- Drink water before, during, and after exercise or work.
- Use a sports drink if you will be working or exercising for more than an hour and will be sweating a lot.
- Don't take salt tablets. Most people already have enough salt in their diets. Use sports drinks instead.
- Avoid caffeine. It makes you urinate more often, which makes you dehydrate faster.
- Do not drink alcohol.
- Wear one layer of lightweight, light-colored clothing. Change into dry clothing if your clothes get soaked with sweat.
- If you start to feel dehydrated, stop what you are doing. Try to find a cool spot to rest in, and drink plenty of fluids.

Eye (Object in)

When to Call a Doctor

Call 911 if the eyeball seems to be punctured.

Call a doctor if:

- The object is over the colored part of the eye or is stuck in the eye. Do not try to remove the object.
- There is blood over or in front of the colored part of the eye.
- You can't remove an object that is over the white of the eye or on the eyelid.
- You have removed the object but:
  - The pain is severe or does not go away.
  - It feels like there is still something in your eye.
  - Light hurts your eye.
  - Your vision does not return to normal.

Your cornea may be scratched. Keep your eye closed as much of the time as you can until you visit the doctor.

More

Eye (Object in)

A speck of dirt or a small object in the eye will often wash out with your tears. If the object does not come out, it may scratch the surface of the eye, called the cornea. Most corneal scratches will heal on their own in 1 or 2 days.

If an object is thrown forcefully into the eye (from a machine, for example), it may puncture the eyeball. This needs emergency care.

Always wear safety glasses or other protective eyewear when you work with machines or tools, mow the lawn, or ride a bike or motorcycle.

Home Treatment

- Wash your hands before you touch the eye.
- Do not rub the eye. You might scratch the cornea.
- Do not try to remove an object that is over the colored part of the eye or stuck in the white of the eye. Try flushing it out with water or saline.
- If the object is at the side of the eye or on the lower lid, moisten a cotton swab or the tip of a twisted piece of tissue and touch the end to the object. The object should cling to the swab or tissue. Your eye may be a little irritated afterward.

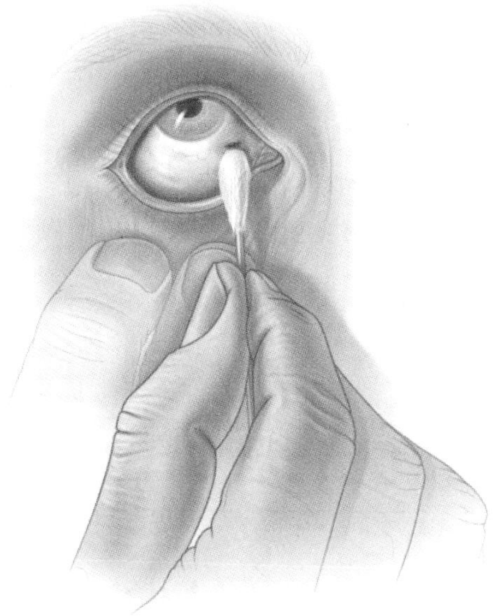

Use a moist cotton swab.

- Gently wash the eye with cool water. An eyedropper helps.
- Never use tweezers, toothpicks, or other hard items to remove an object from the eye.

Fainting and Unconsciousness

When to Call a Doctor

Call 911 if:

- A person is unconscious for more than a few seconds.
- A person faints and has bleeding from the rectum or in the stools, blood in the urine, or unexpected vaginal bleeding.

Call a doctor if:

- A person faints for a second or two and is now awake.
- A person with diabetes faints, even if he or she is now awake. This could be a low or high blood sugar emergency.
- Fainting has occurred more than once.

If the person has a head injury, see page 36.

A person who is unconscious is completely unaware of what's going on and cannot make purposeful movements.

When you faint, you lose consciousness briefly—usually only a few seconds. This is most often caused by a brief drop in blood flow to the brain. When you fall or lie down, blood flow improves and you "wake up." Stress or injury can also make you faint.

Fainting usually is not a cause for concern. But if it happens often, there may be a problem.

Staying unconscious for more than a few seconds usually is a sign of a serious problem. There are many reasons why this might happen. These include stroke, epilepsy, very low or very high blood sugar, head injury, not being able to breathe, alcohol or drug overdose, shock, bleeding, heartbeat problems, and heart attack.

Home Treatment

- Make sure the person can breathe. If the person is not breathing, start rescue breathing. See page 20.
- Lay the person on his or her side.
- Look for a medical alert bracelet, necklace, or card that says the person has a problem like epilepsy, diabetes, or a drug allergy.
- Treat any injuries.
- Do not give the person anything to eat or drink.

Falls

When to Call a Doctor

Call 911 if:

- A person is unconscious for more than a few seconds after a fall. See page 33.
- A person who fell has a seizure. See page 45.
- A person cannot get up at all after a fall.
- You can see a bone after a fall, or a body part is the wrong shape now.

Call a doctor if:

- You passed out after a fall but are now conscious again. See page 33.
- A fall caused severe bleeding or bruising. See Bleeding Emergencies on page 17 and Bruises on page 22.
- You think you might have broken a bone. See page 49.
- You have pain in your hips, lower back, or wrist after a fall.
- You think you fell because of a medicine or a health problem.

If you fall and you are not badly hurt, you may be able to treat yourself at home. To get up safely:

- Roll to your hands and knees.
- Crawl to a piece of furniture that will support your weight, such as a sofa or sturdy table.
- Use the furniture to pull yourself up.
- Sit for a minute before you try to stand.

If you have a minor injury, such as a bruise, strain, or sprain, look up the right home treatment in the index at the back of this book.

Avoiding Falls

Falls can cause serious injuries, especially in older adults who may have weak bones. And the damage may take longer to heal than it would in a younger person.

Do what you can to prevent falls. This means things like making your home safer, staying active, and being aware of medicines and health problems that can affect your balance or movement. See page 364 to learn what steps you can take today to protect yourself.

Frostbite

When to Call a Doctor

- The skin is white or blue and hard, rubbery, and cold. These are signs of severe frostbite. You need careful rewarming and antibiotics to prevent permanent tissue damage and infection.
- Blisters form. Do not break them. The risk of infection is very high.
- You have signs of infection. These may include increased pain, swelling, warmth, or redness; red streaks leading from the area; pus; or fever.

Frostbite is freezing of the skin and, if it is severe, the tissues beneath it. Frostbite is most likely to occur on the feet, hands, ears, nose, and face.

How severe the frostbite is depends on how long you were in the cold and how cold it was. Wind and damp air can make things worse.

With mild frostbite (sometimes called frostnip):

- The skin may be pale or red and may tingle or burn.
- If you rewarm the area soon, it will probably not blister or get worse.

As frostbite gets worse:

- The skin may feel hard, frozen, and numb. Later you may feel burning, throbbing, or shooting pain.
- Blisters may form as the skin warms. In severe cases, blisters may appear as small bloody spots under the skin.
- The tissue beneath the skin may freeze and harden.
- At its worst, the skin may turn dry, black, and rubbery. You may also have deep, aching pain in your joints.

Home Treatment

- Get inside, or at least take shelter from the wind.
- Check for signs of hypothermia, such as violent shivering, clumsy movement and speech, and confusion. Treat those before treating frostbite. See Hypothermia on page 41.
- Protect the frozen body part from further cold.

More

- To warm small areas (ears, face, nose, fingers, toes), breathe on them or tuck them inside warm clothing next to bare skin.
- Do not rub or massage the frozen area. This can further damage the skin and tissue beneath it. Do not walk on frostbitten feet unless you have no choice.
- Keep the area warm, and prop it up above the level of your heart. Wrap it with blankets or soft clothing to prevent bruising. If possible, soak it in warm water (104°F to 108°F) for 15 to 30 minutes.
- If blisters form, do not break them.
- Take ibuprofen (Advil, Motrin) or acetaminophen (Tylenol) for pain.

Head Injury

When to Call a Doctor

Call 911 if:

- The person is unconscious for more than a few seconds.
- Severe bleeding does not slow down or stop after 15 minutes of direct pressure. See page 17.
- The person has a seizure. See page 45.
- The person feels weak or numb on one side of the body.
- Double vision or trouble speaking lasts more than a minute or two.
- The person seems confused, does not remember being hurt, or keeps asking the same questions.
- You have trouble waking the person at any time in the next 24 hours.

Call a doctor if:

- The person fainted for a second or two and is now awake.
- Vomiting occurs after the first 2 hours, or violent vomiting goes on after the first 15 minutes. (Vomiting once or twice right after the injury is common and usually is not serious.)
- The person has a severe headache.
- Blood or clear fluid drains from the ears or nose and clearly was not caused by a cut or direct hit to the ears or nose.
- There is bruising around the eyes or behind one ear.
- There is a new "dent" or deformity in the skull.
- The wound needs stitches. See page 29.
- The person takes blood thinners such as warfarin (Coumadin).

Most bumps on the head are minor and heal as easily as bumps anywhere else.

Minor cuts on the head often bleed a lot, because the blood vessels of the scalp are so close to the skin's surface. In these cases, the injury may look worse than it is.

But a head injury may also be worse than it looks. An injury that doesn't bleed on the outside may still have caused dangerous bleeding and swelling inside the skull. The more force involved in the injury, the more likely it is serious.

Anyone who has had a head injury should be watched carefully for 24 hours for signs of a serious problem.

Avoid Head Injuries

- Wear your seat belt every time you get in a car.
- Wear a helmet when you bike, ski, and do other activities like these.
- Take steps to prevent falls. See page 364. This is especially important if you have balance problems or take medicines that might make you unsteady.

Home Treatment

- If the person is unconscious, assume he or she has a spinal injury. Do not move the person without first protecting the neck from movement.
- If there is bleeding, put firm pressure directly over the wound with a clean cloth for 15 minutes. If the blood soaks through, put another cloth over the first one. See Stopping Severe Bleeding on page 17.
- Check for injuries to other parts of the body. The panic from seeing a head injury may cause you to miss other injuries that need attention.
- Use ice or cold packs to reduce the swelling. A "goose egg" lump may appear anyway, but ice will help ease the pain.
- For the first 24 hours after a head injury, watch the person closely for signs of a severe head injury: every 2 hours, check for the symptoms listed in When to Call a Doctor.
- Avoid contact sports until cleared by a doctor.

Heart Attack

Signs of a Heart Attack

- Chest pain or pressure. This is the most common symptom. But some people—especially women, older adults, and people with diabetes—may not have chest pain during a heart attack.
- Sweating
- Shortness of breath
- Nausea or vomiting
- Pain or discomfort in the upper back, upper belly, neck, jaw, or arms
- Feeling dizzy or lightheaded
- A fast or uneven heartbeat

The symptoms of a heart attack usually last longer than 5 minutes and do not go away with rest.

When to Call a Doctor

Call 911 if you think you may be having a heart attack. Do not wait to see if you will feel better. After calling 911, chew 1 adult aspirin (unless you are allergic to it).

If you can't get an ambulance, have someone drive you to the hospital. Do not drive yourself.

Call a doctor if you have mild chest pain that does not stop or keeps coming back, and there is no obvious cause. See Chest Pain on page 114.

The coronary arteries carry blood to the heart (see the picture on page 287). A heart attack occurs when one or more of the arteries are blocked and blood cannot reach the heart. Sometimes this happens when plaque inside an artery breaks open and a blood clot forms.

Many people mistake a heart attack for another problem, such as heartburn or a pulled muscle. It is important to recognize the signals your body sends during the early stages of a heart attack and get help. Quick treatment may reduce the damage caused by a heart attack and may save your life.

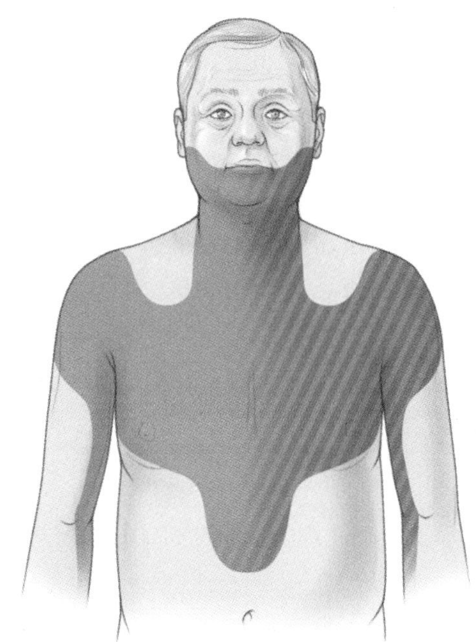

A heart attack may cause discomfort in any of the shaded areas as well as the upper back.

Heat Sickness

When to Call a Doctor

Call 911 if:

- Body temperature reaches 102.3°F and keeps rising.
- A person has signs of heat stroke, such as confusion, fainting, or seizure. The skin may be red, hot, and dry, or the person may be sweating a lot.

Call a doctor if the person still has symptoms of heat exhaustion (headache, fatigue, dizziness, or nausea) after cooling off.

Heat sickness occurs when your body does not stay cool enough in hot temperatures. Older adults tend to be at higher risk for heat sickness because they do not sweat easily. And some have health problems or take medicines that affect how their bodies deal with heat.

Heat exhaustion usually occurs when you are sweating a lot and do not drink enough to replace lost fluids. It often happens when you are working or exercising in hot weather. (See If You Exercise or Work in the Heat on page 31 for tips on how to prevent this.)

Heat stroke can quickly follow if you don't correct the problem. It occurs when your body cannot control its own temperature and your temperature keeps rising, often to 105°F or higher. This can lead to death.

Home Treatment

- Have the person stop and rest. Get the person out of the sun to a cool spot.
- Have the person drink lots of cool water, a little at a time. If the person is nauseated or dizzy, have him or her lie down.

More

Symptoms of heat exhaustion	Symptoms of heat stroke
◆ Sweating a lot ◆ Skin is cool, moist, pale, or red ◆ Fatigue, weakness, headache, dizziness, or nausea	◆ Sweating may be heavy or may have stopped ◆ Skin may be red, hot, and dry, even in the armpits ◆ Confusion, fainting, or seizure

- Take the person's temperature. If it is over 102.3 °F (or if you don't have a thermometer but think the person may have a high fever), call for help and try to lower the temperature quickly:
  - Remove the person's clothing.
  - Apply cool (not cold) water to the whole body. Then fan the person.
  - Put ice packs on the groin, neck, and armpits.
  - Do not put the person in an ice-water bath.
  - When the temperature is down to 102 °F, take care to avoid overcooling. Stop cooling the person as soon as body temperature is back to normal or the person's skin feels the same temperature as yours.
  - Do not use medicine, such as aspirin or acetaminophen (Tylenol), to reduce the temperature.
- Watch for signs of heat stroke (confusion or unconsciousness; red, hot, dry skin).
- If the person stops breathing, start rescue breathing. See page 20.

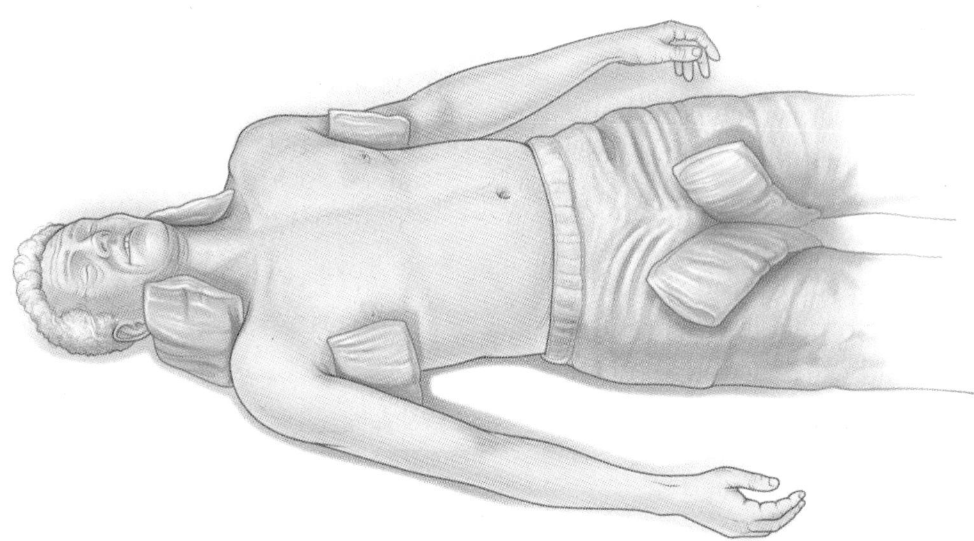

Put ice packs on the groin, neck, and armpits.

Hypothermia

When to Call a Doctor

Call 911 if a person is very confused, stumbles a lot, or faints, and you suspect hypothermia.

Call a doctor if:

- The person's temperature is still below 96°F after 2 hours of warming.
- The person is a frail older adult. It is a good idea to call even if the symptoms seem mild.

Hypothermia is below-normal body temperature that happens when the body loses heat faster than it can produce heat. It is an emergency that can quickly lead to death.

It does not have to be that cold for a person to get hypothermia.

- You can get it at temperatures of 50°F or even higher in wet and windy weather.
- It can happen in water that is 60°F to 70°F.
- It can happen indoors.

Chronic health problems like diabetes or heart disease, some medicines, and normal aging may make you less likely to notice that you're cold or may affect your body's ability to stay warm. Frail or inactive older adults may have an especially hard time.

Do not ignore early warning signs. Often a person will lose a lot of heat before you notice something is wrong. If someone starts to shiver fiercely, stumble, or respond strangely to questions, suspect hypothermia and warm the person quickly.

More

If You Live Alone

If you are an older adult who lives alone, it's a good idea to check in with someone every day when the weather is cold. Ask a friend or family member to check on you once a day to make sure you're okay.

Early warning signs	Advanced warning signs
◆ Shivering	◆ A cold belly
◆ Cold, pale skin	◆ Stiff, hard muscles. Shivering may stop if the person's temperature drops below 90°F.
◆ Lack of interest or concern	◆ Slow pulse and slow breathing
◆ Poor judgment	◆ Weakness or drowsiness
◆ Clumsy movement and speech	◆ Confusion

Home Treatment

The goal of home or "in-the-field" treatment is to stop heat loss and safely rewarm the person.

- Get the person out of the cold and wind. If you are indoors, turn up the heat or move to a warmer spot.
- Remove cold, wet clothes first, and give the person dry or wool clothing to wear. Or warm the person with your own body heat by wrapping a blanket or sleeping bag around both of you.
- Give the person warm drinks and high-energy foods, such as candy. But do not give food or drink if the person is confused or has fainted. Do not give the person alcohol or caffeine.
- If home treatment is not working and you cannot get help, put the person in a warm (100°F to 105°F) bath. This can cause shock or heart attack, so do it only as a last resort.

Stay Warm

If you plan to be out in cold weather:

- Dress warmly, and wear windproof, waterproof clothing. Wear fabrics that stay warm even when wet, such as wool, fleece, or polypropylene.
- Wear a warm hat.
- Keep your hands and feet dry.
- Head for shelter if you get wet or cold.
- Eat well before you go out, and carry extra food.
- Do not drink alcohol while in the cold. It makes your body lose heat faster.

To stay warm indoors:

- Keep the thermostat above 65°F. If heating the whole house is a problem, keep just a few rooms heated and close off the others.
- Eat regularly. Your body needs food to make heat.
- Move around often. If you can't move around well, do chair exercises or other things that will get your blood moving.
- Dress warmly. Wear warm clothes to bed, and use warm bedding.

Nosebleeds

When to Call a Doctor

- Your nose is still bleeding after 30 minutes of pinching it.
- Blood runs down the back of your throat even when you pinch your nose.
- Your nose looks or feels broken.
- You get lots of nosebleeds—4 or more a week, for instance.
- You take blood thinners (such as warfarin or Coumadin) or high doses of aspirin and have more than one nosebleed in a day.

Most nosebleeds are not serious. You may get one because of dry air or high altitude, an injury to the nose, or medicines (especially aspirin). Blowing or picking your nose can also cause a nosebleed.

People who have allergy problems may get nosebleeds a lot because the inside of the nose is irritated. Allergy medicines may help with this, but they can make the problem worse if you use them too often. Talk to your doctor about how best to use these medicines.

Home Treatment

- Sit up straight, and tip your head slightly forward. Tilting your head back may cause blood to run down your throat, which may make you vomit.
- Blow your nose gently to remove any blood clots. Then pinch your nose shut with your thumb and index finger for 10 minutes.
- After 10 minutes, check to see if your nose is still bleeding. If it is, pinch it shut for 10 more minutes. Most nosebleeds will stop after you do this for 10 to 30 minutes.
- Do not blow your nose for at least 12 hours after the bleeding has stopped.
- If your nose is very dry, breathe moist air for a while (such as in the shower). Then put a little petroleum jelly on the inside of your nose. A saline nasal spray may also help. See page 229.

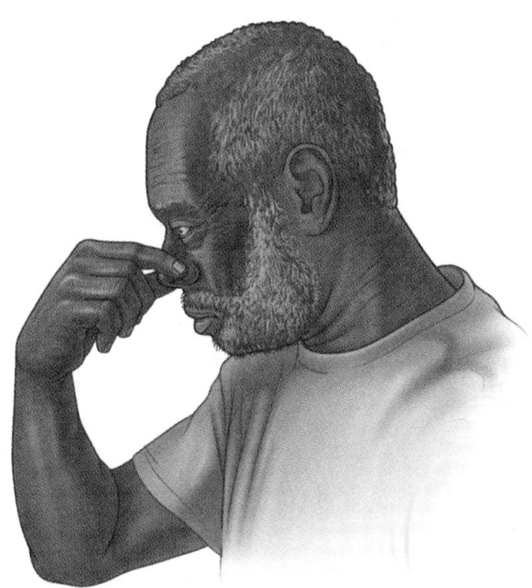

To stop a nosebleed, tip your head forward and pinch your nose shut.

Scrapes

When to Call a Doctor

- The scrape is still bleeding after 30 minutes of pressure.
- You cannot clean the scrape well because it is too large, deep, or painful, or because dirt and other matter is stuck under the skin.
- You have not had a tetanus shot in the past 5 years. If you need a shot, make sure to get it within 2 days.
- You have signs of infection. These may include increased pain, swelling, warmth, or redness; red streaks leading from the scrape; pus; or fever.

Most scrapes are not deep. But your skin gets thinner as you age, and it may tear or peel away more easily if you get a scrape. Open wounds like these can get infected easily (especially if you have diabetes), so be sure to take good care of the scrape.

Home Treatment

- Scrapes are often very dirty. Remove large pieces of dirt and gravel with tweezers. Then scrub well with soap and water and a washcloth. Scrubbing may cause some minor bleeding. Using a water sprayer from a sink is a good way to wash a scrape.
- Apply steady pressure with a clean cloth to stop any bleeding. If the bleeding is heavy, see Bleeding Emergencies on page 17.
- Use ice or a cold pack to reduce swelling and bruising. Put a thin cloth between the ice and your skin.
- If the scrape is large or in an area where clothing may rub on it, apply an antibiotic ointment (such as bacitracin or Polysporin) and cover the scrape with a nonstick bandage. If the skin has peeled away in a thin layer but is still attached, try to smooth it over the area before you bandage it. Change the bandage once a day and anytime it gets wet.

Seizures

When to Call a Doctor

Call 911 if:

- A person is having a seizure for the first time.
- A person having a seizure stops breathing for longer than 30 seconds.
- A seizure lasts longer than 3 minutes.
- More than one seizure occurs within 24 hours.
- A seizure occurs with any signs of stroke. These may include sudden numbness, paralysis, or weakness; sudden problems with walking or balance; sudden vision changes; sudden problems speaking to or understanding others; or sudden, severe headache.
- A seizure occurs with signs of serious illness, such as fever, severe headache, stiff neck, trouble breathing, or an unexplained rash.
- A seizure follows a head injury.
- A person has a seizure after using drugs or drinking a lot of alcohol.
- A person with diabetes has a seizure.

Call a doctor if you have been diagnosed with epilepsy and notice a change in your seizures (for instance, they happen more often or are worse than they used to be).

The brain controls how the body moves by sending electrical signals through the nerves to the muscles. You can have a seizure if the normal signals from the brain change.

- Your whole body may stiffen or jerk violently, or you may have only slight shaking of a hand or other body part.
- You may briefly lose touch with your surroundings and appear to stare into space.
- You may or may not faint.
- You may not remember the seizure afterward.

Any normally healthy person can have a single seizure under certain conditions. For instance, being hit in the head may cause a seizure. Certain medicines can cause seizures in some people. But a seizure may also be a sign of a more serious problem, so see a doctor to find the cause.

More

Home Treatment

No matter what causes the seizure, there are things you can do to help a person during and after a seizure.

During a seizure:

- Protect the person from injury. If you can, keep him or her from falling. Try to move furniture or other objects out of the way.
- Don't force your fingers or anything else into the person's mouth.
- Don't try to hold down or move the person.
- Try to stay calm.
- Pay close attention to what the person is doing so you can describe the seizure to doctors.
- Time the seizure if you can.

After a seizure:

- Check for injuries.
- Turn the person onto his or her side once he or she is more relaxed.
- If the person has trouble breathing, use your finger to gently clear the mouth of any vomit or saliva.
- Loosen tight clothing around the person's neck and waist.
- Provide a safe area where the person can rest.
- Do not give the person anything to eat or drink until he or she is fully awake and alert.
- Stay with the person until he or she is awake and aware of the surroundings. Most people will be sleepy or confused after a seizure.

Shock

When to Call a Doctor

Call 911 if you think someone is in shock. Signs of shock include:

- Weakness, dizziness, and fainting.
- Cool, pale, moist skin.
- A weak, fast pulse.
- Shallow, fast breathing.
- Low blood pressure.
- Extreme thirst, nausea, or vomiting.
- Confusion or anxiety.
- Trouble staying alert or waking up.

Shock means that your body and its functions are shutting down. The body goes into shock when it cannot get enough blood to vital organs like your heart and brain. This may be caused by sudden illness, injury, or bleeding. Sometimes even a mild injury will lead to shock.

Prompt home treatment of shock can save the person's life.

Home Treatment

- **Call 911.**
- Have the person lie down. If there is an injury to the head, neck, or chest, keep the legs flat. Otherwise, raise the person's legs at least 12 inches.
- If the person vomits, roll him or her to one side to let fluids drain from the mouth. Use care if there could be an injury to the back or neck.
- Stop any bleeding (see page 17) and splint any broken bones (see page 53).
- Keep the person warm but not hot. Put a blanket under the person, and cover him or her with a sheet or blanket, depending on the weather. If the person is in a hot place, try to keep the person cool.
- Take the person's pulse in case medical staff on the phone need to know what it is. See page 48. Take it again if the person's condition changes.
- Try to keep the person calm.

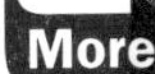

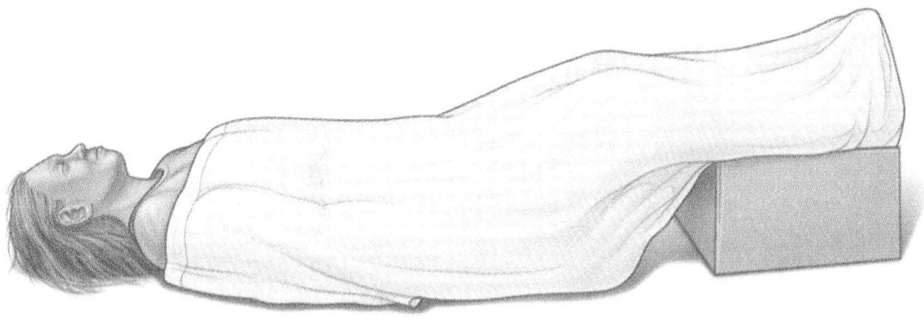

Raise the legs, and keep the person warm but not hot.

How to Take a Pulse

Your pulse is the rate at which your heart beats. It is measured in beats per minute.

As the heart pumps blood through the arteries to the rest of the body, you can feel a throbbing wherever the arteries come close to the skin's surface, such as at the wrist.

To take a pulse:

- Place two fingers gently against the wrist to find the heartbeat. Do not use your thumb.
- Count the beats for 30 seconds. Then double the number of beats to know the beats per minute.

Resting pulse

To get a resting pulse, take the pulse after you have been resting quietly for at least 10 minutes. Certain illnesses can raise your pulse, so it helps to know what your resting pulse rate is when you are well. The pulse rate rises about 10 beats per minute for every degree of fever.

Normal resting pulse for an adult is 50 to 100 beats per minute.

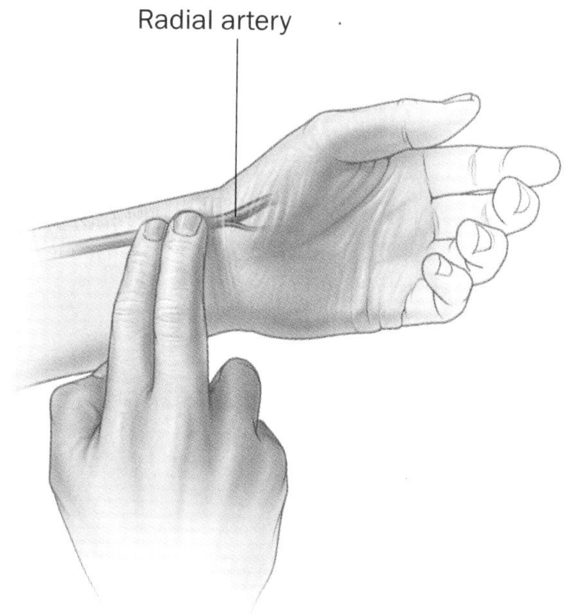

Taking a pulse at the wrist

Splinters

When to Call a Doctor

- A splinter is very large or deep in the skin, and you cannot easily remove it.
- The splinter is in the eye.
- You have signs of infection. These may include increased pain, swelling, warmth, or redness; red streaks leading from the wound; pus; or fever.

To remove a splinter:

- Try Scotch tape first. Put a piece of tape over the splinter and pull it up.
- If that doesn't work, grip the end of the splinter with tweezers, and try to gently pull it out.
- If the splinter is not sticking out where you can reach it, clean a needle with rubbing alcohol and make a small hole in the skin over the end of the splinter. Then lift the splinter with the tip of the needle until you can grab it with the tweezers.

After you have removed the splinter, wash the area with soap and water. Use a bandage if the wound is in an area that might get dirty.

Strains, Sprains, and Broken Bones

When to Call a Doctor

- A bone is poking through the skin.
- The hurt limb or joint looks odd, is a strange shape, or is out of its normal position.
- You have signs of nerve or blood vessel damage, such as:
  - Numbness, tingling, or a pins-and-needles feeling.
  - Skin that is pale, white, or blue, or feels colder than the skin on the limb that is not hurt.
  - Not being able to move the limb normally because of weakness, not just pain.
- The skin over the site of an injury is broken.
- You cannot bear weight on or straighten a hurt limb, or a joint wobbles or feels unstable.
- You have severe pain.
- You have a lot of swelling within 30 minutes after the injury.
- Swelling and pain do not improve after 2 days of home treatment.
- You have signs of infection. These may include increased pain, swelling, warmth, and redness; red streaks leading from the area; or fever.

More

A **strain** is caused by overstretching or tearing a muscle or tendon. Tendons connect muscle and bone.

A **sprain** is an injury to the ligaments or soft tissues around a joint. Ligaments connect one bone to another.

A broken bone is called a **fracture**.

A **dislocation** occurs when one end of a bone is pulled or pushed out of its normal position.

All of these injuries cause pain and swelling. Unless a broken bone is obvious, it may be hard to tell whether you have a strain, sprain, break, or dislocation. Rapid swelling often means you have a more serious injury.

You can treat most minor strains and sprains at home. Bad sprains, broken bones, and dislocations need medical care. Do home treatment while you wait to see your doctor.

Home Treatment

The first steps in home treatment are usually the same no matter what the injury. They are known as "RICE," which stands for rest, ice, compression, and elevation. Start the RICE process right away.

1. Rest (**R**ICE)

- Do not put weight on the injury for at least 24 to 48 hours.
- Use crutches for a badly sprained knee or ankle.
- Support a sprained wrist, elbow, or shoulder with a sling. See page 52.
- Rest a sprained finger by taping it to the healthy finger next to it. This also works for toes. Always put padding between the two fingers or toes that you tape together. See page 53.

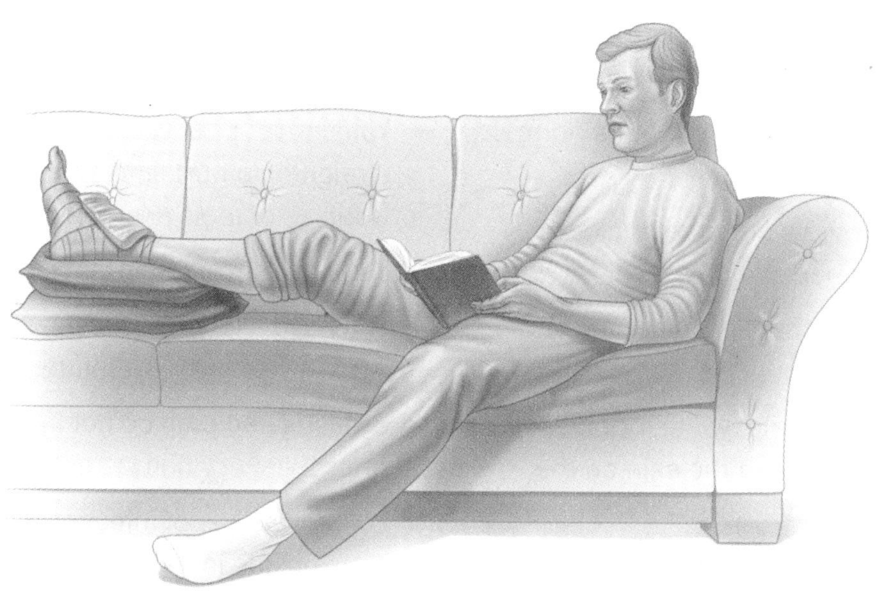

RICE: Rest, ice, compress (wrap), and elevate

2. Ice (R**I**CE)

- Put ice or cold packs on the injury right away to reduce pain and swelling and help it heal. For the first 48 to 72 hours, use ice for 10 to 15 minutes at a time once an hour (or as often as you can). For hard-to-reach injuries, a cold pack or a bag of frozen vegetables works better than ice. See Ice and Cold Packs on this page.
- Heat feels nice, but it does more harm than good if you use it too soon. You may use heat (warm towel, heating pad) after 48 to 72 hours of cold treatments if the swelling is gone. Some experts say to switch back and forth between heat and cold.

More

Ice and Cold Packs

Ice can relieve pain, swelling, and inflammation from injuries and problems like bursitis and arthritis. You can use any of these items to "ice" an area:

- A cold pack you buy at the drugstore or grocery store. Store the pack in the freezer.
- A homemade cold pack. Seal 1 pint of rubbing alcohol and 3 pints of water in a 1-gallon, heavy-duty, plastic freezer bag. Seal that bag inside a second bag. Mark it "Cold pack: Do not eat," and store it in the freezer.
- A bag of frozen vegetables. Peas or corn work well. Do not eat them once you have used them as a cold pack. Label the bag "Do not eat." You can reuse it several times.
- An ice towel. Wet a towel with cold water, and squeeze it until it is just damp. Fold the towel, place it in a plastic bag, and freeze it for 15 minutes. Take the towel out of the bag, and use it like a cold pack.
- An ice pack. Put about a pound of ice in a plastic bag. Add water to barely cover the ice. Squeeze the air out of the bag and seal it. Wrap the bag in a damp towel and put it on the sore area.

Ice the area at least 3 times a day. For the first 48 hours, try to ice for 10 to 15 minutes once an hour. After that, a good pattern is to ice for 10 to 15 minutes, 3 times a day. Also ice after any long periods of activity or hard exercise.

Always keep a thin cloth between your skin and the cold pack so that the cold does not damage your skin. Press the pack firmly so that it touches all parts of the affected area.

Do not use cold for longer than 10 to 15 minutes at a time, and do not fall asleep with ice on your skin.

3. Compression (RI**C**E)

- Wrap the injured area with an elastic (Ace) bandage or compression sleeve to reduce swelling. Do not wrap it too tightly. If the area below it feels numb, tingles, or feels cool, loosen the wrap.
- A tightly wrapped sprain may fool you into thinking you can keep using the joint. With or without a wrap, the joint needs total rest for 1 to 2 days.

4. Elevation (RIC**E**)

- Prop up the injured area on pillows whenever you use ice and anytime you are sitting or lying down.
- Try to keep the injury at or above the level of your heart to help reduce swelling and bruising.

Stress Fractures

A stress fracture is a weak spot or small crack in a bone caused by overuse or repeated impact. For example, stress fractures in the small bones of the foot may result from long-distance running or heavy training for other sports.

The usual sign of a stress fracture is pain in one spot that keeps coming back or will not go away. The pain may get better while you exercise but will be worse before and after activity. There may not be any swelling you can see.

Stress fractures need 2 to 4 months of rest to heal.

Other Tips

You may prevent further damage and feel better faster if you follow these tips after you get hurt:

- Until you can see your doctor, splint an arm, leg, finger, or toe that you think is broken. See Splinting on page 53. You can also use a sling to protect an injured arm or shoulder until you see a doctor.

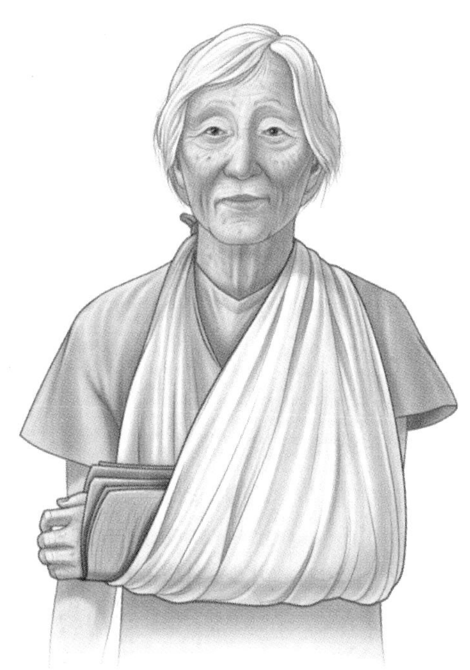

A homemade sling can protect an injured arm until you see a doctor.

- Remove all rings, watches, and bracelets from a hurt finger or hand right away. Swelling may make it hard to remove these items later.
- Take aspirin, ibuprofen (Advil, Motrin), or naproxen (Aleve) to help ease swelling and pain.
- Start gentle exercise as soon as the initial pain and swelling have gone away.

Splinting

These splinting methods are for short-term first aid only. Your doctor will give you a splint or cast that is right for your injury.

If you think a bone is broken, you can splint it so that it doesn't move. This prevents further injury until you can see a doctor. Splinting may also help after a snakebite while you wait for help to arrive.

There are two ways to splint a limb:

Method 1: Tie the injured limb to a stiff object, such as rolled-up newspapers or magazines, a stick, or a cane. You can use a rope, a belt, or anything else that will work as a tie. Do not tie too tightly. Place the splint so the hurt limb cannot bend. Try to splint from a joint above the suspected break to a joint below it. For example, splint a broken forearm from above the elbow to below the wrist.

Method 2: Tape a broken finger or toe to the next finger or toe. Make sure you put padding between them. Tie a hurt arm across the chest to keep it from moving.

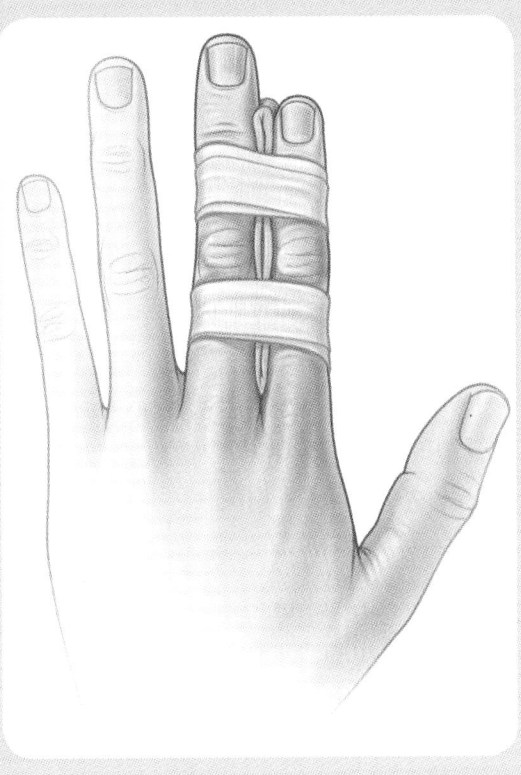

Stroke

Signs of Stroke

- ◆ Sudden weakness, numbness, or loss of movement in your face, arm, or leg, especially on only one side of your body.
- ◆ Sudden loss or change in vision that does not clear when you blink.
- ◆ Sudden trouble speaking or understanding simple statements.
- ◆ A sudden, severe headache that is different from any past headache.
- ◆ Sudden, severe dizziness, loss of balance, or loss of coordination, especially if another warning sign is present at the same time.

When to Call a Doctor

Call 911 if you think you may be having a stroke. If you can't get an ambulance, have someone drive you to the hospital. Do not drive yourself.

Call a doctor if symptoms were definitely there and then went away after a few minutes. This could be a sign that a stroke may soon occur. See What's a TIA? on this page.

A stroke occurs when a blood vessel to the brain bursts or is blocked by a blood clot. Within minutes, the nerve cells in that part of the brain die. As a result, the part of the body controlled by those cells cannot work properly.

The effects of a stroke may range from mild to severe. They may get better, or they may last the rest of your life. A stroke can affect vision, speech, behavior, thought processes, and your ability to move. Sometimes it can cause a coma or death.

Get help as soon as you notice stroke symptoms. Quick treatment may reduce the damage in your brain so that you have fewer problems after the stroke.

If you or a loved one has had a stroke, be sure to see Living Better After a Stroke on page 314.

What's a TIA?

TIAs—transient ischemic attacks—are often called "mini-strokes" because their symptoms are like those of a stroke. The difference is that TIA symptoms usually go away within 10 to 20 minutes. (Rarely, they may last up to 24 hours.)

A TIA is a warning that you may soon have a stroke. It can occur months before a stroke occurs. You may have one or more TIAs before you finally have a stroke. If you think you have had a TIA, see your doctor right away.

Suicide

When to Call a Doctor

Call 911 if you or someone you know is about to attempt or is attempting suicide.

Call a doctor, your local suicide hotline, or the national suicide hotline at 1-800-784-2433 (1-800-SUICIDE) if:

- You are thinking about suicide.
- You think or know that someone has made suicide plans.

If you are very depressed or feel hopeless, you may sometimes think of taking your own life. Occasional, fleeting thoughts of death are normal. But if thoughts of suicide continue, or if you have made suicide plans, you need help today.

The suicide rate among older adults is higher than in any other age group. Though it comes with many great things too, life as an older adult can pose real challenges—the death of loved ones, serious illness or disability, new money worries, and basic changes in your day-to-day life. Some older adults either don't have or don't know where to find the support that can help them cope with these changes.

Older adults may not give you many warning signs that they are thinking about suicide. Pay attention if an older adult you know seems depressed. With help and compassion, that person may choose to live.

Warning Signs of Suicide in Older Adults

- Spending lots of time alone. A suicidal person may stop seeing or calling friends and stop doing his or her normal activities.
- Talking about killing oneself.
- Giving away favorite things.
- Talking about death and dying a lot.
- Heavy use of alcohol or drugs.

Home Treatment

For yourself:

- Do not use alcohol or illegal drugs. They may make you more likely to do things you would not do when sober. It's also important to take your medicines as directed.
- Talk about your thoughts with someone you trust—a friend or family member, a clergy member, or a doctor. Or call a suicide hotline.
- If you think you are in a moment of crisis, ask someone you trust to stay with you until the crisis has passed or until you can get help.

More

If you are worried about someone else:

- Do not ignore warning signs, thinking that the person will "snap out of it."
- Talk about the problem as openly as you can. Show understanding and compassion. Do not argue with or challenge the person.
- Encourage the person to get professional help today. Do what you can to make it happen. Help the person set up the appointment, and make sure the person has a way to get there. Follow up to find out how the treatment is going.
- Use common sense and a direct approach to find out if the suicide risk is high. Ask the person:
  - Do you feel there is no other way?
  - Do you have a suicide plan?
  - How and when do you plan to do it?
- If you think the risk is high, do not leave. Stay with the person until the crisis has passed or until you can get help.

Sunburn

When to Call a Doctor

Call 911 if you are sunburned and have signs of heat stroke, such as confusion or fainting. See page 39.

Call a doctor if:

- You have symptoms of heat exhaustion (dizziness, nausea, headache) even though you have cooled off.
- Symptoms of mild dehydration (dry mouth, dark urine, not much urine) get worse even with home treatment.
- You have bad blisters from a sunburn.
- You have severe pain with fever, or you feel very sick.
- You have a fever of 102°F or higher.

Unless a sunburn is severe, it's usually something you can treat at home. Bad sunburns can be serious in older adults.

Home Treatment

- Drink plenty of water, and watch for signs of dehydration. See page 29. Also watch for signs of heat sickness. See page 39.
- Take a cool bath or use a cool, wet cloth to soothe the skin. Take acetaminophen (Tylenol) or aspirin for pain or mild fever.
- Use a moisturizing lotion to help with itching. There is nothing you can do to prevent peeling. It's part of the healing process.

Common Health Problems

Symptom Guides 59
Chest, Heart, and Lung Problems . 59
Digestive Problems 60
Skin Problems 61
Eye and Vision Problems 62
Ear and Hearing Problems 63
Nose and Throat Problems 63
Headaches 64
Urinary Problems 65
Abdominal Pain 66
Abuse and Violence 68
Alcohol and Drugs 70
Allergies 73
Anger and Hostility 76
Anxiety and Panic 77
Back Pain 79
Bladder and Kidney Infections 90
Bladder Control 92
Blisters 95
Blood Clots in the Leg 96
Boils 98
Breast Problems 99
Breathing Problems 101
Bronchitis 102
Bunions and Hammer Toes 103
Bursitis and Tendinosis 105
Calluses and Corns 109
Canker Sores 109
Carpal Tunnel Syndrome 110
Cataracts 113
Chest Pain 114
Cold Hands and Feet 117
Cold Sores 118
Colds 119
Colorectal Cancer 121
Confusion and Memory Loss 122
Constipation 124
Cough 126
Diarrhea 127
Diverticular Disease 129
Dizziness and Vertigo 130
Dry Mouth 133
Dry Skin 134
Ear Infections 135
Earwax 137
Erection Problems 138
Eye Problems 140
Pinkeye 140
Dry Eyes 143
Blood in the Eye 143
Eyelid Problems 144
Fatigue and Weakness 145

More

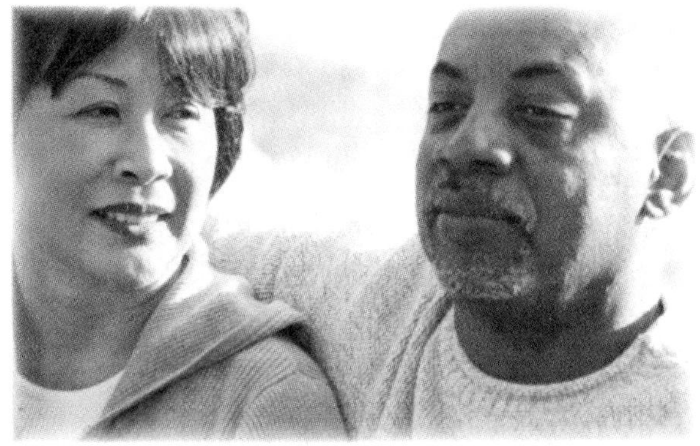

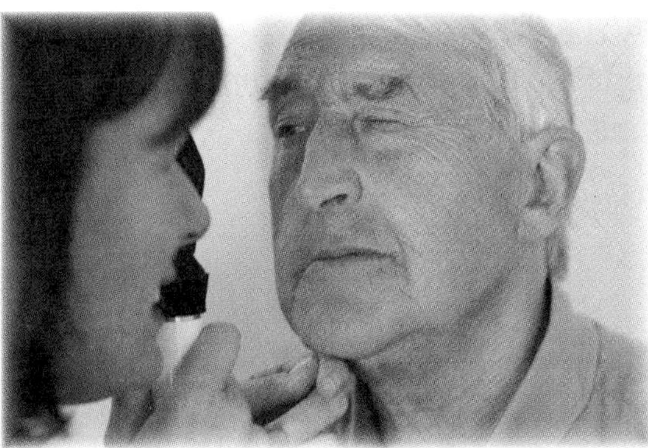

Female Pelvic Problems. 148
Fever 150
Fibromyalgia 152
Flu 153
Food Poisoning 155
Fungal Infections 157
Gallstones 159
Gas. 161
Glaucoma 162
Gout 163
Gum Disease 164
Hair Loss. 165
Headaches. 166
Hearing Problems 170
Hearing Loss. 171
Ringing in the Ears 173
Heartbeat Changes 174
Heartburn 176
Heel Pain and Plantar Fasciitis . . . 178
Hemorrhoids and Rectal Problems. 180
Hernia 182
High Blood Pressure 183
High Cholesterol. 186
Hives 188
Ingrown Toenail 189
Irritable Bowel Syndrome 190
Jaw Pain and Temporomandibular Disorder . . 192
Kidney Stones 193
Knee Problems 194
Laryngitis 196
Leg Pain and Muscle Cramps. . . . 197
Lung Cancer 200
Menopause 201
Neck Pain 204
Osteoporosis. 207
Peripheral Artery Disease. 208
Pneumonia 210
Polymyalgia Rheumatica 212
Pressure Sores 213
Prostate Cancer 214
Prostate Enlargement. 215
Prostatitis 217
Rashes. 218
Rosacea 221
Sexually Transmitted Diseases (STDs). 222
Shingles 225
Sinusitis 227
Skin Cancer 230
Skin Growths and Spots 231
Sleep Problems 232
Sore Throat 235
Swollen Lymph Nodes. 236
Thyroid, Low (Hypothyroidism) . . . 238
Toothache 240
Tooth Injury 241
Tremor (Shaking) 241
Ulcers 243
Vaginitis 245
Varicose Veins 247
Vision Changes 248
Vomiting 253
Warts. 254

Symptom Guides

Look on the left side of the chart to find the symptoms that most closely match yours. Then look on the right to see examples of what can cause those symptoms and where to go to learn more. The charts do not include all possible causes for each symptom.

Chest, Heart, and Lung Problems	
Symptoms	**Possible Causes**
Wheezing or fast, shallow, or troubled breathing	- Allergies, p. 73 - Asthma, p. 271 - Bronchitis, p. 102 - COPD, p. 282 Also see Breathing Problems, p. 101.
Cough, fever, yellow-green or rust-colored sputum, and trouble breathing	- Bronchitis, p. 102 - Pneumonia, p. 210
Chest pain or pressure with sweating or quick pulse	- Heart attack, see p. 38. **This may be an emergency.** Also see Chest Pain, p. 114.
Shortness of breath and coughing	- Asthma, p. 271 - Bronchitis, p. 102 - COPD, p. 282 - Heart failure, p. 303 - Pneumonia, p. 210 Also see Breathing Problems, p. 101.
Burning, pain, or discomfort behind or below the breastbone	- Heartburn, p. 176 Also see Chest Pain, p. 114.
Coughing	See Cough, p. 126.
Pounding or racing heartbeat; heart skipping or missing a beat	- Heart arrhythmia, p. 174 - Anxiety, p. 77
Chest pain when you cough or breathe deeply	- Pneumonia, p. 210 - Pleurisy, p. 116 Also see Chest Pain, p. 114.
Pain when you press on the chest	- Strained chest muscles, p. 116 - Costochondritis, p. 116 Also see Chest Pain, p. 114.

Digestive Problems	
Symptoms	**Possible Causes**
Increasing pain in one part of the belly, with fever, nausea, and vomiting	- Appendicitis, p. 67 - Gallstones, p. 159 - Kidney stone, p. 193 **You may need urgent care.** See Abdominal Pain, p. 66.
Belly pain, possibly with fever or vomiting	- Gallstones, p. 159 - Diverticular disease, p. 129 - Appendicitis, p. 67 Also see Abdominal Pain, p. 66.
Bloody or black stools	- Ulcer, p. 243 - Diarrhea, p. 127 - Rectal problem, p. 180 **Also see Bleeding Emergencies, p. 17.**
Feeling sick to your stomach; vomiting (throwing up)	See Vomiting, p. 253. - Food poisoning, p. 155 - Drug reaction, p. 369
Frequent, watery stools	- Diarrhea, p. 127 - Food poisoning, p. 155 - Irritable bowel syndrome, p. 190
Stools that are dry and hard to pass	- Constipation, p. 124 - Irritable bowel syndrome, p. 190
Pain during bowel movements; bright red blood on surface of stool or on toilet paper	- Hemorrhoids or other rectal problem, p. 180 - Constipation, p. 124
Painless or mildly painful lump or swelling in groin that comes and goes	- Hernia, p. 182
Burning or discomfort behind or below breastbone or in upper belly	- Heartburn, p. 176 - Ulcer, p. 243 Also see Chest Pain, p. 114.
Bloating and gas with diarrhea, constipation, or both	- Irritable bowel syndrome, p. 190
Women only: Lower belly cramps, bloating, diarrhea or constipation	See Female Pelvic Problems, p. 148. - Irritable bowel syndrome, p. 190 Also see Abdominal Pain, p. 66.

Skin Problems	
Symptoms	**Possible Causes**
Change in the shape, size, or color of a mole, or a persistently irritated mole; a sore that does not heal	- Skin cancer, p. 230
Raised, red, itchy welts or fluid-filled bumps after an insect bite or taking a drug	- Allergy, p. 73 - Hives, p. 188 - Insect or spider bite, p. 13
Red, painful, swollen bump under the skin	- Boils, p. 98
Red, flaky, itchy skin	- Dry skin, p. 134 - Fungal infection, p. 157 Also see Rashes, p. 218.
Rash that develops after wearing new jewelry or clothing, being exposed to plants, eating a new food, or taking a new drug	- Allergy, p. 73 Also see Rashes, p. 218.
Red, itchy, blistered rash	- Poison ivy, oak, or sumac, p. 219 - Shingles, p. 225
Painful blisters in a band around one side of the body	- Shingles, p. 225
Cracked, blistered, itchy, peeling skin between the toes	- Athlete's foot (see Fungal Infections, p. 157)
Red, itchy, moist rash on the groin or thighs	- Jock itch (see Fungal Infections, p. 157)
Scaly, itchy, bald spots or sores on the scalp	- Ringworm (see Fungal Infections, p. 157) Also see Hair Loss, p. 165.
Sandpapery skin rash with sore throat and a "raspberry" tongue	- Scarlet fever (see Sore Throat, p. 235)
Sores on the lip or in the mouth	- Canker sores, p. 109 - Cold sores, p. 118
Reddish yellow, scaly patches on scalp, forehead, sides of nose, eyebrows, behind ears, or center of chest	- Sebborheic dermatitis, p. 219
Rash between folds of skin in armpit or groin or under breasts	- Intertrigo (chafing), p. 219
Red or dark spot on skin that does not turn white when you press on it and still looks discolored 30 minutes or more after you take pressure off the area	- Pressure sore, p. 213

Eye and Vision Problems	
Symptoms	**Possible Causes**
Sudden vision loss that does not clear	- Stroke, p. 54 - Closed-angle glaucoma, p. 162 - Retinal detachment, p. 251 - Temporal arteritis, p. 169 **You may need urgent care.**
Sudden onset of severe eye pain, blurred vision, reddened eyeball	- Closed-angle glaucoma, p. 162 - Chemical burn, p. 25 - Object in the eye, p. 31 **You may need urgent care.**
Sudden increase in floaters (dark spots, specks, or lines); new flashes of light that do not go away; shadow or "curtain" across your field of vision	- Retinal detachment, p. 251. **You may need urgent care.** (If you have had a few floaters or flashes for a while, mention it at your next eye exam.)
New blank or dark spot in the center of your vision; straight lines look wavy	- Macular degeneration, p. 250
Gradual loss of side vision; tunnel vision	- Glaucoma, p. 162
Gradual onset of cloudy, filmy, or fuzzy vision	- Cataract, p. 113 - Presbyopia, p. 249
Halos around lights	- Cataract, p. 113 - Glaucoma, p. 162
Red, itchy, watery eyes	- Allergies, p. 73. Think about allergy to eye care products, makeup, or smoke. - Contact lens problem, p. 142
Discharge from or crust in eye; red, swollen eyelids; sandy feeling	- Pinkeye, p. 140 - Contact lens problem, p. 142 - Blepharitis (eyelid inflammation), p. 144
Pimple or swelling on eyelid	- Stye, p. 144
Pain in the eye	- Object in the eye, p. 31 - Contact lens problem, p. 142 - Pinkeye, p. 140 - Chemicals or fumes, p. 25 - Migraine headache, p. 167, or cluster headache, p. 168 - Sinusitis, p. 227
Red spot or blood on white of eye	- Blood in the eye, p. 143
Dry, scratchy eyes	- Dry eyes, p. 143 - Allergies, p. 73 - Pinkeye, p. 140

Eye and Vision Problems—continued

Symptoms	Possible Causes
Eye twitches	- Stress or fatigue. Call a doctor if twitching affects other face muscles or lasts longer than a week.
Black eye	- Bruises, p. 22

Ear and Hearing Problems

Symptoms	Possible Causes
Earache and fever	- Ear infection, p. 135
Ear pain when you chew, with headache	- TM disorder, p. 192
Itching or burning in ear; pain when you wiggle your ear or chew	- Swimmer's ear, p. 136
Feeling of fullness in ear, with runny or stuffy nose, cough, fever	- Cold, p. 119 - Ear infection, p. 135
Hearing loss	- Hearing loss, p. 171 - Earwax buildup, p. 137
Ringing or noise in the ears	- Tinnitus, p. 173

Nose and Throat Problems

Symptoms	Possible Causes
Stuffy or runny nose with watery eyes, sneezing	- Allergies, p. 73 - Cold, p. 119
Cold symptoms with fever, headache, severe body aches, fatigue	- Flu, p. 153
Thick green, yellow, or gray nasal discharge with fever and facial pain	- Sinusitis, p. 227
Bloody nose	See Nosebleeds, p. 43.
Sore throat	See Sore Throat, p. 235.
Sore throat with white spots on tonsils, swollen lymph nodes, fever of 101°F or higher	- Strep throat, p. 235
Swollen lymph nodes in the neck	See Swollen Lymph Nodes, p. 236.
Hoarseness, loss of voice	- Laryngitis, p. 196

Headaches

If Headache Occurs:	Possible Causes
Suddenly (like an explosion) and is very severe	- Bleeding in the brain (aneurysm or stroke). **This may be an emergency.** Also see Stroke on p. 54.
With dizziness and vomiting, and everyone in the household feels the same	- Carbon monoxide poisoning. **This may be an emergency.**
With severe eye pain or sudden vision changes	- Acute closed-angle glaucoma, p. 162 - Temporal arteritis, p. 169 **This may be an emergency.**
With fever, stiff neck, nausea and vomiting, and confusion	- Encephalitis or meningitis, p. 151
Right when you wake up	- Tension headache, p. 167 - Allergies, p. 73 - Sinusitis, p. 227 - Neck pain, p. 204 - TM disorder, p. 192
In jaw area or in both temples	- TM disorder, p. 192 - Tension headache, p. 167 - Temporal arteritis, p. 169
With new medicine	- Drug allergy. Call your doctor.
Each afternoon or evening; after hours of desk work; with sore neck and shoulders	- Tension headache, p. 167 - Neck pain, p. 204
On one side of the head, with vision problems or runny nose	- Migraine headache, p. 167 - Cluster headache, p. 168 - Temporal arteritis, p. 169
With sudden, sharp pain on one side of the face	- Trigeminal neuralgia, p. 169 - Shingles, p. 225
After exposure to chemicals (paint, varnish, insect spray, smoke)	- Chemical headache. Get into fresh air. Drink water to flush poisons. Call a doctor if headache does not get better.
With fever, runny nose, or sore throat	- Flu, p. 153 - Sore throat, p. 235 - Cold, p. 119 - Sinusitis, p. 227
With runny nose, watery eyes, and sneezing	- Allergies, p. 73

Headaches—continued

If Headache Occurs:	Possible Causes
With fever and pain in the cheekbones or over the eyes	- Sinusitis, p. 227
When you drink less caffeine than usual	- Caffeine withdrawal. Cut back slowly. See p. 168.
After a stressful event	- Tension headache, p. 167

Urinary Problems

Symptoms	Possible Causes
Pain or burning when you urinate	- Urinary tract infection, p. 90 - Prostatitis, p. 217 - Sexually transmitted disease, p. 222 - Kidney stone, p. 193
Men only: Trouble urinating or weak urine stream	- Prostate enlargement, p. 215 - Prostatitis, p. 217
Leaking urine or loss of bladder control	- Bladder control problem, p. 92 - Prostate enlargement, p. 215 - Prostatitis, p. 217
Blood in urine (Eating beets, blackberries, or foods with red food coloring can briefly turn your urine pink or red. Some medicines can also change the urine's color.)	- Urinary tract infection, p. 90 - Kidney stone, p. 193 - Injury to the groin or genital area - Very hard exercise (such as running a marathon) Call your doctor if you think you have blood in your urine.

Abdominal Pain

When to Call a Doctor

If you are vomiting, see page 253.
If you have diarrhea, see page 127.

Call 911 if:

- You have belly pain and you faint.
- You have pain in your upper belly with chest pain or pressure, especially if it occurs with any other symptoms of a heart attack. See page 38.
- You have severe pain after a blow or injury to the belly.
- You vomit a lot of blood or what looks like coffee grounds.
- You have severe rectal bleeding. Severe means you are passing a lot of stool that is maroon or mostly blood.

Call your doctor if:

- You have a blow or injury to the belly.
- You have new, severe belly pain for several hours or more.
- You have steady or increasing pain in just one area of your belly for more than 4 hours.
- You have belly pain and a fever.
- You have pain throughout the belly or cramping pain that has lasted longer than 24 hours and is not getting better.
- Pain gets worse when you move or cough and does not feel like a pulled muscle.
- Any new belly pain lasts longer than 3 days.

If you did not find your symptoms here, check the index or the Digestive Problems chart on page 60.

Abdominal pain—pain in the belly—is very common. Usually it is not serious. You can get clues about the cause of pain and how serious the problem may be by asking:

- **How bad is the pain?** People usually need to see a doctor when severe belly pain comes on suddenly and continues, or when new or different pain gets worse over several hours or days.
- **Does it hurt all over or just in one spot?**
  - When your belly hurts all over and you cannot point to a specific spot that hurts, there is usually no reason to worry. This type of pain is very common and will usually go away on its own. Heartburn, stomach flu, food poisoning, and other common illnesses can cause this type of bellyache.

- When your belly hurts in just one spot, it can be a sign of a more serious problem. This is especially true if the pain is bad, starts suddenly and does not go away, or gets worse when you move or cough. It may be a sign of a problem such as appendicitis, pancreatitis, diverticulitis, an ovarian cyst, or gallbladder disease.

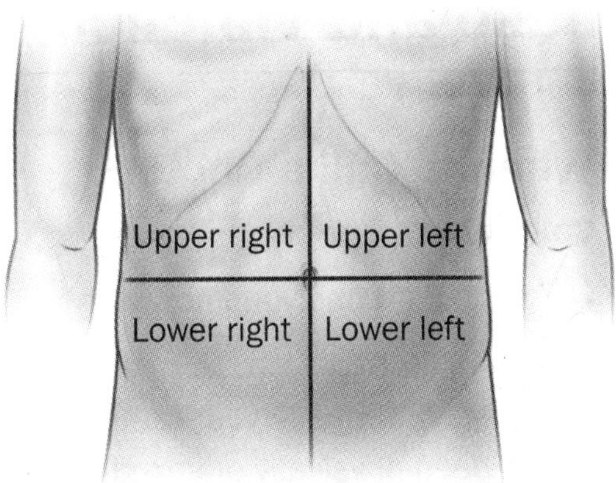

If you have belly pain, your doctor may ask you where it hurts. Lower right? Upper left? All over?

Home Treatment

Most of the time, belly pain goes away on its own. The best home treatment may depend on what other symptoms you have, such as diarrhea or vomiting. Be sure to review the home treatment for any other symptoms you have. Use the index to find what you need, or check the Digestive Problems chart on page 60.

If you have mild belly pain without other symptoms, these tips might help:

- Rest until you feel better.
- Drink plenty of fluids to avoid dehydration (see page 29). Taking many small sips may be easier on your stomach than drinking a lot at once.
- Do not eat solid foods until the pain starts to go away. Then try 5 or 6 small meals instead of 2 or 3 large ones.
- Avoid spicy foods, alcohol, caffeine, and high-fat or high-sugar foods until 48 hours after all symptoms have gone away.

Appendicitis

The appendix is a small sac attached to the large intestine. (See the picture on page 159.) If the appendix gets blocked, it can swell and get infected. This is called appendicitis.

Symptoms may include:

- Pain that begins around the belly button or a little higher and then gets worse and moves to the lower right part of your belly. The pain is steady and gets worse when you walk or cough.
- Loss of appetite, nausea, vomiting, and constipation.
- Fever.
- A hard, swollen belly.

Call your doctor if you have these symptoms. You may need to have your appendix taken out right away so that it doesn't burst and spread infection all through your belly.

Abuse and Violence

When to Call a Doctor

Call 911 if:

- You or someone you know is in danger right now.
- You or someone in your family has just been physically or sexually abused or has been the victim of violence. Abuse is a crime no matter who does it.

Call a counselor or doctor if:

- You are worried about violence or abuse in your own relationship or that of a family member or friend.
- You need help controlling your anger, or someone in your family needs help. Also see Anger and Hostility on page 76.
- You suspect abuse or neglect of an older adult. You may also call Adult Protection Services or the Department of Social Services or Aging Services in your state. Or call the Eldercare Locator toll-free at 1-800-677-1116.
- You suspect abuse or neglect of a child, or a child reports this kind of treatment to you. You may also call local child protective services or the police.

Anger and disagreement are normal parts of healthy relationships. Threats and violence are not normal or healthy.

Abuse is an all-too-common problem. It often starts with threats, name-calling, and slamming doors or breaking dishes. It then gets worse with pushing, hitting, and other violent acts. Every year thousands of people are hurt or killed by their partners, spouses, or other family members.

Signs of Abuse

If you are not sure whether your relationship is abusive, there are signs to look for. This can be the first step in solving the problem. Ask yourself:

- Does my partner limit where I can go, what I can do, and whom I can talk to?
- Does my partner call me names or tell me that I'm crazy?
- Does my partner criticize what I do and say or criticize how I look?
- Does my partner "check up on me" at work, home, or school?
- Does my partner hit, shove, slap, kick, punch, or choke me?
- Does my partner blame me for the abuse he or she commits?
- Does my partner force me to have sex?

- Does my partner hurt my pets or destroy things that are special to me?
- Does my partner threaten to hurt or kill me?

If you answered yes to any of these questions, or if your partner could answer yes, you may be in an abusive relationship.

What You Can Do

Physical, verbal, or sexual abuse is never okay. There is no excuse for it. No one deserves to be abused.

- Know that there are people who can help you—friends, family, neighbors, police, health professionals, social workers, clergy. Talk to someone you trust. Do not feel that you have to hide what's going on. Everyone has the right to be safe.
- Be alert to warning signs, such as threats or heavy drinking. This may help you avoid danger.
- If you can, make sure there are no guns or weapons in the house.
- Have a plan for how to leave your house and where to stay in case of an emergency. Put some money aside if you can, or at least make sure you will be able to get to your money after you leave. Do not tell the person who has been abusing you about your plan. You can find out about shelters and safe homes near you from your local YMCA, YWCA, police station, hospital, or clinic. Or call the National Domestic Violence Hotline toll-free at 1-800-799-7233.

Elder Abuse

The abuse of older adults is a very real and disturbing problem. It may include:

- Physical or sexual abuse. This includes hitting, shaking, or pinching the person, or performing sexual acts without the person's consent.
- Psychological abuse. This can include threats, name-calling, or keeping the older person away from other people.
- Financial abuse. This may include stealing a person's money or things.
- Neglect, or not providing the food, shelter, or care a person needs.

Most often, elder abuse is committed by family members. But it can also occur at the hands of hired caregivers. The stress of caring for an older adult, especially one with serious health problems, is often a factor. But no matter who does it or why it happens, elder abuse is wrong and should be stopped.

If you suspect that an older adult is being abused or neglected, call Adult Protection Services or the Department of Social Services or Aging Services in your state. Or call the Eldercare Locator toll-free at 1-800-677-1116.

Alcohol and Drugs

When to Call a Doctor

Call 911 if:

- A person is unconscious or has trouble breathing after drinking alcohol or taking drugs.
- A person who has been drinking alcohol or using drugs threatens to hurt himself or herself or someone else.
- A person who suddenly stops using alcohol has trembling, hallucinations, seizures, or other severe withdrawal symptoms.

Call a counselor or doctor if:

- You are worried about an alcohol or drug problem in someone close to you.
- You think you have an alcohol or drug problem and are ready to get help. (See Are You a Problem User? on page 71.) Treatment can help you quit.

Alcohol and drug problems are common and costly. They increase your risk of serious car accidents, depression, and falls that can lead to hip fractures. Abusing alcohol or drugs can also make existing health problems worse. Combining alcohol or drugs with prescription medicines may keep the medicines from working the way they should. In some cases the results can be deadly.

But too often, drug and alcohol problems in older adults are overlooked or ignored. Doctors may mistake changes they see for the results of normal aging. If you or someone you know has an alcohol or drug problem, it's important to talk to a doctor and get help. With treatment and support, you can overcome your problem.

Alcohol Problems

People abuse alcohol in different ways. Some people get drunk every day. Some drink large amounts of alcohol at once (binge). Others may be sober for a long time and then go on drinking binges for weeks or months. All of these are problems.

Long-term heavy drinking causes high blood pressure, depression, stomach problems, sexual problems, and cancer. And it damages your liver, nerves, heart, and brain.

Alcohol can cause even more problems for older adults. As you get older, it takes longer for your body to break down alcohol. Drinking the same amount you did 20 years ago can cause a lot more damage.

You have an alcohol problem if you keep drinking even though it's interfering with your health or your daily life.

Signs of an alcohol problem:

- Not remembering what happened while you were drinking (blackouts).
- Drinking more and more for the same high.
- Being uncomfortable when you can't drink alcohol.
- Gulping or sneaking drinks.
- Drinking alone or early in the morning.
- Getting "the shakes."

If your body is dependent on alcohol and you suddenly stop drinking, you may have severe withdrawal symptoms (such as trembling, delusions, hallucinations, sweating, and seizures). It's very hard to stop drinking without help if you are dependent on alcohol. You may need to go through "detox" under medical care.

Drug Problems

Drug abuse includes the use of marijuana, cocaine, meth, heroin, and other illegal drugs. It also includes the abuse of legal prescription drugs. People most often misuse pain medicines, tranquilizers, sedatives, and amphetamines, but not always on purpose. Some people turn to drugs as a way to get a high or deal with stress.

Are You a Problem User?

Answer the questions below honestly. They ask about your use of alcohol and drugs, including prescription and illegal drugs.

- Have you ever felt that you ought to cut down on your drinking or drug use?
- Have you ever been annoyed when others criticized your drinking or drug use?
- Have you ever felt guilty about your drinking or drug use?
- Have you ever taken an early-morning drink or used drugs first thing in the morning to steady your nerves or get the day started?

If you answer yes to 2 or more of these questions, you may have a problem with alcohol or drugs. Talk about it with your doctor or a counselor.

Signs of a drug problem:

- Constant red eyes, sore throat, dry cough, and fatigue. This can also just be allergies.
- Major changes in sleeping or eating habits
- Being moody, hostile, or abusive
- Work problems, especially being absent a lot

More

- Losing interest in favorite activities
- Withdrawing from friends or family

Drug dependence or addiction occurs when you develop a physical or psychological need for a drug. You may not know you are dependent on a drug until you suddenly try to stop taking it. Withdrawing from the drug can cause muscle aches, diarrhea, depression, and other symptoms.

The usual treatment for drug dependence is to reduce the dose of the drug slowly until it can be stopped. This often needs to be done under a doctor's care.

Home Treatment

- Pay attention to early signs that alcohol or drug use is becoming a problem. See Are You a Problem User? on page 71.
- Go to an Alcoholics Anonymous (AA) or Narcotics Anonymous (NA) meeting. These support groups help members get sober and stay sober.
- If you are worried about a friend's or family member's alcohol or drug use:
  - Don't ignore it. Discuss it as a health problem.
  - Build up the person's self-esteem. Help the person see that he or she can succeed without alcohol or drugs. Offer your support.
  - Ask if the person will accept help. If the person agrees, **act that very day** to get help. Call a doctor, AA, or NA for an immediate appointment. Make it easy for the person to get help. If the person says no to help, keep trying.
  - Go to a few meetings of Al-Anon, a support group for family and friends of alcoholics. Read some 12-step program information. Many programs use the 12-step approach for dealing with addiction.

Allergies

When to Call a Doctor

Call 911 if you have any signs of a severe allergic reaction soon after you take a drug, eat a certain food, or are stung by an insect. For example:

- You faint or feel like you may faint.
- You have swelling around your lips, tongue, or face that is causing breathing problems or is getting worse.
- You start wheezing or have trouble breathing.

Call a doctor if:

- Your face, tongue, or lips are swollen, even if you do not have trouble breathing and the swelling is not getting worse.
- There is a lot of swelling around the site of an insect sting. (For instance, the entire arm or leg is swollen.)
- You get a skin rash, itching, a feeling of warmth, or hives. Also see Hives on page 188.
- Allergy symptoms get worse over time, and home treatment does not help. Your doctor may recommend stronger medicine or allergy shots. See page 75.

Most allergies are caused by pollen, dust, and other things in the air. You can often find the cause of an allergy by noting when symptoms occur:

- Symptoms that happen at the same time each year are often caused by tree, grass, or weed pollen. You are most likely to have problems during spring, early summer, or early fall.
- Allergies that last all year may be caused by dust, dust mites, cockroaches, mold, or animal dander.
- An animal allergy is often easy to spot: Your symptoms clear up when you stay away from the pet or its bedding.

Allergies to pollen or grass often cause **hay fever**. If you have hay fever, you already know the symptoms: itchy, watery eyes; sneezing; runny, stuffy, or itchy nose; and fatigue. You may also get dark circles under your eyes.

Home Treatment

Decongestants and antihistamines may help with some allergies. Talk to your doctor about the best choice for you, and use caution when you take these drugs. Make sure they are safe to take with any other medicines you are taking.

If you know what you are allergic to, the best treatment is to avoid it whenever you can. Keep a record of your

More

symptoms and the plants, animals, foods, medicines, or chemicals that seem to trigger them.

In general:

- Avoid yard work, which stirs up both pollen and mold. If you must do yard work, wear a mask, and take an antihistamine before you start.
- Do not smoke. If you need help quitting, see page 351.
- Do not use aerosol sprays, perfumes, room deodorizers, or cleaning products that trigger allergy symptoms.

For seasonal symptoms caused by pollen or grass:

- Keep your house and car windows closed. Do not open your bedroom windows at night.
- Limit the time you spend outside when pollen counts are high.
- Wash dogs and other pets often, or leave them outside. They can bring lots of pollen into your house.

For year-round symptoms caused by dust:

- Keep your bedroom and other places where you spend a lot of time as dust-free as you can. Remove "dust collectors," such as wall hangings, books, knickknacks, and artificial flowers.
- Dust and vacuum 1 or 2 times a week. This stirs up dust and makes the air worse until the dust settles, so wear a mask if you do the cleaning yourself. Damp-mop tile, wood, or stone floors.

Life-Threatening Allergic Reactions

A few people have severe allergies to insect stings, nuts or other foods, or drugs, especially antibiotics such as penicillin. The reaction is sudden and severe. It may cause dangerous swelling in the throat and mouth, trouble breathing, and a drop in blood pressure. This is called anaphylaxis. It needs emergency care.

If you have ever had a severe allergic reaction, your doctor may suggest that you carry an allergy kit. These kits include pills and a shot (such as EpiPen) that you can give yourself in case you are exposed to the same thing that caused your severe reaction before. The shot can help prevent a bad reaction and give you time to get help. To learn how to give yourself the shot, go to the Web site on the back cover and enter **Q994** in the search box.

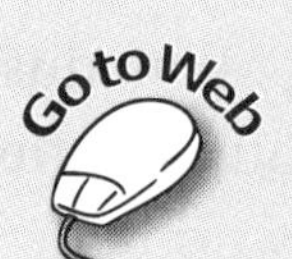

If you have ever had an allergic reaction to a drug, wear medical alert jewelry that lists your allergies.

- Try not to use carpets, upholstered furniture, and heavy drapes that collect dust. Vacuum cleaners pick up dust but not dust mites. Use leather, vinyl, or plastic furniture that you can wipe clean and small rugs that you can wash.

- Cover your mattress and box spring with dustproof cases, and wipe them clean weekly. Do not use wool or down blankets or feather pillows. Wash all bedding in hot water once a week.
- Use an air conditioner or air purifier with a special HEPA filter. Rent one before you buy it to see if it helps.
- Change or clean heating and cooling system filters often.

For year-round symptoms caused by mold or mildew (worse when weather is damp):

- Keep your home aired out and dry. Keep the humidity below 50 percent. Use a dehumidifier when the weather is humid.
- Use an air conditioner, which removes mold from the air.
- Change or clean heating and cooling system filters often.
- Clean bathroom and kitchen surfaces often with bleach.
- Use exhaust fans in the bathrooms and kitchen.

If you are allergic to a pet:

- Keep the animal outside, or at least out of your bedroom.
- If your symptoms are severe and your efforts to reduce pet dander do not help, the best answer may be to find a new home for the pet.

Looking for the Alzheimer's Disease topic? See page 261.

What About Allergy Shots?

Allergy shots can reduce or prevent symptoms for many people who have allergies to insect stings, pollen, dust and dust mites, mold, animal dander, or cockroaches.

You will need skin and blood tests to find out what you are allergic to. Allergy shots don't work for all types of allergies. For example, they help with allergies to insect stings, but they don't help with many food allergies.

Shots may take 3 to 5 years to complete. It may take up to a full year of weekly or monthly shots before you see any change in your symptoms.

Getting allergy shots takes time and money. But they work for many people and may be worth it for you if:

- Your allergies bother you a lot, and medicines don't help enough.
- You can't avoid the things you are allergic to, and your efforts to control them don't solve the problem.
- You have had a severe reaction to an insect sting, or your reactions have gotten worse over time.

Go to Web

For help deciding whether to try allergy shots, go to the Web site on the back cover and enter **H126** in the search box.

Anger and Hostility

When to Call a Doctor

Call 911 if you or someone you know is in danger right now.

Call a counselor if:

- Anger has led or could lead to violence or harm to you or someone else.
- Anger or hostility upsets your work, family life, or friendships.

Anger tells your body to prepare for a fight. It can be a normal response to daily events. And it is a healthy response to any situation that's a real threat. You can sometimes use anger as a positive force to help you take action.

Hostility is being ready for a fight all the time. Hostile people often have an "attitude" or are stubborn, impatient, or hotheaded.

Feeling angry and hostile all or much of the time is not good for you. It keeps your blood pressure high and may make you more likely to have a heart attack, stroke, or other health problem. Constant anger also cuts you off from the people in your life. It may lead to abuse and violence (see page 68).

Home Treatment

- Try to understand why you are angry. Is something happening now that's making you angry, or is it something that happened earlier?
- Notice when you start to get angry, and take steps to deal with your anger in a healthy way. Do not ignore your anger until you "blow up."
  - Think before you act. Count to 10 or use some other form of mental relaxation. When you have calmed down, you'll be better able to deal with the problem.
  - Give yourself a "time-out." Go someplace quiet so you can calm down.
  - Go for a short walk or jog.
  - Talk with a friend about your anger.
  - Draw or paint to release the anger, or write about it in a journal.
- If you are angry with someone, listen to what the other person has to say. Try to understand his or her point of view. Use "I" statements, not "you" statements, to discuss your anger. Say "I feel angry when my needs are not being met" instead of "You make me mad when you take me for granted."
- Learn to forgive and forget. Forgiving lowers your blood pressure and eases muscle tension so you can feel more relaxed.
- Focus on the things in your life that make you happy.
- Read books about how to handle anger, see a counselor, or look for classes or groups that teach anger management.

Anxiety and Panic

When to Call a Doctor

Call a counselor or your doctor if:

- Anxiety or fear upsets your daily life.
- Sudden, severe attacks of fear or anxiety seem to occur for no reason.
- Symptoms of anxiety are still severe after 1 week of home treatment.
- You have nightmares or flashbacks to traumatic events.
- You cannot feel sure about things (for example, whether you unplugged the iron) no matter how many times you check, especially if it interferes with your daily life.

Feeling worried, anxious, and nervous is a normal part of life. Everyone frets or feels anxious from time to time.

Your body tells you when you are anxious:

- You may tremble, twitch, or shake.
- You may feel lightheaded or dizzy.
- You may feel "butterflies" in your stomach.
- Your breathing and heartbeat may speed up.
- Your throat or chest may feel full.
- You may sweat, and your muscles may get tense.
- You may have sleep problems.

Anxiety also affects your emotions:

- You may feel hyper, annoyed, or on edge.
- You may worry a lot or fear that something bad is going to happen.
- You may not be able to concentrate.
- You may feel sad all the time.

A specific situation or fear can cause these symptoms for a short time. When the situation passes, the symptoms go away.

When you have an **anxiety disorder**, you get these symptoms for no clear reason or for reasons that don't make sense. This type of anxiety is not normal and can be overwhelming. People with an anxiety disorder may have fears, called **phobias**, of common places, objects, or situations.

Panic disorder is a problem related to anxiety. People with panic disorder have periods of sudden, intense fear and anxiety when there is no clear cause or danger. These panic attacks can cause scary (but not dangerous) symptoms, such as a pounding heart, shortness of breath, and a sense that you are about to lose control or die.

More

People who have had panic attacks may try hard to avoid anything that might trigger another attack. This often causes even more anxiety.

You can learn ways to manage your anxiety and panic. Many people get help from counseling and medicines. The right medicines — especially when you use them along with counseling—can help prevent anxiety or panic attacks and may help reduce your fear. They usually start to work within a few weeks, but you may need to take the medicines for a year or more to get long-lasting results.

For help deciding if medicines are right for you, go to the Web site on the back cover and enter **B817** in the search box.

Home Treatment

Try these tips to relieve anxiety. They can also help if you are getting treatment for anxiety or panic disorder.

- Accept your anxiety. When a situation makes you feel anxious, say to yourself, "This is not an emergency. I feel uneasy, but I'm not in danger. I can keep going even if I feel anxious."
- Be kind to your body:
  - Relieve stress and tension with exercise, massage, warm baths, walks, or whatever works for you.
  - Learn and use a relaxation technique. See page 358.
  - Get enough rest. If you have trouble sleeping, see Sleep Problems on page 232.
  - Avoid alcohol, caffeine, and nicotine. They can increase your anxiety, cause sleep problems, or trigger a panic attack.
- Use your mind. Do things you enjoy, like going to a funny movie or taking a walk or a hike.
- Plan your day. Having too much or too little to do can make you more anxious.
- Keep a daily record of your symptoms. Discuss your fears with a good friend or family member, or join a support group. Talking to others about the problem sometimes relieves stress.
- Get involved in social groups, or volunteer to help others. Being alone may make things seem worse than they are.

Looking for the Arthritis topic? See page 266.

Looking for the Asthma topic? See page 271.

Back Pain

When to Call a Doctor

Call 911 if:

- Back pain occurs with chest pain or other symptoms of a heart attack (see page 38).
- A person has signs of damage to the spine after an injury (such as a car accident, fall, or direct blow to the spine). Signs may include:
  - Being unable to move part of the body.
  - Severe back or neck pain.
  - Weakness, tingling, or numbness in the arms or legs.
  - Loss of bladder or bowel control.

Call a doctor if:

- You cannot walk or stand at all. If this is because of weakness and not just because it hurts too much, you need medical care right away.
- You suddenly lose bowel or bladder control. This could be a sign of a serious problem.
- You have new numbness in the buttocks, genital or rectal area, or legs.
- You have leg weakness that is not solely due to pain. Many people with low back pain say their legs feel weak. See your doctor if your leg is so weak that you cannot bend your foot upward, get out of a chair, or climb stairs.
- You have new or increased back pain with fever, painful urination, or other signs of a urinary tract infection. See page 90.
- You have long-term back pain that suddenly gets much worse, and you did not cause it by being more active.
- You have a history of cancer or HIV infection, and you have new or increased back pain.
- You have severe pain that does not improve after a few days of home treatment.
- Pain wakes you from sleep.
- Pain does not improve after 2 weeks of home treatment.

Your back is the whole area from your neck to your tailbone. It includes the bones (vertebrae) and joints of the spine, the spinal discs that separate and cushion the bones, and the muscles and ligaments that hold them all together. You can stress or hurt any of these parts of your back.

What causes most back pain?

- Repeating movements or staying too long in positions that strain the back
- Making sudden or awkward movements that twist the back

More

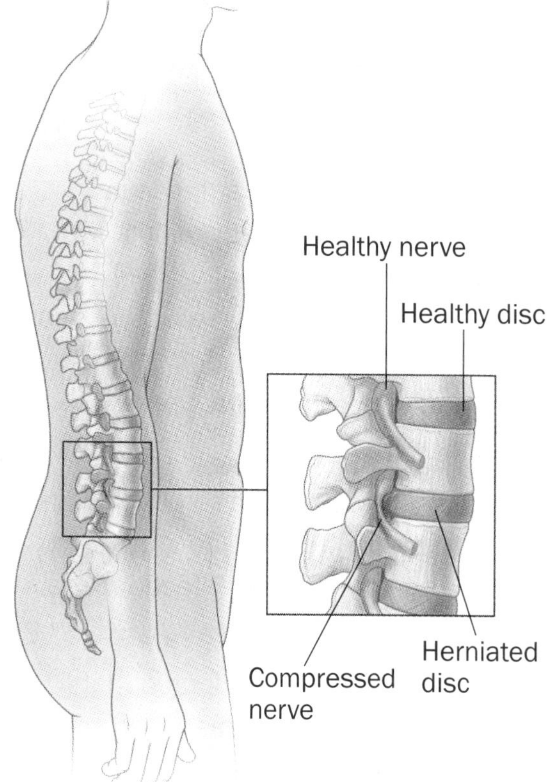

A bulging (herniated) disc can press on a nerve, causing pain.

These kinds of movements or postures can strain or sprain the ligaments, muscles, or the joints between the spine and the pelvic bones (sacroiliac joints).

You can injure a disc in your back the same way, causing it to bulge or tear (rupture). This is called a **herniated disc**. If the tear is large enough, the gel inside the disc may leak out and press against a nerve.

A sprain or strain can cause several days of severe pain, followed by a gradual decrease in pain as the injury heals. Pain from a herniated disc may last much longer. You may feel the pain in your low back, in your buttocks, or down your leg.

With good self-care, most of these back injuries will heal in 6 to 12 weeks. Home treatment can help relieve pain, promote healing, and prevent reinjury.

Back pain can also be caused by problems that affect the bones and joints of the spine.

- **Osteoporosis** can weaken the bones of the spine and cause them to break or collapse. See page 207.

Sciatica

Sciatica is an irritation of the sciatic nerve. The sciatic nerve starts in the lower part of your spine and runs down the back of each leg, from your buttocks to your foot. Sciatica often occurs because a damaged disc in the lower spine is pressing on the sciatic nerve.

The main symptom is pain, numbness, or weakness that extends from your back down into your leg. The pain is usually worse in the leg.

For relief, see Home Treatment on page 81, and follow these tips:

- Do not sit for long periods of time. Take breaks to walk and stretch.
- Switch between sitting, standing, lying down, and taking short walks. You can slowly increase how far you walk as long as it does not cause pain.
- Put ice or a cold pack on the middle of your lower back for 10 to 15 minutes once an hour. Put a thin cloth between the ice and your skin.

- **Arthritis** pain may be a steady ache, unlike the sharp, sudden pain of back strain and disc injuries. If you think arthritis may be causing your back pain, combine the home treatment for back pain with the treatment for arthritis on page 266.
- **Spinal stenosis** can cause pain, numbness, or weakness in the legs and feet. See page 83.

Home Treatment

- Follow the First Aid for Back Pain guidelines on page 82. These include rest, ice, pelvic tilts, and short walks.
- Sit or lie in positions that feel good and reduce your pain, especially any leg pain.
- Avoid sitting for long periods of time. Do not sit up in bed, and avoid soft couches and twisted positions. Follow the tips for good body mechanics on page 84.
- Bed rest can help relieve back pain but may not speed healing. Unless you have severe leg pain, 1 to 2 days of bed rest should relieve pain. Do not stay in bed for more than 3 days unless your doctor tells you to.
- For bed rest, try one of the following positions (see pictures on page 85):
    - Lie on your back with your knees bent and supported by large pillows. Or lie on the floor with your legs on the seat of a sofa or chair.
    - Lie on your side with your knees and hips bent and with a pillow between your legs.
    - Lie on your stomach if it does not make the pain worse.
- Take aspirin, ibuprofen (Advil, Motrin), or naproxen (Aleve) for pain and swelling. If your doctor has told you not to take these medicines, try acetaminophen (Tylenol) instead. Do not take more than the maximum dose. If you mask the pain completely, you may be tempted to move in ways that could make your back worse.
- Relax your muscles. See page 358.

Then, 2 to 3 days after the injury, you can try the following:

- Put heat on your sore back for 20 minutes at a time. Moist heat (hot packs, baths, showers) works better than dry heat. Some people like switching between heat and ice packs or using ice only. Do what works for you.
- Keep taking short walks. Increase to 5 to 10 minutes, 3 to 4 times a day.
- Try swimming. It may hurt right after a back injury, but lap swimming or kicking with swim fins often helps keep pain from coming back.
- When your pain has improved, try easy exercises that don't increase your pain. One or two of the exercises described on pages 86 to 89 may be a good place to start. Start with 5 repetitions, 3 or 4 times a day, and increase to 10 repetitions if it does not cause pain.

More

Be patient. It can take from a few weeks to a few months for a back injury to get better. Increase your activity level as your pain decreases. Being more active may cause a temporary increase in pain, but that doesn't mean you are damaging your back. It is better to be active than to rest too much. Being inactive can lead to stiffness, weakness, and more pain in your back.

Once you have hurt your back, you are more likely to have back pain in the future. But you can take steps to prevent it. See How to Have a Healthy Back on page 84.

First Aid for Back Pain

When you first feel a strain in your back, try these steps to avoid or reduce pain. These are the most important home treatments for the first few days of back pain.

1. Relax: Lie down in a comfortable position. This will let your back muscles relax.

2. Ice: Put ice or a cold pack on your back for 10 to 15 minutes every hour. Using cold for the first 3 days reduces pain and speeds healing. Put a thin cloth between the ice and your skin.

3. Pelvic tilts: This exercise gently moves the spine and stretches the lower back.

- Lie on your back with knees bent and feet flat on the floor.
- Slowly tighten your stomach muscles and press your lower back against the floor. Hold for 10 seconds (don't hold your breath). Slowly relax.

4. Walk: Take a short walk (3 to 5 minutes) on a flat, level surface every 3 hours. Walk only as far as you can without pain. If your back or legs hurt, stop.

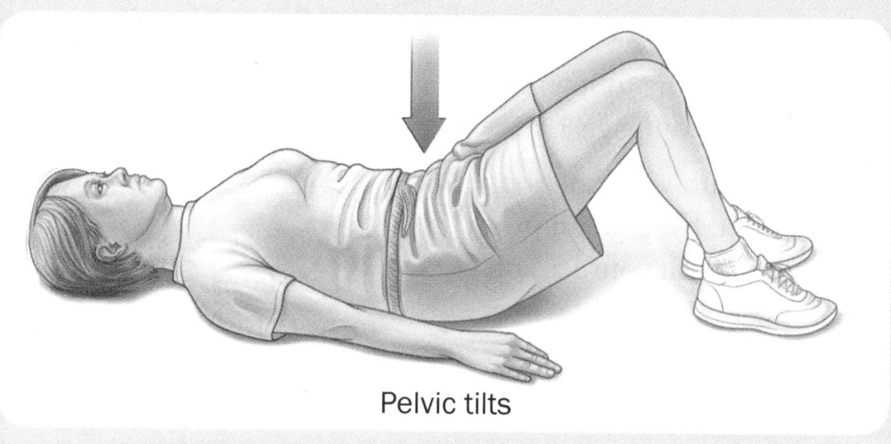

Pelvic tilts

Who to See for Back Pain

Medical doctors

A doctor (MD or DO) can:

- Diagnose the cause of back pain and assess an injury.
- Help you make an exercise and home care plan or a modified work plan if you need it.
- Prescribe muscle relaxants, anti-inflammatory drugs, and pain medicines. (If you get a strong pain medicine or muscle relaxer, be extra careful to avoid postures and activities that could reinjure your back.)
- Suggest physical therapy.
- Help you decide if you need back surgery.

Physical therapists

After basic first aid, a physical therapist with training in orthopedic treatment can:

- Identify muscle or disc problems.
- Provide hands-on therapy.
- Design an exercise program to help you recover and teach you how to prevent future problems.

Chiropractors and osteopaths

Chiropractors and osteopaths can relieve some types of back pain through spinal manipulation. (If you have a herniated disc, this may make your problem worse.) Spinal manipulation usually works best if you have had symptoms for less than 4 weeks. If your symptoms do not improve after 1 month of treatment, stop the treatment and see your doctor.

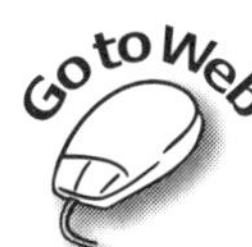

For help deciding whether to see a chiropractor, go to the Web site on the back cover and enter **C245** in the search box.

Other health professionals

Acupuncturists, massage therapists, and others can also provide treatments that may give short-term relief.

Spinal Stenosis

Spinal stenosis is narrowing of the spinal canal. The spinal canal is the opening in the bones of the spine that the spinal cord runs through. When the spinal canal is narrowed, it can squeeze and irritate the spinal cord and the spinal nerves. This can cause pain, numbness, or weakness, most often in the legs, feet, and buttocks.

Spinal stenosis is most often caused by changes in the spinal canal as people age. It can happen anywhere along the spine, but it is most common in the lower back or the neck.

- You may be able to control your symptoms with pain medicines such as ibuprofen (Advil, Motrin) and naproxen (Aleve), exercise, and physical therapy.
- Your doctor may also give you cortisone pills or a cortisone shot in your spine to reduce swelling of the nerves.
- You may need surgery if your symptoms get worse or limit what you can do.

More

How to Have a Healthy Back

The keys to preventing back pain are to:

- Use your body in ways that reduce stress on your back.
- Stretch and strengthen your back.
- Practice good health habits. These include getting regular exercise, staying at a healthy weight, and not smoking. (Nicotine weakens the discs in your back.)

Some of the tips presented here are things you'll want to do every day. Not only are they good for your back, but they're good for your overall health. The rest will come in handy if you ever have back pain. They include:

- Ways to protect your back by using good body mechanics.
- Exercises to make your back stronger and more flexible.
- Exercises to avoid.

Good Body Mechanics

The goal of good body mechanics is to sit, stand, sleep, and move in ways that reduce the stress on your back. Use good body mechanics all the time, not just when you have back pain.

Sitting

- Try not to sit in the same position for more than an hour at a time. Get up or change positions often.
- If you must sit a lot, the extension exercises starting on page 86 are very important.
- If you work at a desk or computer, set up your workstation to reduce stress on your back and neck.
  - Use a chair that you can adjust and that does not upset the normal curve of your back.
  - Keep your feet flat on the floor or on a footrest.
  - Keep your screen at or just below eye level so you do not have to tilt your head or look sideways.

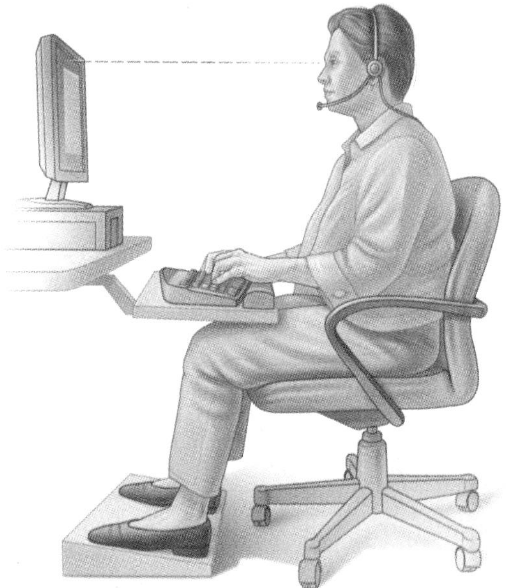

Adjust your chair, keyboard, and screen to reduce back and neck stress.

- If your chair does not give enough support, use a small pillow or rolled towel to support your lower back.
- When you drive, pull your seat forward so that you can easily reach the pedals and steering wheel. Stop often to stretch and walk around. A small pillow or towel roll behind your lower back might help too.

Lifting

- Keep your back straight. Do not bend forward at the waist.
- Bend your knees, and let your arms and legs do the work. Tighten your buttocks and belly to support your back.
- Keep the load as close to your body as you can, even if the load is light.
- While holding a heavy object, use your feet to turn, not your back. Try not to turn or twist your body.

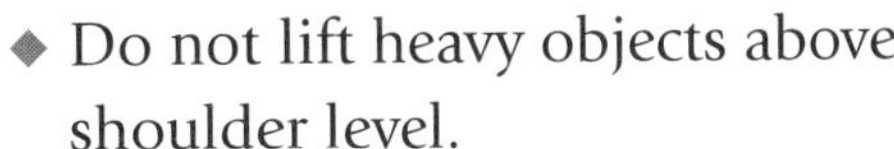

- Do not lift heavy objects above shoulder level.
- For very heavy or awkward items, use a hand truck or ask someone to help you.

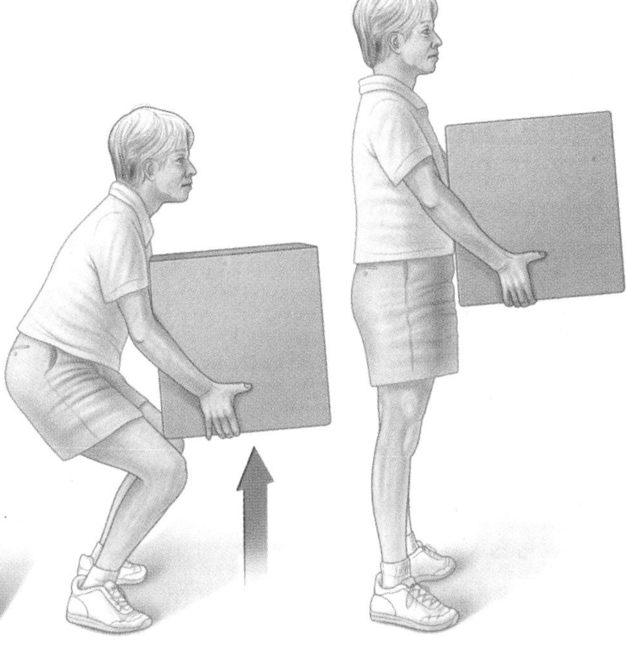

When you lift heavy objects, keep your back straight, bend your knees, and keep the load close to your body.

Lying down

- If you sleep on your back, you may want to use a towel roll to support your lower back, or put a pillow under your knees.
- If you sleep on your side, try placing a pillow between your knees.
- Sleeping on your stomach is fine if it does not cause back or neck pain.

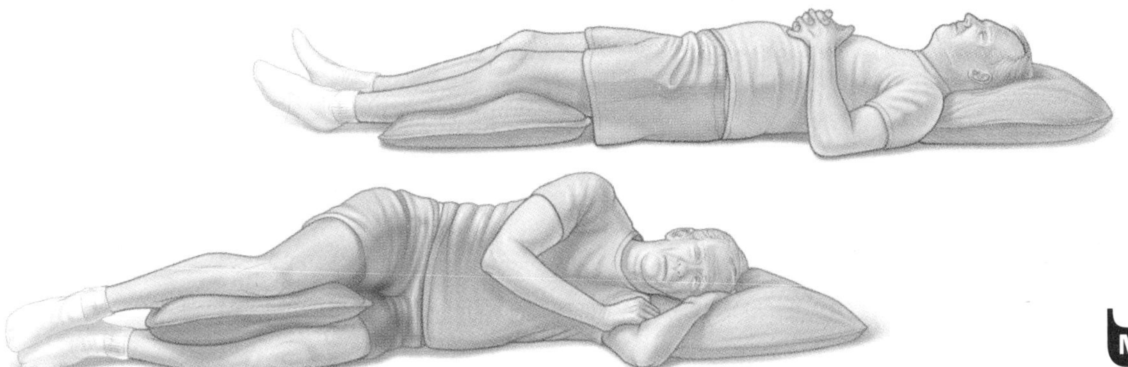

Try placing pillows between or under your knees to relieve back pain while lying in bed.

More

Exercise

Regular exercise helps you stay fit and flexible, and it strengthens the muscles that support your back. It also helps you stay at a healthy weight, which reduces the strain on your lower back.

Although there is no proof that specific exercises can help prevent back pain, the exercises described here are a common, practical way to help you stay strong and flexible. You may want to make them a part of your regular fitness routine.

Do not do these exercises if you have just hurt your back. Instead, see First Aid for Back Pain on page 82.

It helps to do both extension exercises and flexion exercises. Extension exercises strengthen your lower back muscles and stretch the stomach muscles. Flexion exercises stretch the lower back muscles and strengthen the stomach muscles—they are the reverse of extension exercises.

- You do not need to do every exercise. Do the ones that help you the most.
- If any exercise makes your back pain worse, stop it and try something else. Stop any exercise that makes the pain spread into your buttocks or legs, either during or after the exercise.
- Start with 5 repetitions, 3 or 4 times a day. Bit by bit, work up to 10 repetitions. Do all exercises slowly.

Extension Exercises

Press-ups

This is a good exercise to start and end with.

- Lie facedown with your arms bent and your palms flat on the floor.
- Lift yourself up on your elbows, keeping the lower half of your body relaxed. Press your chest forward.
- Keep your hips pressed to the floor. Feel the stretch in your lower back.
- Lower your upper body to the floor. Repeat slowly.

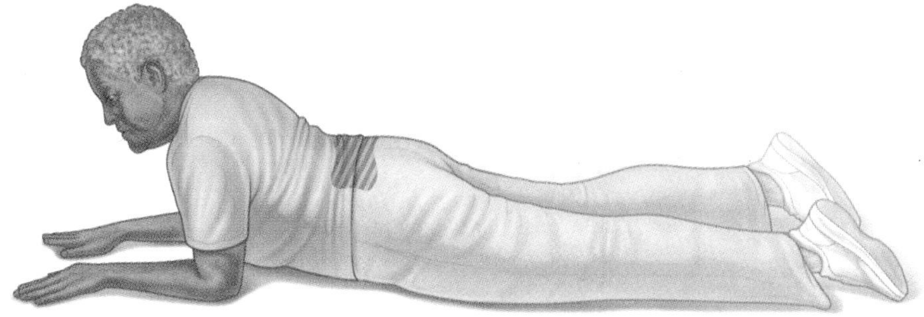

Press-up (shading shows where you should feel the stretch)

Shoulder lifts

These strengthen the back muscles.

- Lie facedown with your arms beside your body.
- Lift your shoulders straight up from the floor as high as you can without pain. Keep your chin down and your eyes facing the floor. Keep your belly and hips pressed to the floor.

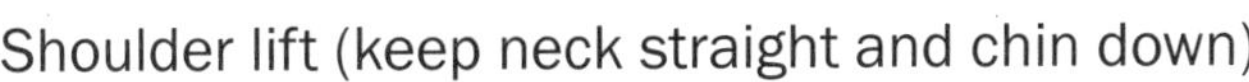

Shoulder lift (keep neck straight and chin down)

Backward bends

These help a lot if you work in a bent-forward position.

- Stand with your feet slightly apart. Back up to a countertop if you want extra support.
- Place your hands in the small of your back, and gently bend backward. Don't lock your knees, and bend only at the waist. Hold the backward stretch for 1 to 2 seconds.

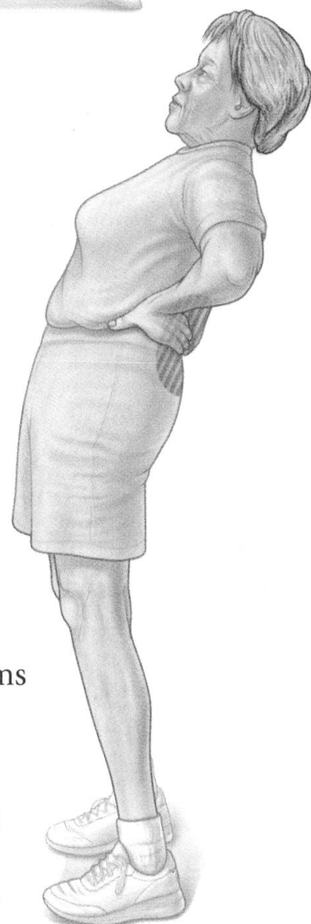

Backward bend (keep neck straight and chin down)

Flexion Exercises

Curl-ups

These strengthen your stomach muscles, which help support your spine.

- Lie on your back with knees bent, feet flat on the floor, and arms crossed on your chest. Do not hook your feet under anything.
- Slowly curl your head and shoulders up until your shoulder blades barely rise from the floor. Keep your lower back pressed to the floor. To avoid neck problems, remember to lift your shoulders, and do not force your head up or forward. Hold for 5 to 10 seconds (don't hold your breath), and then curl down very slowly.

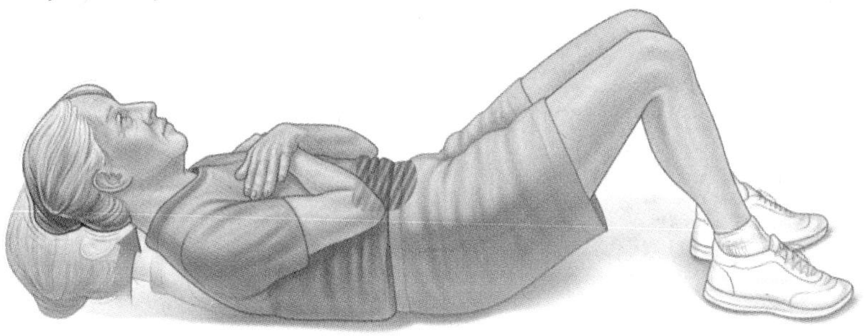

Curl-up (keep neck straight and chin tucked in)

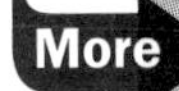

Knee-to-chest stretch

This stretches the lower back and butt muscles and relieves pressure on the joints in your spine.

- Lie on your back with knees bent and feet close to your buttocks.
- Bring one knee to your chest, keeping the other foot flat on the floor (or the other leg straight, if that is more comfortable for your lower back). Keep your lower back pressed to the floor. Hold for 5 to 10 seconds.
- Relax, and lower your knee to the starting position. Repeat with the other leg.

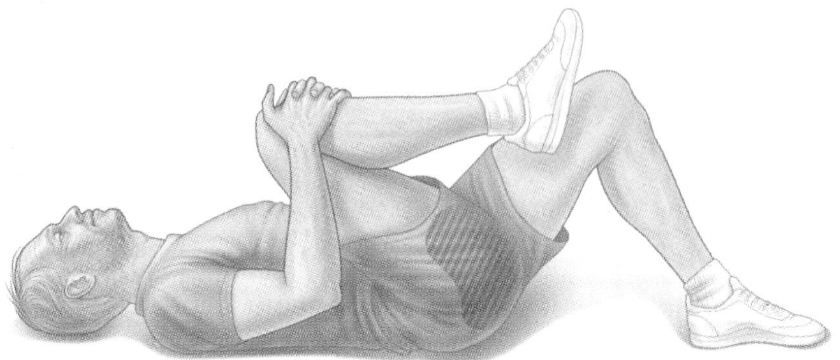

Knee-to-chest stretch (shading shows where you should feel the stretch)

Hamstring stretch

This stretches the muscles in the back of your thigh, which will let you bend your legs without stressing your back.

- Lie on your back in a doorway. Extend the leg you want to stretch straight up, resting the heel on the wall next to the doorway. Keep the other leg resting on the floor.
- Keep the leg straight, and slowly move your heel up the wall until you feel a gentle pull in the back of your thigh. Stretch as far as you can without pain.
- Relax in this position for 30 seconds. Then bend the knee to relieve the stretch. Repeat with the other leg.

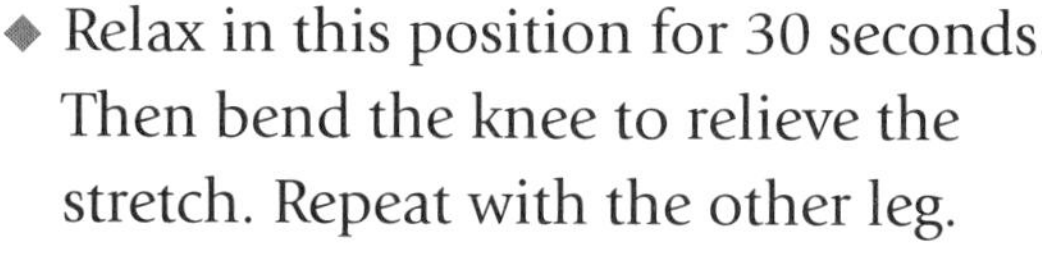

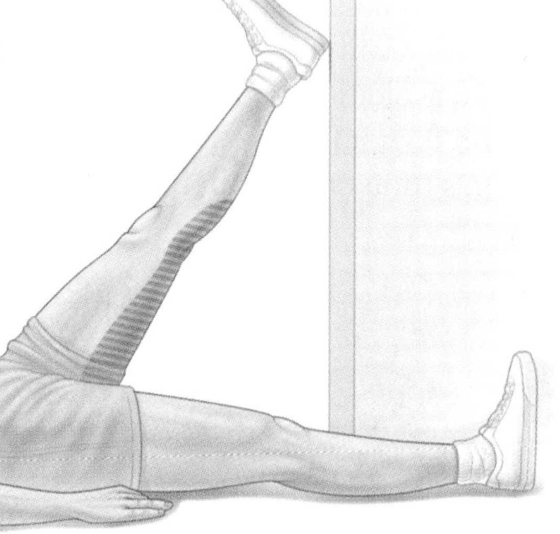

Hamstring stretch (shading shows where you should feel the stretch)

Other Strengthening and Stretching Exercises

Prone buttocks squeeze

This strengthens the butt muscles, which support the back and help you lift with your legs. You may need to place a small pillow under your stomach for comfort.

- Lie flat on your stomach with your arms at your sides.
- Slowly tighten your buttocks muscles and hold for 5 to 10 seconds. Do not hold your breath. Relax slowly.

Pelvic tilts

See First Aid for Back Pain on page 82.

Exercises to Avoid

These common exercises actually increase the risk of low back pain:

- Sit-ups with your legs straight out in front of you
- Bent-leg sit-ups when you have back pain
- Lifting both legs while lying on your back
- Lifting heavy weights above the waist (military press, biceps curls while standing)
- Any stretching done while sitting with the legs in a V
- Toe touches while standing

Hip flexor stretch

This stretches the muscles in the front of your hip.

- Kneel on one knee with your other leg bent in front of you.
- Slowly sink your hips so your weight shifts onto your front foot. The knee of your forward leg should be in a straight line with your ankle. Hold for 10 seconds. You should feel a stretch in the groin of the leg you are kneeling on. Repeat with the other leg.

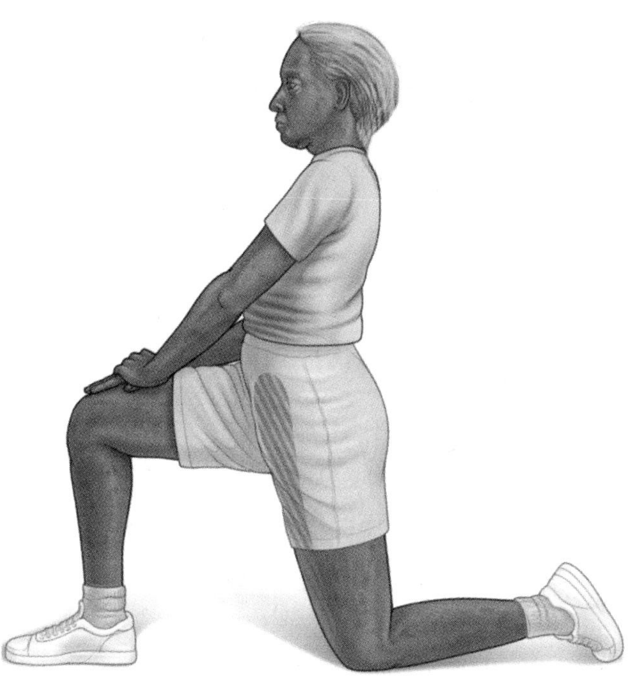

Hip flexor stretch (shading shows where you should feel the stretch)

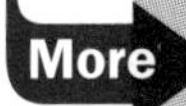
More

Back Surgery

Rest, pain medicines, and exercise can relieve almost all back problems. And back pain usually gets better within 6 to 12 weeks.

Most back surgeries are done to treat problems that have not improved with time. You may need surgery if you have a broken bone in your spine, a spinal infection, or another serious problem. Or you may think about surgery if you have a disc problem that has not improved with time and other treatment.

If you are thinking about having surgery to treat your back pain, get all the facts. Find out how much it will cost, what the risks are, and how likely it is to help your problem in the short term and over time.

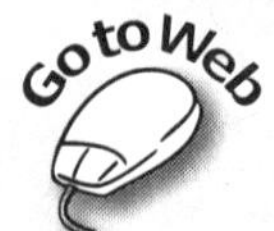

For help deciding if surgery is right for you, go to the Web site on the back cover and enter **D606** in the search box.

If you do plan to have surgery, it is very important to use good body mechanics and do exercises for your back. Having a strong, flexible back will help you recover more quickly after surgery.

Bladder and Kidney Infections

When to Call a Doctor

- Painful urination occurs with:
  - Fever and chills.
  - Not being able to urinate when you feel the urge.
  - Pain in the back, side, groin, or genital area.
  - Blood or pus in the urine, or cloudy urine.
  - Unusual discharge from the vagina or penis.
  - Nausea and vomiting.
- Urinary symptoms do not improve after 1 or 2 days, or they get worse even with home treatment. You may need treatment to help prevent a kidney infection.
- You have diabetes and you have symptoms of a bladder or kidney infection.

Bladder and kidney infections are types of **urinary tract infections**, or **UTIs**. They are usually caused by bacteria that live in the body all the time. Most UTIs are bladder infections. A bladder infection that is not treated can spread to your kidneys. A kidney infection is serious and can cause permanent damage.

Symptoms of a bladder or kidney infection may include:

- Burning or pain when you urinate, as well as itching or pain in the urethra.
- Cloudy or reddish urine that smells strange.
- Pain in the lower belly or back.
- Often having the urge to urinate but not being able to pass much urine.
- Fever and chills if the infection is bad, especially if it has spread to the kidneys.

Urinary pain or burning may also be a symptom of a sexually transmitted disease. See page 223.

Men with symptoms like those of a bladder infection may have a prostate infection (see page 217) or epididymitis. See a picture of the prostate and epididymis on page 218.

Home Treatment

Start home treatment at the first sign of a bladder infection. A day or two of self-care may clear up a minor infection.

- Drink extra fluids as soon as you notice symptoms and for the next 24 hours.

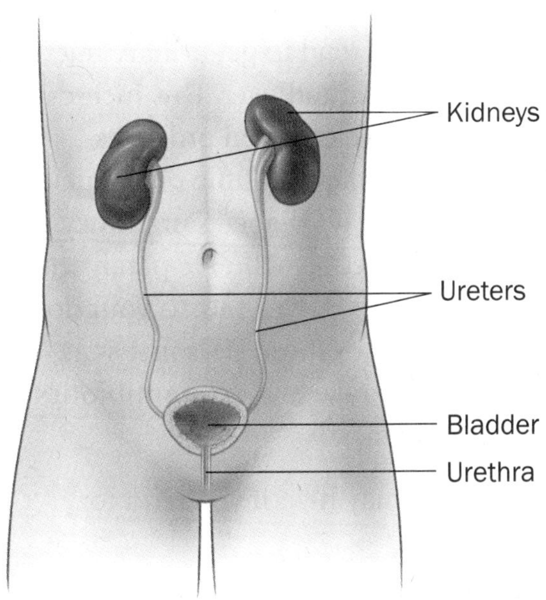

The kidneys filter the blood, and the waste products from the blood become urine. Urine travels through the ureters to the bladder and then leaves the body through the urethra.

- Urinate often, and follow the other tips in Preventing UTIs.
- Watch for fever. A fever may mean you have a more serious infection.
- Use a heating pad or take a hot bath to help relieve pain. Do not use bubble bath or harsh soaps.
- Do not have sex until symptoms improve.

If your symptoms last longer than 1 or 2 days or get worse, call your doctor. You may need to start taking antibiotics.

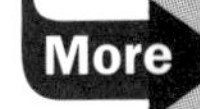

Preventing UTIs

Some people tend to get urinary tract infections over and over. This includes men who have enlarged prostates, women who had multiple pregnancies, people who have diabetes or kidney stones, and people who are paralyzed from the waist down. Talk to your doctor if you have 3 or more UTIs in 1 year. You may need to take low-dose antibiotics to prevent them.

These tips may help if you tend to get UTIs:

- Drink plenty of water and other fluids.
- Urinate often.
- Do not use douches, vaginal deodorants, or perfumed feminine hygiene products.
- Wash your genitals once a day with water and a mild soap. Rinse and dry well.
- Urinate right after you have sex.
- Drink cranberry and blueberry juice.

Some people feel the tips below may also help prevent urinary problems:

- Wear cotton underwear, cotton-lined panty hose, and loose clothing.
- Avoid alcohol, caffeine, and carbonated drinks. These can irritate the bladder.
- Avoid bubble baths.

Bladder Control

When to Call a Doctor

- You have a sudden change in bladder control. This could be a sign of a serious problem.
- You have to urinate often but cannot pass much urine.
- Your bladder does not feel empty after you urinate.
- You have trouble urinating even when your bladder feels full.
- It burns or hurts when you urinate. See Bladder and Kidney Infections on page 90.
- Your urine has blood in it.
- Your urine smells strange.
- You want help with your bladder control problem.

If you sometimes cannot control your bladder, you are not alone. This problem (called **urinary incontinence**) happens to many people, especially older adults.

The two most common bladder control problems are stress incontinence and urge incontinence.

If you have **stress incontinence**:

- Small amounts of urine leak out when you exercise, cough, laugh, or sneeze. This is more common in women.
- Kegel exercises may help. See page 94.
- Other treatments, including medicines or surgery, may help reduce your symptoms. To decide what treatment option might be right for you, go to the Web site on the back cover and enter **F581** in the search box.

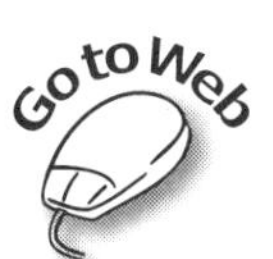

If you have **urge incontinence**:

- The need to urinate comes on so fast that you don't have time to get to the toilet.
- An illness or disease may be causing the problem. This can include a bladder infection, an enlarged prostate, tumors that press on the bladder, and nerve problems such as those caused by Parkinson's disease, multiple sclerosis, and stroke.

Bladder control problems often can be controlled or cured if you can find and fix the cause. Water pills (diuretics) and other common medicines can cause short-term problems. Constipation, urinary tract infections, kidney stones, childbearing, and being overweight are other causes.

Try not to let a bladder control problem embarrass you. Work with your doctor to treat it.

Home Treatment

- Avoid caffeine. It can make symptoms worse.
- Do not cut down on fluids. You need them to stay healthy. If having to get up at night bothers you, cut down on fluids before bed.
- Practice "double-voiding." Empty your bladder as much as you can, relax for a minute, and then try to empty it again.
- If you have trouble controlling your bladder when you laugh, sneeze, cough, or exercise, try doing Kegel exercises every day. See page 94.
- Urinate on a schedule, perhaps every 3 to 4 hours during the day, whether you have the urge or not. This may help you regain control.
- Wear clothing that you can take off quickly, such as pants with an elastic waist.

More

- Clear a path from your bed to the bathroom, or place a portable toilet by your bed.
- Use absorbent pads or briefs, such as Attends or Depend. No one will know you're wearing them.
- Keep skin in the genital area dry to prevent rashes. Use Vaseline or Desitin ointment to help keep urine from irritating the skin.
- Ask your doctor or pharmacist whether any medicines you take, including nonprescription drugs, can affect bladder control. Do not stop taking your medicine without first talking to your doctor.
- If you smoke, quit. This may reduce your coughing, which may help with bladder control. If you need help quitting, see page 351.
- Lose weight if you need to. See page 326.

Kegel Exercises

Kegel exercises strengthen the pelvic muscles that control the flow of urine. This can help cure or improve some bladder control problems.

- To find the muscles, repeatedly stop your urine in midstream and start again.
- Practice squeezing these muscles while you are not urinating. If your belly or buttocks move, you are not using the right muscles.
- Hold the squeeze for 3 seconds, and then relax for 3 seconds.
- Repeat 10 to 15 times.

Try to do Kegel exercises at least 3 times each day. You can do them anywhere, anytime. No one else will know you're doing them.

Blisters

When to Call a Doctor

- You have signs of infection. These may include increased pain, swelling, redness, or warmth; red streaks leading from the blister; pus; or fever.
- You get blisters often and don't know why.
- You have a band of painful blisters on one side of your body or face. See Shingles on page 225.
- You have diabetes or peripheral artery disease, and you get blisters on your hands, feet, or legs.

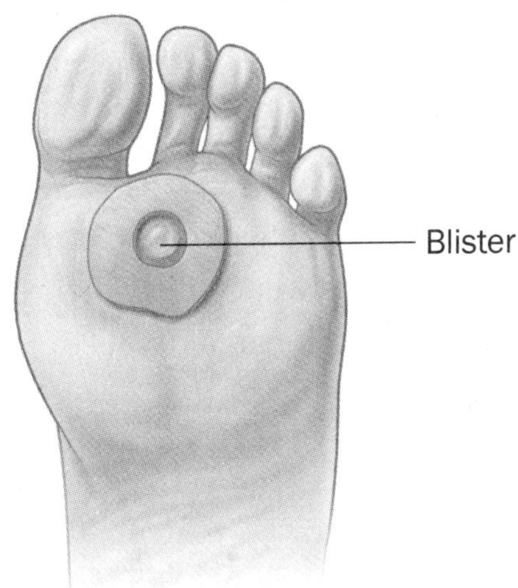

Use a doughnut-shaped pad to protect the blister.

Blisters are usually caused by something rubbing against the skin.

Home Treatment

- If a blister is small and closed, leave it alone. Use a loose bandage to protect it. Avoid the activity or shoes that caused the blister.
- If a small blister is in a weight-bearing area like the bottom of the foot, protect it with a doughnut-shaped moleskin pad. (Moleskin has soft felt on one side and a sticky backing on the other.) Leave the area over the blister open.
- If a blister is large and painful, it is usually best to drain it.
    - Wash your hands.
    - Wipe a needle or straight pin with rubbing alcohol.
    - Gently poke a hole in the edge of the blister.
    - Press the fluid in the blister toward the hole so it can drain out.

After you have opened a blister, or if it has torn open:

- Wash the area with soap and water. Do not use alcohol, iodine, or any other cleanser.

More

- Do not remove the flap of skin over a blister unless it is very dirty or torn or there is pus under it. Gently smooth the flap flat over the tender skin.
- Apply an antibiotic ointment and a clean bandage.
- Change the bandage once a day or anytime it gets wet or dirty. Remove it at night to let the area dry.

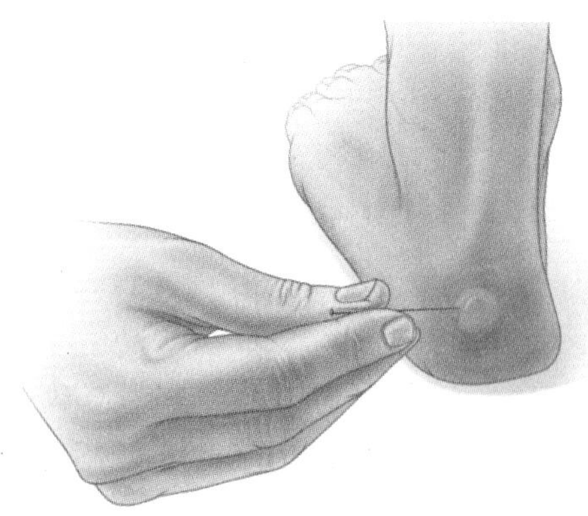

Use a needle or straight pin to puncture a large blister.

Blood Clots in the Leg

When to Call a Doctor

Call 911 if you have a history of blood clots and:

- You have sudden chest pain or shortness of breath.
- You cough up blood.
- You faint.
- You vomit a lot of blood or what looks like coffee grounds.
- You have severe rectal bleeding. Severe means you are passing a lot of stool that is maroon or mostly blood.

Call your doctor if:

- You have a new hard, red, or tender area in your leg.
- You have signs of a blood clot, such as pain in your calf, back of the knee, thigh, or groin, or your leg or groin is red and swollen.
- You are taking a blood thinner such as warfarin (Coumadin) and:
  - Your stools have blood in them, or they are black or look like tar.
  - Your nose bleeds, or your gums bleed when you brush your teeth.
  - You have blood in your urine.
  - You have new bruises or blood spots under your skin, and you don't know why.

Thrombophlebitis means a blood clot (thrombus) has formed in a vein, and the vein has become inflamed (phlebitis). Thrombophlebitis is most common in the lower leg veins. Doctors use different names to describe whether the clot is near the skin or deep inside it.

- **Superficial thrombophlebitis** means a blood clot has formed in a vein close to the surface of the skin. You may be able to feel the clot as a firm lump. The skin over the clot can become red, warm to the touch, and tender. A blood clot close to the skin's surface is usually not serious.
- **Deep vein thrombosis (DVT)** means a blood clot has formed in a vein that lies deep beneath the skin. DVT may not cause symptoms, or it may cause swelling, warmth, or pain. DVT can be dangerous, because these clots can break loose and travel to the lung (pulmonary embolism). This can be deadly.

You are more likely to have blood clots in your legs if:

- You are inactive for a long period of time. This can happen if you are confined to bed or have to sit during a long ride in a plane or car.
- You have had surgery or a major injury, such as a broken leg.
- You have cancer or take a medicine (such as estrogen) that increases the chance that you will form blood clots.
- Others in your family have had problems with blood clots.

Superficial thrombophlebitis can often be treated at home. If you have DVT, you will need to take blood thinners (anticoagulants) for 3 to 6 months or longer. This can keep clots from growing and can prevent future blood clots.

Home Treatment

- If you take blood-thinning (anticoagulant) medicine, be sure you know how to take it safely. To learn more about how to take these medicines, go to the Web site on the back cover and enter **J953** in the search box.

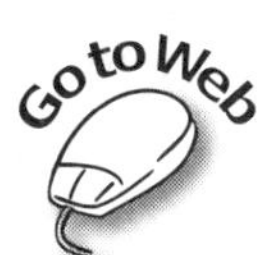

- Do not rub or massage the painful leg. This could cause the clot to come loose and travel through your bloodstream.
- Use a heating pad set on low or a warm cloth on the painful area. Put a thin cloth between the heating pad and your skin.
- Prop up the sore leg on a pillow or footstool anytime you sit or lie down.
- While you are sitting, try this exercise to improve blood flow: Point your toes toward your head so you stretch your calf muscles, and then relax. Repeat.
- Try not to sit or stand for long periods.
- Do gentle exercise, such as walking.
- Ask your doctor about compression stockings. They can reduce pain and swelling and may keep blood from pooling in your legs. You can buy them with a prescription at medical supply stores and some drugstores.
- Do not smoke. If you need help quitting, see page 351.

Boils

When to Call a Doctor

If needed, your doctor can drain the boil and treat the infection. **Call your doctor if**:

- The boil is on your face, near your spine, or in the anal area.
- You have any other lumps near the boil, especially if they hurt.
- You are in a lot of pain or have a fever.
- The area around the boil is red or has red streaks leading from it.
- You have diabetes and you get a boil.
- The boil is as large as or larger than a Ping-Pong ball.
- The boil has not improved after 5 to 7 days of home treatment.
- You get many boils over several months.

A boil is a red, swollen, painful bump under the skin. It may look like an overgrown pimple. Boils are often caused by infected hair follicles. A boil can become large and cause severe pain.

Boils occur most often where there is hair and rubbing. The face, neck, armpits, breasts, groin, and buttocks are common sites.

Home Treatment

- Do not squeeze, scratch, drain, or open the boil. Squeezing can push the infection deeper into the skin. Scratching can spread the infection.
- Wash with an antibacterial soap. Dry the area well.
- Put hot, wet cloths on the boil for 20 to 30 minutes, 3 or 4 times a day. Do this as soon as you notice a boil. The heat and moisture can help bring the boil to a head, but it may take 5 to 7 days. A hot pack or a waterproof heating pad placed over a damp towel may also help.
- Keep using heat for 3 days after the boil opens. Apply a bandage so the draining fluid does not spread. Change the bandage every day.
- Do not wear tight clothing over the area.

Breast Problems

When to Call a Doctor

- ◆ You find a lump in your breast, armpit, or chest area that concerns you, especially if it is hard and not like the rest of your breast tissue.
- ◆ You find a breast lump after menopause.
- ◆ You have a bloody or greenish discharge from a nipple, or a watery or milky discharge that occurs without pressing on the nipple or breast.
- ◆ You have a change in a nipple, such as crusty or scaly skin or a nipple that now turns in rather than points out.
- ◆ One of your breasts changes shape or seems to pucker or pull when you raise your arms.
- ◆ The skin looks dimpled like an orange peel.
- ◆ You have a change in the color or feel of the skin of a breast or the darker area around a nipple.
- ◆ You have new pain in one breast that lasts longer than 1 or 2 weeks and was not caused by an injury.
- ◆ You have any signs of infection in a breast, such as pain, redness, warmth, or swelling.
- ◆ You are a man and you find a lump in your chest area.

Breast Lumps

Breast lumps are common, especially in women who still have periods. Breast lumps usually go away after menopause, but they may occur in women who take hormones after menopause.

Most breast lumps are not cancer. Still, you should have a doctor check any lump or thickness that is not like the rest of your breast tissue. (It may be bigger or harder or feel different.)

How dense or lumpy a woman's breasts are tends to run in the family. If your mother had lumpy breasts, you probably will too. It is also common for one breast to be denser than the other. The important thing is to watch for a change in the breast tissue.

You doctor may want to do tests to check a lump in your breast, such as a mammogram, ultrasound, or MRI. A mammogram is usually done first, but ultrasound or MRI may be used for women who have dense breasts or breast implants.

More

Breast Cancer

Here are a few things you should know:

- Breast cancer can often be cured if you find it early.
- Regular mammograms and breast exams done by a health professional can help find breast cancer early and save lives.
- Self-exams can help you learn what is normal for your breasts and may make you aware of changes sooner. See page 325.
- Your risk for breast cancer goes up after age 50. Most women over 50 should have a mammogram every 1 to 2 years.
- If your mother or a sister had breast cancer before menopause, you are at increased risk for breast cancer. Talk with your doctor. You may need to have a mammogram every year.

What You Can Do to Prevent Breast Cancer

- Do not have more than 1 alcohol drink a day. Moderate to heavy drinking increases your risk for breast cancer.
- Eat a low-fat diet (see page 333). It has not been proven that a diet low in fat will prevent cancer. But women in populations that eat a high-fat diet are more likely to die of breast cancer than those that eat a low-fat diet.
- Have a breast exam by a health professional every year.
- Have a mammogram every 1 to 2 years. See page 324.
- If you have a strong family history of breast cancer, you may need to have a mammogram every year. Also talk with your doctor about medicines or other treatments that may lower your risk of breast cancer.

Breathing Problems

When to Call a Doctor

Call 911 if:

- You cannot breathe, or you have severe trouble breathing. For signs of severe trouble breathing, see page 19.
- You have shortness of breath with chest pain or pressure or other symptoms of a heart attack. See page 38.
- Your tongue or throat swells quickly and makes it very hard to breathe. This can be caused by an allergic reaction. See page 74.

Call your doctor if:

- You wheeze when you breathe. Wheezing is a high-pitched sound you may make if you have a problem in your airways.
- You tire quickly when you talk or eat, or you often have to stop to catch your breath.
- You wake up in the night short of breath.
- You have trouble breathing or cough a lot when you exercise.
- You have any trouble breathing that lasts longer than an hour and is not related to a cold, flu, or other illness.

Be sure to check the Chest, Heart, and Lung Problems chart on page 59 if you do not find your symptoms here.

Breathing problems have many possible causes, from asthma to anxiety to heart problems. A breathing problem can be a sign of something serious, though this is not always the case. Use the When to Call a Doctor list to decide if you need medical care and how soon.

If you have already been diagnosed with allergies, asthma, COPD (chronic obstructive pulmonary disease), or heart failure, one of these topics may help:

- Allergies, page 73
- Living Better With Asthma, page 271
- Living Better With COPD, page 282
- Living Better With Heart Failure, page 303

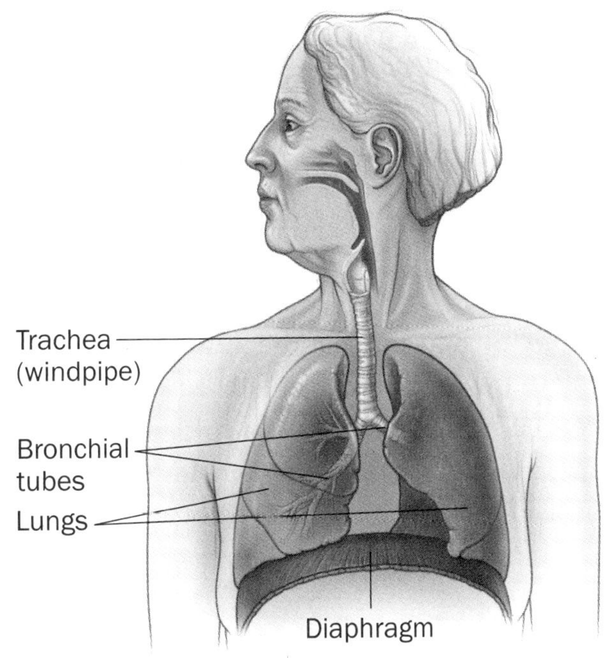

The respiratory tract

Bronchitis

When to Call a Doctor

- A cough occurs with new wheezing or new trouble breathing.
- You cough up blood.
- You cough up yellow, green, or rust-colored mucus from your lungs (not from your nose or the back of your throat) for more than 2 days, and you have a fever.
- You have a fever of 104°F or higher.
- You have a fever higher than 101°F with shaking chills and a cough that brings up mucus.
- You still have a fever after using home treatment. Bronchitis may cause fevers of 102°F or higher for up to a day. But call a doctor if the fever stays high. See the fever guidelines on page 150.
- Your breathing is fast or shallow, and you are short of breath.
- You have pain in the muscles of your chest (chest-wall pain) when you cough or breathe.
- You are more tired than you would be with a typical cold.
- You cannot drink enough fluids and are dehydrated, or you cannot eat at all.
- You have lung problems or another long-term disease, and you have symptoms of bronchitis (cough, fever, tightness in your chest).
- A cough lasts more than 7 to 10 days after other symptoms have gone away, especially if it brings up mucus. (It is normal for a dry, hacking cough to last a few weeks after a cold.)
- Any cough lasts longer than 2 weeks.

Bronchitis means that the airways leading to the lungs are irritated. It is usually caused by a virus, such as a cold, and may start 3 to 4 days after a cold goes away. But bronchitis can also be caused by bacteria, cigarette smoke, or air pollution.

You may have a dry cough, a mild fever, fatigue, pain or tightness in your chest, and wheezing. As your cough gets worse, it may bring up mucus (sputum).

If you get bronchitis often—especially if you smoke—you may reach a point where your airways are inflamed and irritated all the time. This is called chronic bronchitis. If you smoke, you are also at high risk for emphysema. Chronic bronchitis, emphysema, and other lung diseases are known as **chronic obstructive pulmonary disease (COPD)**. If you have COPD, see page 282.

Home Treatment

- If your doctor prescribes medicine, take it as directed. But don't be surprised if your doctor does not prescribe medicine. Bronchitis often goes away without it.
- Drink plenty of fluids.
- Get some extra rest.
- Try a nonprescription cough suppressant with dextromethorphan, such as Robitussin-DM or Vicks Dry Hacking Cough. Some people find that this helps quiet a dry, hacking cough so they can sleep. Read the label on the bottle, and don't take cough medicines that have more than one active ingredient.
- Take aspirin, ibuprofen (Advil, Motrin), or acetaminophen (Tylenol) for fever and body aches. But do not take aspirin if you have asthma.
- Breathe moist air from a humidifier, a hot shower, or a sink filled with hot water to relieve a stuffy nose and head.
- Do not smoke. If you need help quitting, see page 351.
- If you have classic flu symptoms, see Flu on page 153.

Bunions and Hammer Toes

When to Call a Doctor

- You have sudden, severe pain in your big toe. See page 163.
- Your big toe starts to partly cover your second toe.
- You have diabetes, poor blood flow, peripheral artery disease, or a weak immune system, and you develop any kind of foot problem. Irritated skin over a bunion or hammer toe can easily get infected.
- You have a sore over a bunion or hammer toe.
- Pain does not get better after 2 to 3 weeks of home treatment.

A **bunion** is a bump on the outside of the joint at the base of your big toe. You get a bunion when the big toe bends toward and sometimes partly covers the second toe.

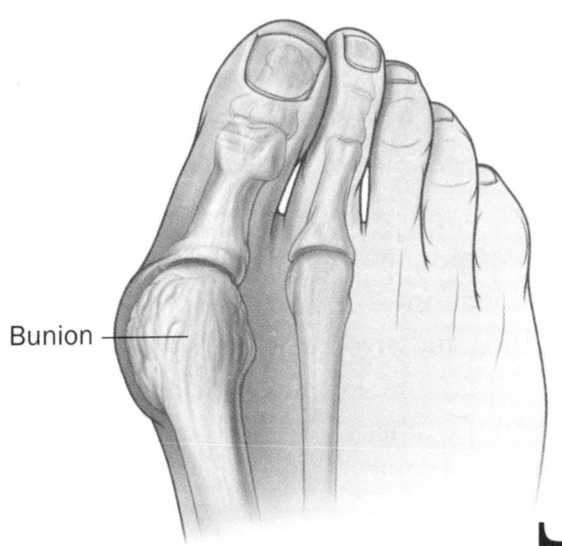

More

A **hammer toe** is a toe that bends up at the middle joint.

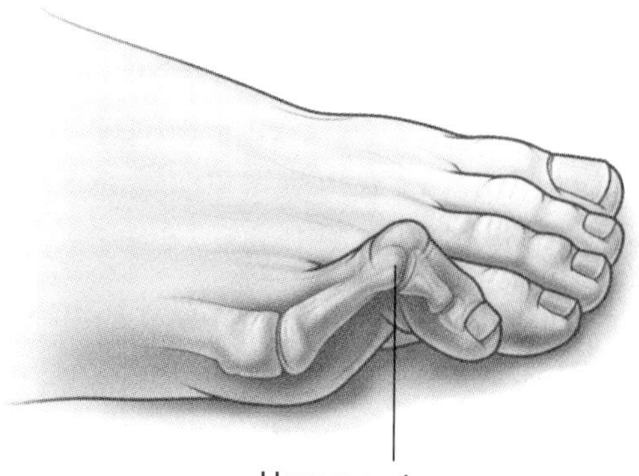

These foot problems sometimes run in families. Tight or high-heeled shoes increase the risk of both. If you already have a foot problem, wearing tight shoes or high heels may make it worse.

Home Treatment

Once you have a bunion or a hammer toe, there is usually no way to get rid of it. But home treatment will help relieve pain and keep the problem from getting worse.

- Wear roomy, low-heeled shoes that have wide, deep toe areas and good arch support. To find the best footwear for your problem, go to the Web site on the back cover and enter **H581** in the search box.
- Cushion the joint with moleskin or a doughnut-shaped pad to prevent rubbing and pressure. (Moleskin has soft felt on one side and a sticky backing on the other.)
- Take an old pair of shoes, and cut out the area over the toe. Wear these shoes around the house. Or wear comfortable sandals that do not press on the area.
- Try ibuprofen (Advil, Motrin) or acetaminophen (Tylenol) to relieve pain. Ice or cold packs may also help. See page 51.
- Ask your doctor about bunion pads, arch supports, or custom-made supports called orthotics. These can hold your foot in a healthy position and take pressure off your big toe.

What About Foot Surgery?

If you have tried home treatment but you still have severe pain or an oddly shaped joint that affects your walking, you may want to think about surgery.

- Surgery can help reduce pain and help you walk better, but it may not cure the problem.
- If you want surgery to improve how your foot looks rather than to relieve pain, you may not be happy with the result.
- Surgery can sometimes cause other problems.
- Surgery costs a lot.

For help deciding if surgery is worth the cost and risks, go to the Web site on the back cover and enter **C531** in the search box.

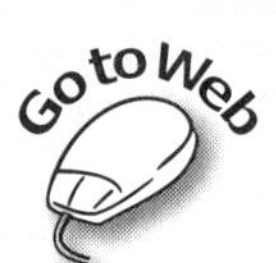

Bursitis and Tendinosis

When to Call a Doctor

Call 911 if shoulder pain occurs with chest pain or other symptoms of a heart attack (see page 38).

Call a doctor if:

- You have fever with sudden joint swelling or redness.
- You cannot use a joint at all.
- You have severe pain when the joint is at rest.
- Pain lasts longer than 2 weeks even with home treatment. Your doctor or a physical therapist can help you create a plan for exercise and home treatment.

If you have had a sudden injury, see Strains, Sprains, and Broken Bones on page 49.

Bursitis and tendinosis are common reasons for pain and swelling in the legs, knees, hips, wrists, elbows, and shoulders.

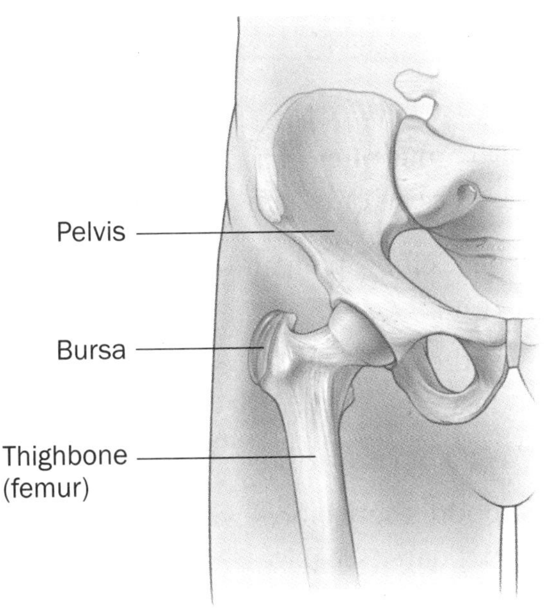

The fluid-filled bursa helps cushion a joint like the hip.

A bursa is a small sac of fluid that helps the tissues around a joint slide over one another easily. Injury, overuse, or constant direct pressure on a joint can cause pain, redness, heat, and swelling of the bursa. This is called **bursitis**.

Tendons are tough, ropelike fibers that connect muscles to bones. **Tendinosis** develops when wear and tear or overuse of a tendon causes tiny tears in the tissue. This leads to pain, inflammation, and breakdown in the tendons or the tissues surrounding them.

Both bursitis and tendinosis can be caused by jobs, sports, or things you do around the house that require a lot of twisting or fast moving of the joints or constant pressure on a joint (kneeling, for example).

The same home treatment is good for both problems.

More

Home Treatment

Bursitis or tendinosis will usually get better in a few days or weeks if you avoid the activity that caused it. But the mistake many people make is thinking that the problem is gone when the pain is gone.

To keep the problem from coming back, you will need to strengthen and stretch the muscles around the joint and change the way you do some activities.

- Rest the area. Change the way you do the activity that causes pain so that you can do it without pain. See the guidelines for specific joints later in this topic. To stay fit, try activities that do not stress the area.
- As soon as you notice pain, use ice or cold packs for 10 to 15 minutes at a time, 3 times a day. Always put a thin cloth between the ice and your skin. See Ice and Cold Packs on page 51. Keep using ice as long as it relieves pain. Heating pads or hot baths may feel good, but they don't help you heal.
- Take aspirin, ibuprofen (Advil, Motrin), or naproxen (Aleve) to ease pain and swelling. But do not use the medicine to control the pain while you keep overusing the joint.
- To prevent stiffness, gently move the joint through as full a range of motion as you can without pain. As the pain gets better, keep doing range-of-motion exercises, and add exercises that strengthen the muscles around the joint.
- When you are ready to try the activity that caused the pain, start slowly and do it for short periods only or at a slower speed. Increase the intensity slowly and only if the pain does not come back.
- Warm up before and stretch after the activity. Use ice after exercise to prevent pain and swelling.

Along with the home treatment information for bursitis and tendinosis above, the following tips will help for problems with a specific joint.

Wrists

Wrist pain may be caused by tendinosis. Although this is not the same as carpal tunnel syndrome, the same home care may help. See page 111.

Elbows

Elbow pain is often caused by tendinosis in the forearm or bursitis in the elbow.

To relieve elbow pain and prevent further injury:

- Rest the elbow and give it time to heal.
- Wear a brace or elbow sleeve.
- Support a sore elbow with a sling for 1 to 2 days (see page 52). Do range-of-motion exercises daily.

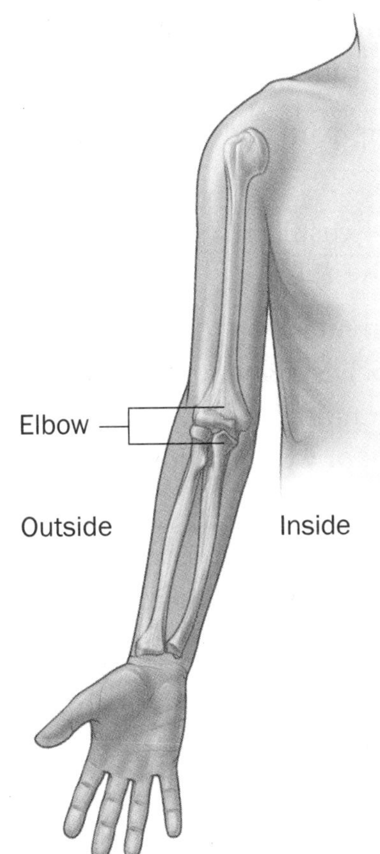

Tennis elbow causes pain on the outside of the elbow. Golfer's elbow hurts on the inside.

- Strengthen the wrist, arm, shoulder, and back muscles.
- Avoid activities that make you repeat a wrist motion many times.
- Make changes in your activities so you don't irritate the tendon:
  - Use tools with larger handles.
  - Avoid leaning on the point of your elbow for long periods.
  - Switch hands during activities such as raking, sweeping, or gardening.

Shoulders

Shoulder pain that occurs on the outside of the upper arm is often caused by bursitis or tendinosis around the shoulder joint. Pain on the top of the shoulder or in the neck may be caused by tension in the trapezius muscles, which run from the back of the head across the back of the shoulders. See Neck Pain on page 204.

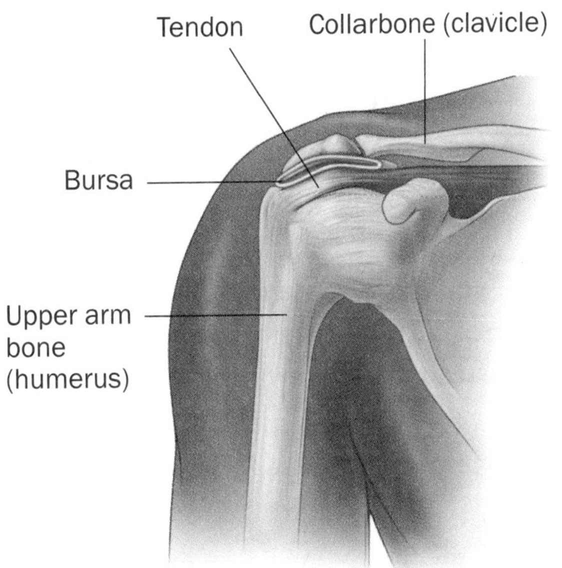

Bursitis, tendinosis, and muscle tension are common causes of shoulder pain.

Common symptoms of shoulder bursitis or tendinosis are pain, pinching, and stiffness when you raise your arm. The symptoms are often brought on by doing repeated overhead movements. Pain and swelling can occur when you keep using your shoulder without giving it time to rest.

More

To relieve shoulder pain and stiffness:

- Avoid activities that involve overhead reaching, but keep using your shoulder.
- Try the "pendulum" exercise: Bend forward and hold the back of a chair with the hand of your healthy arm. Let the other arm hang straight down from the shoulder. Move the hanging arm in circles; start with small circles and slowly make them bigger. Then switch directions. Again, go from small circles to large ones. Next, swing the arm forward and backward, then from side to side. Do this exercise 10 times a day.
- If you swim, use a different swim stroke. Try breaststroke or sidestroke instead of the crawl or butterfly.
- Put your shoulder through its full range of motion every day.

Hips

Hip pain may be caused by tendinosis or bursitis. You may feel it at the side of your hip when you rise from a chair and take the first few steps, while you climb stairs, or while you drive. If pain is severe, sleeping on your side may also hurt.

Pain in the front of the hip may also be caused by arthritis (see page 266).

Hip pain can also cause knee or thigh pain. This is called referred pain.

To relieve hip pain and avoid further problems:

- Wear well-cushioned shoes. Do not wear high heels.
- Avoid activities that force one side of your pelvis higher than the other, such as running in only one direction on a track or working sideways on a slope.
- Sleep on your "good" side with a pillow between your knees or on your back with pillows under your knees.
- Try the hip stretch on page 89. Stretch after activity, when your muscles are warm.

Knees

Knee pain may be caused by bursitis or tendinosis. Also see Knee Problems on page 194.

Legs and Feet

Heel or foot pain may be caused by plantar fasciitis or Achilles tendinosis. See page 178. Pain in the front of the lower leg may be shin splints. See page 198.

Calluses and Corns

When to Call a Doctor

- A callus or corn breaks open and starts to hurt.
- A callus or corn bleeds or looks red or black.

Calluses and corns are areas of skin that have gotten thick and hard because of rubbing and pressure.

Calluses are common on the soles of the feet, the heels, and the hands. Corns are often on the toes.

Home Treatment

- If you have diabetes or peripheral artery disease, talk to your doctor before you try to remove a callus or corn on your own.
- If a callus or corn hurts, soak your foot in warm water for 5 to 10 minutes. Then rub the callus or corn with a towel or pumice stone. You may need to repeat this a few times over several days.
- You can also use a nonprescription product for removing calluses and corns.
- To prevent pain and rubbing, cushion the area with a doughnut-shaped pad or moleskin patch. (Moleskin has soft felt on one side and a sticky backing on the other.)
- Do not try to cut or burn off a callus or corn.

Canker Sores

When to Call a Doctor

- You have a canker sore and a fever.
- You get canker sores after you start a new medicine.
- A canker sore does not heal in 2 weeks, or you get several sores.
- A canker sore hurts a lot, or it goes away and then comes back.
- You have white spots in your mouth that are not canker sores, and they have not gone away after 1 to 2 weeks.

More

Canker sores are painful, open sores on the inside of the mouth. You can get them because of a mouth injury, an infection, certain foods, hormone changes, and other reasons. Canker sores usually heal in 7 to 10 days.

Home Treatment

- Avoid coffee, spicy and salty foods, nuts, chocolate, and citrus fruits when you have open sores in your mouth.
- Use a nonprescription canker sore medicine, such as Orabase or Anbesol. This can help protect the sore, ease pain, and speed healing. Or put a thin paste of baking soda and water on the sore to relieve pain.
- Rinse your mouth with an antacid (such as Maalox or Mylanta) or with a mixture of 1 tablespoon of hydrogen peroxide in 8 ounces of water.
- Do not smoke or chew tobacco. If you need help quitting, see page 351.
- Use a toothbrush with soft bristles to brush your teeth.

Carpal Tunnel Syndrome

When to Call a Doctor

- You have tingling, numbness, weakness, or pain in your fingers and hand even after 2 weeks of home treatment.
- You often have little or no feeling in your fingers or hand.
- You cannot do simple hand movements, or you drop things a lot because you can't hold on to them.
- You cannot pinch your thumb and first finger together, or you have no thumb strength.
- Your hand muscles (especially the muscles of your thumb) look smaller.
- You have problems at work because of pain in your fingers or hand.

The carpal tunnel is a narrow space in your wrist. The nerve that controls feeling in some of your fingers and controls some of the hand muscles passes through this space.

You get carpal tunnel syndrome when there is pressure on the nerve where it goes through the carpal tunnel. This can cause:

- Numbness or pain in your hand or wrist that wakes you up at night.

- Numbness or tingling in your fingers, except for the little finger and half of the ring finger.
- Numbness or pain that gets worse when you use your hand or wrist, especially when you grip an object or flex your wrist.
- Aching pain in your arm between your hand and your elbow. The pain may come and go.
- A weak grip.
- Loss of muscle mass in your hand, especially below your thumb.

Activities that make you use the same finger or hand movements over and over (especially if you do them with your wrist bent down) can cause carpal tunnel syndrome or make it worse. You may do things at work, at home, or during sports or hobbies that cause this problem.

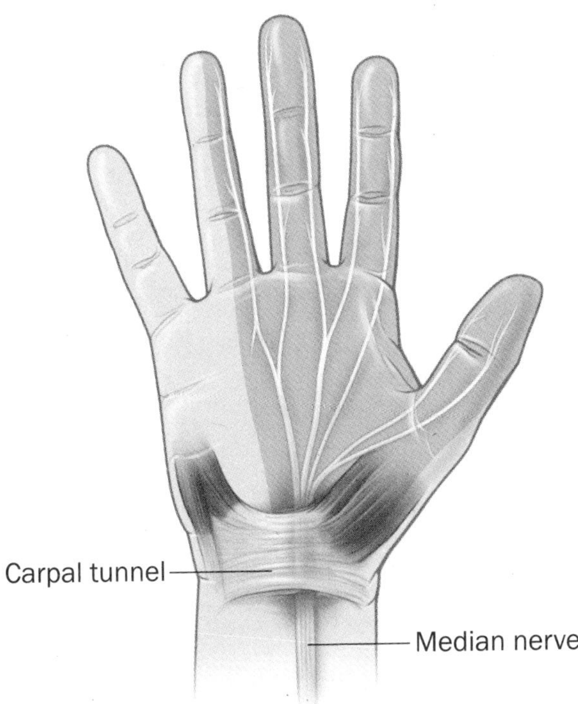

Carpal tunnel syndrome causes pain and tingling in the shaded area.

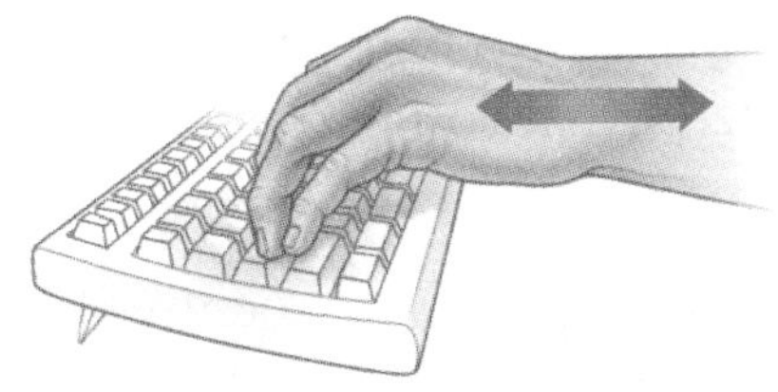

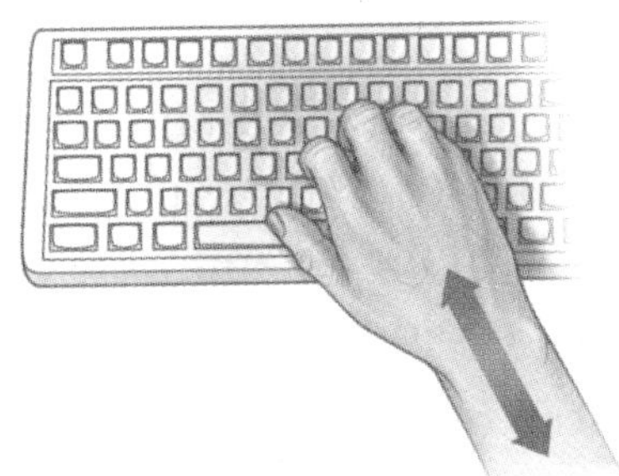

When you type, keep your wrists straight. Your hands will be slightly higher than your wrists.

Home Treatment

- Stop any activity that you think may be causing numbness or pain. If the problem improves when you stop, return to that activity slowly. Try to keep your wrist straight or only slightly bent.
- Watch your posture. When you type, keep your wrists straight, with your hands a little higher than your wrists. A keyboard wrist support and arm supports on your chair may help. When your arms are at your sides, relax your shoulders.
- Use your whole hand (not just your fingers and thumb) to hold objects.
- Reduce the speed and force of repeated hand movements. For instance, type a little slower, and don't hit the keys too hard.

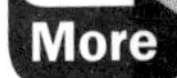
More

- Switch hands and change positions often when you have to repeat the same motions a lot.
- Rest your hands frequently.
- Use ibuprofen (Advil, Motrin) or naproxen (Aleve) to relieve pain and reduce swelling.
- Use ice or a cold pack on the palm side of your wrist. Always put a thin cloth between the ice and your skin. See Ice and Cold Packs on page 51.
- Don't sleep on your hands.
- Ask your doctor about a wrist splint. This can relieve pressure and keep your wrist in a good position when you sleep.
- Do simple range-of-motion exercises with your fingers and wrist to prevent stiffening and keep your muscles strong. Stop if it hurts.

Losing weight, quitting smoking, reducing alcohol and salt, and controlling diabetes and thyroid problems may help reduce swelling in your wrist. Use the index in the back of the book to find information that can help.

What About Surgery?

Most cases of carpal tunnel syndrome can get better without surgery. If you are thinking about surgery, learn as much as you can about its pros and cons, including the cost of the surgery.

To help you decide whether surgery is

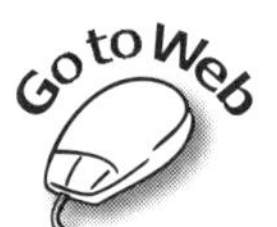

right for you, go to the Web site on the back cover and enter **B566** in the search box.

Preventing Carpal Tunnel Syndrome

You are more likely to get carpal tunnel syndrome if:

- You spend a lot of time doing activities that make you repeat the same finger and hand movements.
- You do lots of activities with your wrists bent downward.
- You work with tools or machines that vibrate in your hand, like sanders or drills.

But there are ways you can reduce your risk as well as any pain or weakness you already have. To learn how to keep your wrists healthy, go to the Web site on the back cover and enter **S503** in the search box.

Cataracts

When to Call a Doctor

- You have severe eye pain.
- You have a change in your vision, such as vision loss, double vision, or blurred vision. A sudden change could be a sign of a serious problem.
- You need to change your eyeglasses prescription often.
- Daytime glare is a problem.
- You have trouble driving at night because of glare from headlights.
- Vision problems are affecting your daily life.

A cataract is a painless, cloudy area in the lens of the eye (see the picture on page 162). By blocking some of the light that comes into the eye, a cataract may cause cloudy, foggy, filmy, or double vision. Glare is also common with cataracts. It can cause lights to look star-shaped or have haloes around them at night.

Cataracts can be caused by:

- Normal changes in your eyes as you get older.
- Eye injury.
- Certain medicines.
- Eye disease and other health problems, especially diabetes.

Home Treatment

Home treatment may help you avoid or delay cataract surgery. There are many things you can do to make the changes in your vision easier to live with.

- Move room lights and use window shades to prevent glare.
- Use more lighting or higher-watt bulbs in your home.

Do You Need Surgery?

For most adults, the need for cataract surgery depends on how much their cataracts affect their quality of life. Most cataracts grow slowly. At first, you may just need stronger glasses. Many people get along very well with the help of glasses, contact lenses, and other vision aids.

Later, if a cataract grows and starts to seriously affect your vision, you can have surgery to remove it. Some cataracts, such as those caused by injury, need to be removed right away.

For most people with cataracts, whether and when to have surgery is up to them. For help with your decision, go to the Web site on the back cover and enter **Z558** in the search box.

Go to Web

More

- Use contrasts in color and brightness to make things easier to find. For example, use dark switch plates on light-colored walls. Use bright labels to "color code" medicines, spices, and stove dials.
- Use a magnifying glass to help you read. Look for large-print books and other reading material. You can often get bank checks, medicine labels, and other items in large print.
- Have your eyes checked regularly. Update your glasses when needed.
- Wear sunglasses to reduce glare and block out harmful sunlight. Buy sunglasses that screen out UVA and UVB rays.
- If you smoke, quit. Smoking can make cataracts worse. If you need help quitting, see page 351.

For other tips on living with reduced vision, see page 251.

Chest Pain

When to Call a Doctor

Call 911 if:

- You think you may be having a heart attack. Do not wait to see if you feel better.
- You have been diagnosed with angina, and you have chest pain that does not go away with rest or is not getting better within 5 minutes after you take a dose of nitroglycerin.

After calling 911, chew 1 adult aspirin (unless you are allergic to it). If you cannot get an ambulance, have someone drive you to the hospital. Do not drive yourself.

Call a doctor if:

- You think you have angina (see page 115) and have not seen a doctor about it.
- You have been diagnosed with angina and are having chest pain more often than usual.
- You have any chest pain and have a history of heart disease or blood clots in the lungs.
- You have mild but constant chest pain that does not go away with rest.
- You have chest pain with other symptoms of pneumonia. See page 210.
- Mild chest pain lasts longer than 2 days without getting better.

Is It a Heart Attack?

You may be having a heart attack if:

- ❑ You have chest pain that feels like pressure, tightness, squeezing, crushing, intense burning, or aching in your chest.
- ❑ The pain or pressure lasts longer than 5 minutes and does not go away with rest or nitroglycerin.

Other signs include:

- ❑ Pain that spreads to your upper back, upper belly, neck, jaw, or arms.
- ❑ Sweating.
- ❑ Shortness of breath.
- ❑ Nausea or vomiting.
- ❑ Feeling dizzy or lightheaded.
- ❑ A fast or uneven heartbeat.

The more boxes you check, the more likely it is that you are having a heart attack. Women and people with diabetes may not have chest pain but may have some of the other symptoms.

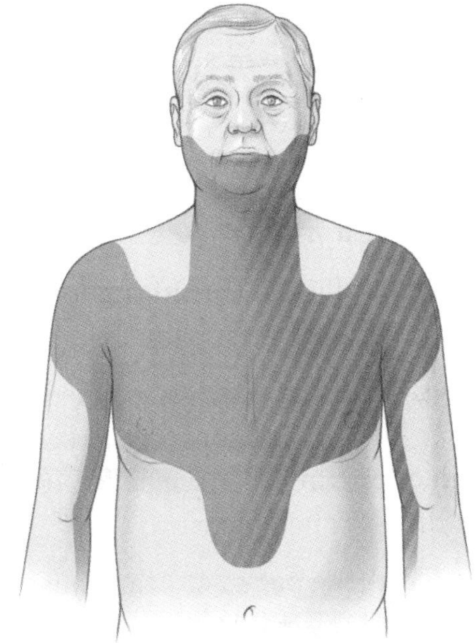

A heart attack may cause discomfort in any of the shaded areas as well as the upper back.

Angina

Angina is pain, pressure, heaviness, or numbness behind the breastbone or across the chest. It occurs when your heart does not get enough oxygen. This can happen during moments of stress, exercise, or anything that works your heart too hard. The pain goes away when you stop and rest or take a medicine called nitroglycerin.

The pain of a heart attack is usually more severe than angina, lasts longer, and does not go away with rest or nitroglycerin. Unlike angina, it's caused by blocked blood flow to the heart muscle, not just lack of oxygen.

Angina is a sign of **coronary artery disease**. Having coronary artery disease means you are at high risk for a heart attack. To learn how to reduce your risk, see page 287.

More

Other Causes of Chest Pain

Chest pain is not always caused by a heart problem.

- Heartburn (see page 176) or gas can cause chest pain.
- Hyperventilation (breathing too fast) can also cause chest pain.
- Chest pain that gets worse when you take a deep breath or cough may be a sign of pneumonia (see page 210) or an illness called pleurisy.
- An ulcer (see page 243) can cause chest pain, usually below the breastbone. The pain may be worse when your stomach is empty.
- Gallstones (see page 159) may cause pain in the right side of the chest or around the shoulder blade. The pain may get worse after a meal or in the middle of the night.
- Shingles (see page 225) may cause a sharp, burning, or tingling pain that feels like a tight band around one side of the chest.

A shooting pain that lasts a few seconds, or a quick pain at the end of a deep breath, is usually not a cause for concern.

Chest-Wall Pain

If you can point to the exact spot in your chest that hurts and it hurts more when you press on it, you probably have chest-wall pain.

If you have chest-wall pain, you may have strained a muscle in your chest or hurt a rib. Or the cartilage in your chest wall could be inflamed for no obvious reason. This is called **costochondritis**. It usually goes away in a few days.

Home Treatment

If you have angina caused by coronary artery disease, there are many things you can do to control it. See Living Better With Coronary Artery Disease on page 287.

For chest-wall pain caused by injury:

- Take aspirin, ibuprofen (Advil, Motrin), or acetaminophen (Tylenol) for pain.
- Use an ice pack to help relieve pain the first 2 to 3 days after an injury. See Ice and Cold Packs on page 51.
- After the first 2 to 3 days (or after the swelling has gone down), you can use heat for the pain. Use a heating pad set on low or heat that is no warmer than bathwater. Don't go to sleep while using a heating pad.
- Use products such as Bengay or Icy-Hot to help soothe sore muscles.
- Avoid any activity that strains the chest. As your pain gets better, slowly return to your normal activities.

Looking for the Chronic Obstructive Pulmonary Disease (COPD) topic? See page 282.

Cold Hands and Feet

When to Call a Doctor

- You have severe pain in your hands or feet.
- Your hands or feet (or any part of them) are pale, white, blue, or black, and normal color does not return within 30 minutes.
- Your hands or feet do not warm up even after home care.

Many older adults have cold hands and feet. Usually this is because of reduced blood flow to the hands and feet. This can be caused by cold weather, blood flow problems, or being inactive. A low thyroid level can make you more sensitive to cold. See Low Thyroid (Hypothyroidism) on page 238.

Some people have a problem called **Raynaud's** that makes the hands and feet overreact to cold. It causes your hands and feet to feel cold and numb and then turn white. As blood flow returns, your fingers and toes may turn blue, then red, and start to throb and hurt.

Raynaud's can be painful, but it usually does not cause serious problems. If you can't keep your hands and feet warm enough, your doctor may prescribe medicine.

Home Treatment

- Do not smoke, and avoid drinks with caffeine, such as coffee and soda. Caffeine and nicotine can reduce blood flow to your skin.
- Keep indoor temperatures at 65°F or higher.
- Wear layers of warm clothing. Wear cotton-blend or wool socks to bed, and wear socks and slippers around the house.
- Wear a hat. You lose more heat from your head than from any other part of your body.
- Wear mittens instead of gloves. Mittens keep fingers warmer than gloves do.
- Move around. Walking briskly or whirling your arms around like a windmill will get your blood moving and warm you up.

Cold Sores

When to Call a Doctor

- You have cold sores and a fever.
- A sore lasts longer than 2 weeks.
- You often have outbreaks of cold sores. Your doctor can prescribe a medicine that may help.
- You have cold sores, and you live or work with someone who has a weak immune system. The virus that causes cold sores can be dangerous for people with weak immune systems.

Cold sores (fever blisters) are small, red blisters on the lips and outer edge of the mouth. They often ooze a clear fluid and scab over after a few days.

Cold sores are caused by a type of herpes virus (another type causes chickenpox). Herpes viruses stay in the body after the first infection. Later, something causes, or triggers, the virus to become active again. A cold, a fever, or stress can trigger a cold sore. Sometimes you get cold sores for no clear reason.

Sunlight can trigger cold sores in some people. Wear lip balm with sunscreen in it when you are going to be outdoors.

Home Treatment

- Do not kiss or have oral sex with anyone while you have a cold sore. This can spread the virus.
- Put ice or a cool, wet cloth on the area 3 times a day. This may help reduce redness and swelling.
- Use petroleum jelly to ease cracking and dryness.
- Use a lip protector such as Blistex or Campho-Phenique to ease the pain. Do not share the product with anyone else.
- Apply vitamin E gel or a product that has aloe vera, goldenseal, or bee propolis.
- Be patient. Cold sores usually go away in 7 to 10 days.

Colds

When to Call a Doctor

- You have trouble breathing.
- You have a high fever. See page 150.
- You cough up yellow, green, or bloody mucus (sputum) from your lungs and have a fever.
- Mucus from your nose is thick (like pus) or bloody.
- You have redness in your face or around your eyes, or you have pain in your face, eyes, or teeth that does not get better with home treatment.
- Your symptoms are worse than what you would expect with a cold, and you don't think you have the flu. See Flu on page 153.
- The person who is sick seems confused or acts odd. Even a small change is important in a person who is old or frail. It may be a sign of delirium. See Confusion and Memory Loss on page 122.

Everyone gets a cold from time to time. Lots of different viruses cause colds, but the symptoms are usually the same:

- Runny nose and sneezing
- Red eyes
- Sore throat and cough
- Headaches and body aches

You will probably feel a cold come on over the course of a couple of days. As the cold gets worse, your nose may get stuffy with thicker mucus. Most colds last a week or two.

There is no cure for the common cold. Antibiotics will not help. If you catch a cold, treat the symptoms.

If you feel like you have a cold all the time, or if cold symptoms last more than 2 weeks, you may have allergies (see page 73) or sinusitis (see page 227). A cold can also lead to a worse infection like bronchitis (see page 102) or pneumonia (see page 210).

Home Treatment

- Get extra rest. Slow down a little from your usual routine. You don't need to stay home in bed, but try not to expose others to your cold.
- Drink plenty of fluids. Hot water, herbal tea, or chicken soup will help relieve a stuffy nose and head.
- Take aspirin, ibuprofen (Advil, Motrin), or acetaminophen (Tylenol) to relieve aches.
- Use a humidifier in your bedroom and take hot showers to relieve a stuffy nose and head.

More

- If you have streaks of mucus in the back of your throat (postnasal drip), gargle with warm water.
- Use throw-away tissues, not handkerchiefs. This will reduce the chance of spreading the cold to others.
- If your nose is red and raw from rubbing it with tissues, put a dab of petroleum jelly on the sore area.
- Do not take cold remedies that use several drugs to treat different symptoms. Treat each symptom on its own. Take a decongestant for a stuffy nose and a pain reliever like ibuprofen (Advil, Motrin) for a headache. See Home Treatment for coughs on page 126.
- If you have high blood pressure or heart disease, do not take decongestants unless your doctor tells you to. Some decongestants are also unsafe if you have thyroid disease, glaucoma, urinary problems, an enlarged prostate, or diabetes.
- Do not use nasal decongestant sprays for more than 3 days in a row. Doing so may lead to a "rebound" effect, which makes the mucous membranes in your nose swell up even more.
- Do not take antihistamines for a cold. They don't help.

How to Avoid Colds

- Wash your hands often! Be extra careful during the winter and when you are around people with colds.
- Keep your hands away from your nose, eyes, and mouth. These are the most likely places for a cold virus to enter your body.
- Eat well, and get plenty of sleep and exercise. This keeps your body's immune system strong.
- Do not smoke. If you need help quitting, see page 351.

Colorectal Cancer

When to Call a Doctor

- Your bowel habits have changed for no clear reason.
- Your stools have blood in them, or they are black or look like tar.
- You often have diarrhea, constipation, or a feeling that your bowel does not empty completely.
- Your stools have become very thin (they may be as thin as a pencil).
- You have frequent belly pain or new problems with gas or bloating.
- You are losing weight and don't know why.
- You have a family member with colon cancer and want to know how to prevent it in yourself.
- You want to talk about what screening test would be best for you.

Cancer of the colon and rectum is one of the leading causes of cancer deaths in the United States. Treatment works very well early in the disease and can cure the cancer. But because the cancer usually does not cause symptoms early on, it is often not found until later.

This is why screening tests are important. These tests can help find cancer early, when treatment works best. They can also find growths and changes in the colon before they turn into cancer.

Screening Tests

Colorectal cancer occurs most often in people over 50, so anyone who is 50 or older needs to be tested. How often you need to be tested depends on whether you are at high risk. You are at high risk if someone in your family has had this cancer or colon polyps, or if you have had colon polyps, ulcerative colitis, or Crohn's disease.

Talk to your doctor about your risk for colorectal cancer, what type of test you should have, and how often you need to be tested. Your doctor may suggest one or more of these tests:

Colonoscopy. For this test, doctors use a flexible lighted tube to view the rectum, the colon, and part of the small intestine. They can remove any growths or polyps at the same time. Colonoscopy is the most thorough screening test. It also costs the most. But if the first result is normal and you are not at high risk, you would only need to have the test every 10 years.

Flexible sigmoidoscopy. As in a colonoscopy, the doctor uses a lighted tube to look for growths and cancers. But the doctor can only view the rectum and part of the colon. If the test finds any growths, you may need a colonoscopy. If the first result is normal and you are not at high risk, you would need to have a sigmoidoscopy every 5 years.

More

Fecal occult blood test. This test can find hidden blood in your stool. It does not cost much and is easy to do at home, but it's only a first step. If the test finds blood in your stool, you will need more tests. If this is your only screening test (not recommended), you need it every year.

Barium enema. This is an X-ray exam of the colon and rectum. The colon is filled with a white liquid called barium so that it shows more clearly on the X-ray. Barium enema is not used very often to screen for colorectal cancer. If you are not at high risk, you would need to have the test every 5 years.

Which Test Should You Have?

Some tests for colorectal cancer may cost less, but you need to have them more often. And in some cases, you may wind up having to have a more expensive test anyway.

For help deciding which tests are right for you and how often you need them,

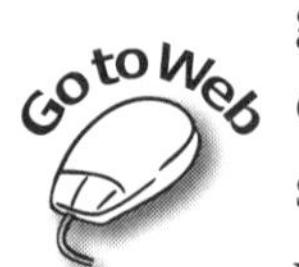

go to the Web site on the back cover and enter **K502** in the search box. Then talk with your doctor.

Confusion and Memory Loss

When to Call a Doctor

Call 911 if:

- Confusion occurs with other signs of a stroke, such as sudden, severe headache; sudden trouble seeing or speaking; sudden weakness or numbness; and sudden loss of balance. See page 54.
- Confusion and memory loss develops quickly, over a few hours or few days. This is called **delirium**. It can be a sign of many serious problems, such as a medicine problem, an infection, an alcohol or drug problem, or the worsening of a long-term illness like heart disease or diabetes.

Call a doctor if:

- You are worried that confusion or memory loss is caused by medicine or a health problem.
- Confusion or memory loss occurs with changes in behavior or personality.
- You have new trouble with familiar things, like how to read or how to tell time, or you get lost in places you know well.
- Confusion or memory loss starts to upset your daily life.

If you are worried that you or a family member has Alzheimer's disease, see the warning signs on page 123.

It's normal to forget a person's name or lose a set of keys from time to time. But more serious confusion or memory loss needs to be checked out by a doctor. If it comes on quickly, it may be caused by something that needs urgent care.

We all forget things as we get older. It also may take a little longer to remember things as you age. This is normal. But if your memory keeps getting worse—especially if you start to have other problems too—see your doctor. See the warning signs of Alzheimer's disease on this page to help you know what to watch for.

If you or a loved one already has Alzheimer's, see Living Better With Alzheimer's Disease on page 261.

Home Treatment

The best way to keep your mind sharp and avoid the problems that can cause confusion is to stay healthy and fit.

- Eat a healthy diet, and drink plenty of water (unless your doctor has told you to limit fluids).
- Get enough sleep. If you have trouble sleeping, see Sleep Problems on page 232.
- Try to reduce stress. Slow down and focus on what you're doing. People often forget things because they have too much on their minds. See Managing Stress on page 356.
- Keep your body active. Try to get some exercise most days of the week.

Warning Signs of Alzheimer's

You may wonder how to tell whether memory loss is normal or related to Alzheimer's disease. Early on, it's not always clear. But there are some warning signs you can look for:

1. Frequent memory loss and confusion. This is more than just forgetting a person's name or missing an appointment now and then.
2. Trouble with familiar tasks like cooking a meal or driving a car
3. Problems with language and finding the right words to say
4. Confusion about time and place
5. Poor or decreased judgment, such as wearing a bathrobe to the store or giving away large sums of money to strangers
6. Problems with abstract thinking, such as doing simple math or solving basic problems
7. Putting things in strange places and then forgetting where they are
8. Fast mood swings or changes in behavior
9. Major changes in personality
10. Loss of interest in one's usual activities at home and work

Adapted from the Alzheimer's Association

More

- Keep your brain active. This is the "use it or lose it" approach. See page 359 for ideas.
- Do not drink alcohol. If you drink, limit it to 1 drink a day.
- Do not use illegal drugs.
- Some people take an herb called ginkgo biloba to help with memory. Talk to your doctor before using this or any other treatment to make sure that it's safe for you. Ginkgo seems to have few side effects, but it can cause bleeding problems and may not react well with other medicines. See page 370.
- If you feel depressed, tell your doctor. Treatment can help. See Are You Depressed? on page 146.

Be Careful With Medicines

Misuse of medicines is a common cause of confusion. This is especially true in older adults.

You can help prevent problems by using medicines safely. See Master Your Medicines on page 367 for lots of good tips on how to make medicine use safer and easier.

Constipation

When to Call a Doctor

- Constipation gets worse or does not improve with home treatment.
- Your stools have blood in them, or they are black or look like tar.
- You have sharp or severe belly pain.
- You still have rectal pain after you pass a stool, or pain keeps you from passing stools at all.
- You have repeated leaking of stool.
- Stools keep getting thinner (they may be no wider than a pencil).
- You cannot pass stools unless you take laxatives.

Constipation means you have trouble passing stools or having a bowel movement. Some people pass stools 3 times a day; others do it 3 times a week. It doesn't matter what your normal schedule is: If your stools pass easily, you are not constipated.

Constipation causes cramping and pain in the rectum that gets worse when you try to pass hard, dry stools. If a stool gets stuck in the rectum, mucus and fluid may leak out around it. This may cause you to go back and forth between constipation and diarrhea.

You may get constipated if you don't get enough fiber and water in your diet, don't get enough exercise, put off having bowel movements, take certain medicines, or use laxatives too often. Irritable bowel syndrome (see page 190) may also cause constipation.

Home Treatment

- Eat more fiber (see page 336).
  - Eat plenty of fruits, vegetables, and whole grains.
  - Eat bran cereal that has at least 10 grams of bran in a serving.
  - Add 2 tablespoons of wheat bran to cereal or soup.
  - Try a fiber supplement, such as Citrucel, FiberCon, or Metamucil. Start with 1 tablespoon or less, and drink extra water to avoid bloating.
- Avoid foods that are high in fat and sugar.
- Drink plenty of water and other fluids.
- Get some exercise every day. A walking program is a good start.
- Set aside a relaxed time for each bowel movement. Urges usually occur sometime after meals. A daily routine (after breakfast, for example) may help.
- Go when you feel the urge. The bowel sends signals when a stool needs to pass. If you ignore it, the urge will go away and the stool will become dry and hard.
- If you need more help, use a stool softener or a very mild laxative such as Milk of Magnesia. Do not use mineral oil or any other laxative for more than 2 weeks unless your doctor tells you to.

Looking for the Coronary Artery Disease topic? See page 287.

Cough

When to Call a Doctor

- You have a fever and a cough that brings up yellow, green, or bloody mucus from the lungs.
- A cough lasts more than 7 to 10 days after other symptoms have cleared, especially if the cough brings up mucus from the lungs. (It is normal to have a dry, hacking cough for several weeks after a cold.)
- You are in poor health, and coughing makes you feel weak or very tired.
- Any cough lasts longer than 2 weeks.

Coughing is the body's way of keeping the lungs clear.

- **Productive coughs** bring up mucus (sputum) from the lungs. If you have this kind of cough, you should not try to stop it with cough medicine.
- **Nonproductive coughs** are dry coughs that do not bring up mucus. You may get a dry, hacking cough after a cold or after being exposed to dust or smoke. A dry cough that follows a viral illness like a cold may last several weeks and get worse at night.

Many longtime smokers have a frequent dry cough. Having a "smoker's cough," means your lungs are always irritated.

A common type of blood pressure medicine can cause a dry cough. Tell your doctor if your cough began after you started taking a medicine called an ACE inhibitor, such as lisinopril (Prinivil, Zestril) or enalapril (Vasotec). You may need to switch to another medicine.

Chronic coughs are often caused by the backflow (reflux) of stomach acid into the throat. If you think acid reflux may be causing your cough, see Heartburn on page 176.

Home Treatment

- Drink plenty of water. Water helps loosen mucus and soothe the throat. Or try hot tea or hot water with honey or lemon juice in it.
- Suck on cough drops or hard candy if your throat hurts. Expensive, medicine-flavored cough drops don't work any better than cheap, candy-flavored ones or hard candy. If you have diabetes, make sure you choose ones that are sugar-free.
- To ease a dry cough at night, use extra pillows to raise your head.
- Do not take cold remedies that use several drugs to treat different symptoms. Treat each symptom on its own.
- Use cough medicines wisely. Coughing can be good, because it brings up mucus from the lungs and helps prevent infection. People with asthma and other lung diseases need to cough. But if you have a dry,

hacking cough that doesn't bring anything up, ask your doctor to suggest a good cough suppressant.

- Do not take anyone else's prescription cough medicine.
- Avoid dust and smoke, or wear a mask to protect yourself.
- If you smoke, quit. See page 351 for help.

Looking for the Depression topic? See page 292.

Looking for the Diabetes topic? See page 296.

Diarrhea

When to Call a Doctor

Call 911 if you have signs of severe dehydration. These include little or no urine for 12 hours; sunken eyes, no tears, and a dry mouth and tongue; skin that sags when you pinch it; feeling very dizzy or lightheaded; fast breathing and heartbeat; and not feeling or acting alert.

Call a doctor if:

- Symptoms of mild dehydration (dry mouth, dark urine, not much urine) get worse even with home treatment.
- Belly pain gets worse or focuses in one area, especially the lower right or lower left part of the belly. This could be a sign of a serious problem.
- You have large, loose bowel movements every 1 to 2 hours for more than 24 hours.
- Your stools have blood in them, or they are black or look like tar.
- You have diarrhea and a fever.
- Diarrhea gets worse or happens more often.
- You get diarrhea after drinking untreated water.
- Diarrhea lasts longer than 2 weeks.

Diarrhea is loose, watery stools or bowel movements. Diarrhea has many causes—stomach flu, food poisoning, antibiotics and other medicines, certain foods, and food additives such as sorbitol and olestra. For some people, stress or anxiety can be a cause. Irritable bowel syndrome (see page 190) may cause frequent or long-term diarrhea.

Drinking untreated water or using ice made with untreated water is another cause. Just because water looks clean

More

doesn't mean it is clean. Untreated water may contain parasites, viruses, or bacteria. You may get diarrhea a few days to a few weeks later.

Home Treatment

- Stop eating food for several hours or until you feel better. Keep taking small sips of water or a rehydration drink such as Gatorade (see page 30).
- Do not take diarrhea medicines like Pepto-Bismol or Imodium during the first 6 hours. After that, use them only if you do not have a fever or bloody stools.
  - Do not take more than the label tells you to.
  - Stop the medicine as soon as stools get firmer.
- Avoid foods high in fat or sugar, spicy foods, alcohol, and caffeine until 48 hours after all symptoms have gone away.
  - Be careful not to get dehydrated. This can happen when your body loses a lot of fluids. See page 29.

Lactose Intolerance

People who are lactose-intolerant have trouble digesting the lactose (sugar) in milk. If you are lactose-intolerant, you may get gas, bloating, cramps, and diarrhea after you drink milk or eat dairy products such as ice cream.

To reduce your symptoms:

- Do not eat or drink large amounts of dairy products all at once.
- Try cheese instead of milk. It may be easier on your stomach, because most of the lactose is removed during processing.
- Eat yogurt made with active cultures. These have enzymes that digest the lactose in milk.
- Drink pretreated milk (such as Lactaid), or try enzyme tablets (such as Lactaid or Dairy Ease).
- You may be able to tolerate milk if you drink it with snacks or meals.

If you have severe lactose intolerance:

- Read food labels to avoid all forms of lactose.
- Be sure to include nondairy sources of calcium in your diet. You can get good calcium from tofu, broccoli, certain greens, and calcium-fortified orange juice.
- Ask your doctor or dietitian if you need to take a calcium supplement. People over 50 need 1,200 mg of calcium a day to help keep their bones strong.
- Plan your diet so it gives you the nutrients that milk products would normally provide.

Diverticular Disease

When to Call a Doctor

Call 911 if:

- You have severe rectal bleeding. Severe means you are passing a lot of stool that is maroon or mostly blood.
- You faint.

Call your doctor if:

- You have severe belly pain or steady pain in just one area of your belly for more than 4 hours. See page 66.
- You have belly pain along with a fever and chills.
- You have cramping pain in your belly that does not get better when you have a bowel movement or pass gas.
- You have any unusual changes in your bowel movements, or your belly is swollen.
- Your stools have blood in them, or they are black or look like tar.
- Your symptoms get worse in spite of home treatment.

Many older adults have diverticular disease. There are two types of this disease.

Diverticulosis means that small pouches (called diverticula) have formed in the wall of the large intestine (colon). Most people who have them don't have symptoms. But sometimes the pouches bleed.

Diverticulitis means that these pouches have gotten infected or inflamed. This often causes pain in the lower left part of the belly. It can also cause nausea and vomiting, constipation, diarrhea, and chills and a fever. If you have an infection, you may need antibiotics.

Eating a diet that is too low in fiber may cause diverticular disease. Making changes in your diet may help prevent future problems.

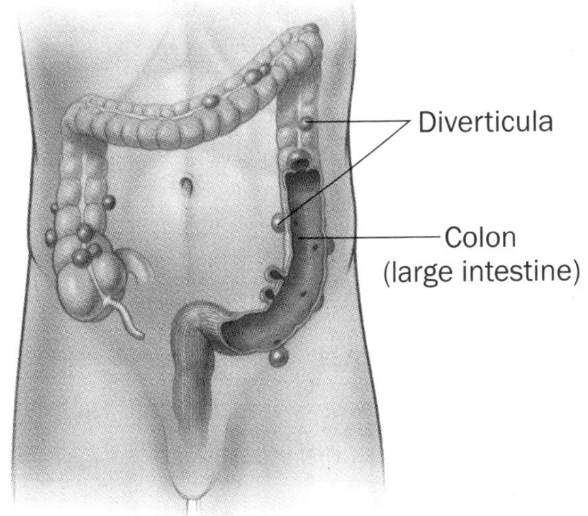

Diverticular disease means that pouches (diverticula) have formed in the lining of the colon.

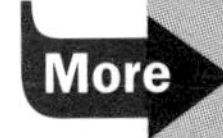

Home Treatment

These tips may help during an attack:

- Drink plenty of water.
- Choose only liquids until you feel better.
- Use a heating pad set on low on your belly to relieve mild cramps and pain.
- Try a nonprescription pain medicine, such as acetaminophen (Tylenol), ibuprofen (Advil, Motrin), or naproxen (Aleve).

To prevent future attacks, eat a high-fiber diet, drink plenty of water, and get regular exercise. Also see the tips for treating constipation on page 125.

Dizziness and Vertigo

When to Call a Doctor

Call 911 if:

- Vertigo occurs with severe headache, confusion, loss of speech or sight, weakness in the arms or legs, or numbness in any part of the body.
- Lightheadedness occurs with chest pain or pressure or any other symptoms of a heart attack. See page 38.
- Someone who is feeling dizzy faints, and you cannot wake the person.
- Vertigo or loss of balance occurs with severe headache, stiff neck, fever, seizure, or confusion.
- Severe lightheadedness lasts a long time and occurs with a sudden change in heart rate.

Call a doctor if:

- You are lightheaded or have vertigo after an injury.
- You have severe vertigo, or you have vertigo with hearing loss.
- You think a medicine may be making you dizzy.
- You have vertigo often and have not seen your doctor about it.
- Vertigo lasts longer than 5 days.
- Your vertigo is a lot different than past attacks.
- You feel lightheaded several times during just a few days.
- You feel lightheaded while at rest, and your pulse is less than 50 or more than 120 beats per minute. See page 48 to learn how to take your pulse.

Dizziness is a word people use for two different feelings: lightheadedness and vertigo. Knowing what these mean may help you and your doctor narrow down the list of possible problems.

Lightheadedness is a feeling that you are about to faint.

- You may feel unsteady but do not feel like you are moving.
- It usually improves when you lie down.

Feeling lightheaded now and then is common. There are many reasons why you might feel lightheaded. Some of the most common ones are in the chart on this page.

Lightheadedness is usually not a cause for concern unless it is severe, happens often, or occurs with symptoms like heartbeat changes or fainting.

Vertigo is the feeling that you or your surroundings are spinning, whirling, or tilting when there is no actual movement. It may make you sick to your stomach. You may have trouble standing or walking and may lose your balance.

Vertigo is often related to an inner ear problem. The most common form is triggered by moving your head. Vertigo may also be caused by a head cold (viral labyrinthitis).

Problem	Possible Causes
Lightheadedness	Drop in blood pressure from getting up too fast Flu, cold, or allergies Dehydration, see p. 29 Medicines Stress or anxiety, see p. 77 Blood loss (could either be visible or hidden inside the body; see Bleeding Emergencies on p. 17) Heart rhythm problem, see p. 174 Heart attack, see p. 38
Vertigo	Inner ear problem (benign positional vertigo, labyrinthitis, Ménière's disease) Migraine headache, see p. 167 Multiple sclerosis or other nerve problems Stroke, see p. 54 Brain tumor (rare)

More

Home Treatment

- If you feel lightheaded, lie down for a minute or two. This lets more blood flow to your brain. Then sit up slowly. Stay seated for a minute or two before you slowly stand up.
- If you are having vertigo, do not lie flat on your back. Propping yourself up slightly may help. Keep your eyes open.
- If you have a cold or the flu, rest and drink extra fluids.
- Do not drive, operate machinery, or do anything else that might be dangerous if you have vertigo or feel lightheaded. You might hurt yourself if you fall or faint.

There are balance exercises that can help if you have problems with vertigo. To learn how to do them, go to the Web site on the back cover and enter **K233** in the search box.

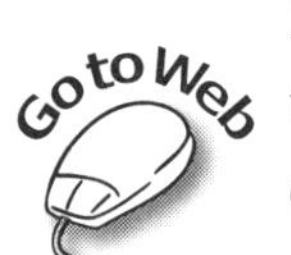

Ménière's Disease

Ménière's disease can cause attacks of vertigo, hearing loss or ringing in your ear, and nausea. The attacks can last hours or days. You may get them as often as once a week or as seldom as once a year. Most experts think the problem is caused by fluid buildup in the inner ear.

If you have Ménière's disease, some of these tips may help:

- Eat less salt. See page 304 for tips on how to reduce the salt in your diet.
- Avoid caffeine and alcohol.
- Don't smoke. If you need help quitting, see page 351.
- Reduce stress. Try the relaxation technique on page 358.

Medicines cannot cure Ménière's disease, but they may help with the symptoms. Talk to your doctor about whether you should try them.

Dry Mouth

When to Call a Doctor

- You have trouble swallowing food because of a dry mouth.
- You have a dry mouth along with a sore throat that won't go away.
- At night, your mouth is so dry that it sometimes wakes you up.
- Your dentures are not comfortable because your mouth is dry.
- You think dry mouth may be caused by medicines you are taking.

Many older adults have a dry mouth. Dry mouth is often caused by:

- Medicines, such as water pills (diuretics), antihistamines, and antidepressants.
- Diabetes.
- Sjögren's syndrome, a problem that is more common in older women.
- Radiation treatments to your head or neck.

Having a dry mouth can lead to tooth decay, mouth infections, and bad breath.

Home Treatment

- Sip water often throughout the day.
- Brush and floss every day to help protect your teeth.
- Suck on sugarless candies or chew sugarless gum. This helps your mouth make more saliva.
- Add extra liquid to foods to make them easier to chew and swallow. Drink water with meals.
- Avoid caffeine, tobacco, and alcohol. These make your mouth dry.
- Try a saliva substitute, such as Xerolube or Optimoist. You can buy these without a prescription.

Dry Skin

When to Call a Doctor

- You itch all over your body, but there is no obvious cause or rash.
- Itching is so bad that you can't sleep, and home treatment does not help.
- You have open sores from scratching, or your skin is red and swollen.

Dry, itchy, flaky skin is the most common skin problem, especially in winter. As you age, your skin makes less of the natural oil that helps it hold moisture. Dry indoor air can make your skin dry. So can taking hot showers or baths.

Home Treatment

- Take baths instead of showers. Baths are much kinder to the skin. If you take showers, keep them short and not too hot.
- Use bath oils when you bathe. Be careful not to slip.
- Use mild soaps, such as Dove or Cetaphil. You may only need to use soap under your arms and in the groin area.
- Use a moisturizing lotion right after you bathe.
- Try not to scratch. It can damage the skin.
- For very dry hands or feet, try this for a night: Apply a thin layer of petroleum jelly, and wear thin cotton gloves or socks to bed.

Relief From Itching

- Keep the itchy area well moisturized. Dry skin may make itching worse.
- Take an oatmeal bath: Wrap 1 cup of oatmeal in a cotton cloth, and boil it as you would to cook it. Use this as a sponge, and bathe in cool-to-warm water without soap. Or try an oatmeal bath product for dry skin, such as Aveeno Dry Skin (Oilated) Formula.
- Use calamine lotion on itchy insect bites or plant rashes.
- Try a nonprescription 1% hydrocortisone cream for small itchy areas. Do not use it on the face or genitals. If itching is severe, your doctor may prescribe a stronger steroid cream or ointment.
- Try nonprescription antihistamine pills. Some types, such as Claritin and Alavert, won't make you sleepy.
- Cut nails short or wear gloves at night to prevent scratching.
- Wear cotton or silk clothing. Do not wear wool and acrylic fabrics next to the skin.

Ear Infections

When to Call a Doctor

- Ear pain is severe or gets worse even with home treatment.
- Ear pain occurs with a headache, a very stiff neck, fever, vomiting, or feeling grouchy or confused. These may be signs of a serious illness. See page 151.
- There is pus or blood draining from the ear.
- You feel dizzy or unsteady.
- Your doctor has prescribed antibiotics for your ear infection, and you are not better after taking them for 48 hours.
- There is redness or swelling around, behind, or inside the ear.
- Ear pain follows a cold.
- Mild ear pain lasts longer than 3 to 4 days.

This topic covers the two most common kinds of ear infections:

- **Swimmer's ear**, which affects the ear canal.
- **Middle ear infections**. These are deeper in the ear than ear canal infections and can cause more problems.

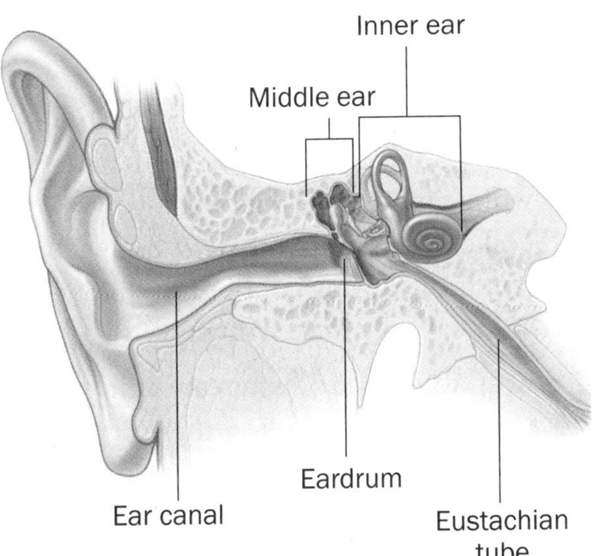

Most ear infections are in the ear canal or middle ear.

Middle Ear Infection

A middle ear infection (otitis media) can develop during a cold. Colds can cause the eustachian tube, which connects the middle ear to the throat, to swell and close. Fluid then builds up in the middle ear. Bacteria or viruses can grow in the fluid, causing an infection.

Symptoms of a middle ear infection include:

- Ear pain.
- Dizziness.
- Ringing or a feeling of fullness in the ear.
- Hearing loss.
- Fever, headache, and runny nose.

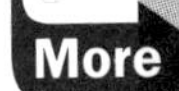

The trapped, infected fluid puts pressure on the eardrum. If there is pus or blood draining from the ear, the eardrum may have ruptured. Ear pain caused by an infection usually improves after the eardrum ruptures. A single eardrum rupture usually is not serious.

Antibiotics can treat an ear infection caused by bacteria, but most ear infections clear up on their own in a couple of days. And if a virus caused the infection, antibiotics won't work.

There are good reasons not to use antibiotics unless you really need them. See page 228.

Home Treatment

- Put a warm, moist cloth on your ear to ease the pain, or use a heating pad set on low. But never use a heating pad in bed. You could fall asleep and burn yourself.
- Take aspirin, acetaminophen (Tylenol), or ibuprofen (Advil, Motrin) for pain.
- Get extra rest.
- Drink plenty of clear liquids.
- If your eardrum ruptures, avoid getting water in your ear for 3 to 4 weeks. Showers or baths are fine, but do not soak your head in the tub. Swimming in pools is fine too, as long as you use earplugs.
- If you feel dizzy, lie down for a minute or two. Sit up slowly and stay seated for 1 or 2 minutes before you stand up slowly.

Swimmer's Ear

Swimmer's ear is an irritation or infection of the ear canal. It often develops after water, sand, or dirt gets in the ear canal.

Other causes include a cut inside the ear or an injury from a cotton swab or other object; too much earplug use; soap or shampoo buildup; and skin problems such as eczema and psoriasis.

If you have swimmer's ear, your ear will probably hurt, itch, and feel full. The ear canal may be swollen. A bad infection can cause discharge from the ear and possibly some hearing loss.

Unlike in a middle ear infection, the pain of swimmer's ear is worse when you press on the "tag" in front of the ear, touch your earlobe, or chew.

Home Treatment

- If there is pus or blood draining from your ear, do not put eardrops or anything else into the ear unless a doctor has told you to.
- Gently rinse your ear using a bulb syringe and a mixture of equal parts white vinegar and rubbing alcohol. Make sure the mixture is at body temperature. Putting cool or hot fluids in your ear may make you dizzy.
- Keep water out of your ear until the irritation clears up. To plug your ear, use cotton that is lightly coated with petroleum jelly. Do not use plastic earplugs.

- If your ear itches, try nonprescription swimmer's eardrops before and after your ears get wet. Warm the drops by rolling the container between your hands. To insert the drops, lie down with your ear facing up, or tilt your head to the side. Place drops on the outer ear near the opening of the ear canal, and gently wiggle the ear until the drops flow in. Pulling your ear up and back will help.
- Put a warm, moist cloth on your ear to ease the pain, or use a heating pad set on low. But never use a heating pad in bed. You could fall asleep and burn yourself.
- Take acetaminophen (Tylenol) or ibuprofen (Advil, Motrin) for pain.

Earwax

When to Call a Doctor

- Earwax is still hard, dry, and packed after 1 week of home treatment.
- Earwax causes ringing in your ears, a full feeling in your ears, or hearing loss.
- You have nausea or balance problems along with earwax.
- You get an earwax problem, and you have had a ruptured eardrum or ear surgery.

Earwax helps keep the ears clean and keeps out dust and water. Normally, earwax drains freely from the ears and does not cause problems.

As a rule, it is best to leave earwax alone. You can avoid most earwax problems by not using cotton swabs in your ears.

Once in a while, earwax will build up, get hard, and cause some hearing loss or discomfort. Poking at the wax with cotton swabs, fingers, or other objects will only push the wax deeper into the ear canal and pack it against the eardrum.

You should be able to take care of most earwax problems with home treatment. But when wax is tightly packed, you may need professional help to remove it.

Home Treatment

Do not use home treatment if you think your eardrum is ruptured or if pus or blood is draining from your ear.

More

To remove earwax safely, try one of these methods:

- Place 2 drops of warm (body temperature) mineral oil in the ear twice a day for 1 or 2 days to soften and loosen the wax. Then use the spray from a warm, gentle shower or a bulb syringe to remove the wax. Spray the water into the ear, and then tip the head to let the wax drain out.
- Use a nonprescription wax softener (such as Debrox or Murine). Then gently flush the ear with warm water from a bulb syringe. Tip your head to let the wax drain out. Repeat the process each night for 1 or 2 weeks.

With either method, be sure the water is warm but not hot. Putting cool or hot fluids in your ear may make you dizzy.

Erection Problems

When to Call a Doctor

- An erection lasts longer than 4 hours after you use an erection-producing medicine such as Viagra, Cialis, or Levitra.
- You took an erection-producing medicine in the past 24 hours, and you are having chest pain. **Do not take nitroglycerin!** See Chest Pain on page 114.
- You cannot have an erection at all, or you think the cause of erection problems may be physical.
- You have erection problems along with urinary problems, pain in your lower belly or lower back, or a fever.
- Your erection problems started after a recent injury.
- You think your erection problems may be caused by a medicine.

Erection problems are more common as men get older. It may take longer to get erections, and they may be less firm. But with the right approach, healthy men can have erections at any age.

From time to time, most men have trouble getting an erection or having one that lasts long enough to have sex. This is normal and is usually nothing to worry about. But if you often cannot get or maintain an erection, you may want to work with your doctor to find the cause.

Erection problems can be caused by:

- Problems with blood vessels, nerves, or hormones. These can be related to diabetes, heart disease, injuries, and other health problems.

- Medicines. Blood pressure medicines, water pills (diuretics), and mood-altering drugs can all have sexual side effects.
- Alcohol.
- Smoking.
- Depression, stress, grief, or relationship problems.

Home Treatment

- Rule out medicines as a cause. Ask your doctor or pharmacist if any medicines that you take can have sexual side effects. But do not stop taking any of your medicines without talking to your doctor.
- Limit alcohol. Have no more than 2 drinks a day.
- If you smoke, quit. Smoking makes it harder for the blood vessels in the penis to relax and let blood flow in. If you need help quitting, see page 351.
- Try to reduce stress. See page 356. Regular exercise may help too.
- Take time for more foreplay.
- Talk to your partner about your concerns. If you and your partner have trouble talking about sex, see a therapist who can help you talk about it together. Reading books about sex with your partner may also help.
- Find out if you can have erections at other times. If you get erections when you masturbate or have them when you first wake up, the cause is more likely emotional than physical.
- Talk to your doctor about medicines that can help, such as Viagra, Levitra, or Cialis.
- There are also devices that can help with erections. Talk to your doctor if you want to learn more about them.

Medicines for Erection Problems

Medicines such as Viagra, Levitra, and Cialis are a popular treatment for erection problems. They are often the first choice, because they are easy to use and have a high success rate.

But they are not right for everyone. They can be dangerous for men who take nitroglycerin or have heart disease or low blood pressure.

For help deciding if these medicines are right for you, go to the Web site on the back cover and enter **R582** in the search box. Then talk to your doctor.

Go to Web

Eye Problems

This topic covers three common problems:

- Pinkeye (conjunctivitis)
- Dry eyes
- Blood in the eye

If your symptoms do not match these problems, be sure to check the Eye and Vision Problems chart on page 62.

Pinkeye

When to Call a Doctor

- There is a new difference between the sizes of the pupils of your eyes.
- The skin around the eye or eyelid is red.
- You have blurring or loss of vision that does not clear at all when you blink.
- You have pain in the eye, rather than irritation.
- Light is very painful for your eye.
- You think you may have an object in the eye. See page 31.
- The eye is red and has a yellow, green, or bloody discharge that does not start to go away in 24 hours. You may need antibiotics.
- Pinkeye lasts longer than 7 days.
- Your eye has not improved within 48 hours after you started using antibiotics.
- You wear contact lenses, and you have had pinkeye more than once.

Pinkeye is inflammation of the conjunctiva, which lines the eyelid and covers the surface of the eye. Pinkeye is also called conjunctivitis.

Pinkeye may be caused by:

- Infection with a virus or bacteria. This kind of pinkeye spreads very easily.
- Dry air, allergies, smoke, and chemicals. This kind of pinkeye does not spread from person to person.

If you have pinkeye, you may have redness in the whites of your eyes, red and swollen eyelids, lots of tears, itching or burning, and a sandy feeling in your eyes. Light may hurt your eyes more than usual. And there may be fluid or pus in your eyes that crusts over and makes your eyelids stick together when you sleep.

Although pinkeye will often clear on its own in 7 to 10 days, pinkeye that is caused by a virus can last many weeks. Antibiotics will help if you have pinkeye that is caused by bacteria. If you have pinkeye because of allergies or chemicals, it will not go away unless you can avoid the cause. But home treatment can reduce your symptoms.

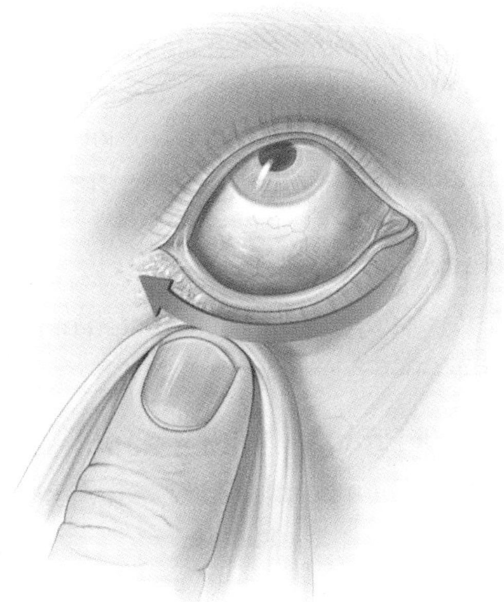

Wipe from the inside corner to the outside to remove crusts.

Home Treatment

Good home care will speed healing and help you avoid spreading pinkeye to others.

- Wash your hands often. Always wash them well before and after you treat pinkeye or touch your eyes or face.
- Put cold or warm wet cloths on your eye several times a day if your eye hurts.
- Use moist cotton or a clean, wet cloth to remove any crust. Wipe from the inside corner (next to the nose) to the outside. Use a clean part of the cloth for each wipe.
- Do not wear contact lenses or eye makeup until the pinkeye is gone. Throw away any eye makeup you were using when you got pinkeye. Clean your contacts and storage case. If you wear disposable contacts, use a new pair when it is safe to wear contacts again.
- If the doctor prescribes eyedrops or ointment, use them as directed. You may need to have someone help you.
    - Pull the lower eyelid down with two fingers to create a small pouch. Squeeze in the drops or ointment. Close the eye for 20 to 30 seconds to let the medicine soak in.
    - Putting ointment in the eye can be tricky. If you have trouble, put it on your eyelashes. The ointment will melt and get into your eye.

More

- Be sure the bottle tip is clean and does not touch the eye, eyelid, or eyelashes. If the tip does touch the eye area, throw the bottle away and replace it.

- Make sure any medicine you buy without a prescription is ophthalmic (for eyes), not otic (for ears).
- Do not share towels, pillows, eye makeup, or contact lens equipment while you have pinkeye.

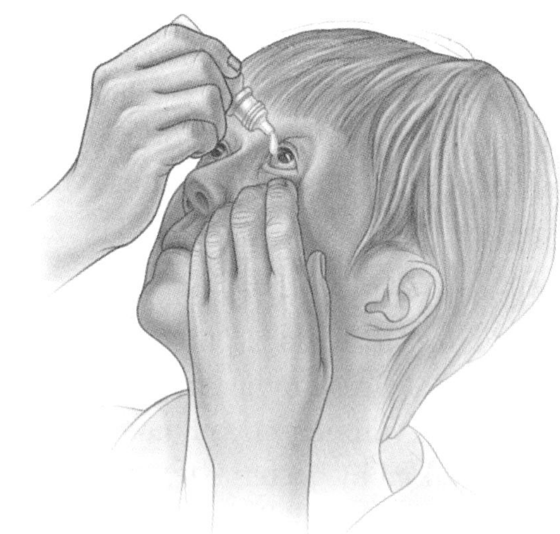

Do not let the bottle tip touch the eye, eyelid, or eyelashes.

Avoiding Problems With Your Contacts

If you wear contact lenses, these tips can help you avoid problems.

- Keep your lenses and anything that touches them (hands, storage cases, makeup) very clean. Wash your hands before you touch your contacts.
- Follow the cleaning instructions for your lenses, and use a store-bought contact lens solution. Generic brands are just as good as name brands, and they cost less. Do not make your own solution. It can get contaminated too easily.
- Never wet your lenses with saliva. It has bacteria that may infect the eye. Don't use tap water either.
- Put in your contacts before you put on eye makeup. Do not put makeup on the inner rim of the eyelid. Replace eye makeup every 3 to 6 months.
- If you use extended-wear contacts, follow the wearing and cleaning schedule your eye care professional recommends. When worn for long periods of time, these lenses are more likely to cause severe eye infections.
- Visit your eye doctor as directed or at least once a year.

Having a Problem With a Contact?

Symptoms of a possible problem with your contacts may include:

- Redness, pain, or burning in the eye.
- Discharge from the eye.
- Blurred vision.
- Extreme sensitivity to light.

Take out your lenses, clean them, and don't put them back in until your symptoms are gone. If symptoms last longer than 2 to 3 hours after you take out your contacts, call your eye doctor.

Dry Eyes

When to Call a Doctor

Call a doctor if dry eyes are a problem and artificial tears do not help.

Eyes that don't have enough moisture in them may feel dry, hot, sandy, or gritty, and your vision may be blurry. Dry air, smoke, aging, and certain diseases can cause dry eyes. Some common medicines also can make your eyes dry. These include antihistamines, decongestants, and some drugs for depression.

Home Treatment

- Rest your eyes. When you read, watch TV, or use a computer, take breaks often and close your eyes. As you work, try to blink your eyes more often.
- Try "artificial tears" eyedrops. Preservative-free tears are the gentlest on your eye.
- Do not use eyedrops that reduce redness (such as Visine) to treat dry eyes. Your eyes may get even worse when you stop using the drops.
- Avoid smoke and fumes from chemicals.

Blood in the Eye

When to Call a Doctor

- You have blood in your eye after a blow to the head or injury to the eye.
- There is blood in the colored part of the eye.
- Your eye is bloody and painful.
- You often get blood spots in your eyes.
- You notice blood in your eye while taking a blood thinner, such as warfarin (Coumadin), or large doses of aspirin.

Sometimes blood vessels in the whites of the eyes break and cause a red spot or speck. This is called a **subconjunctival hemorrhage**. The blood may look alarming, especially if the spot is large. But it usually is not a cause for concern, and the red spot will go away in 2 to 3 weeks.

If you have a black eye, see Bruises on page 22.

Eyelid Problems

When to Call a Doctor

- ◆ Pain, redness, and swelling spread to the entire eyelid or to the eyeball.
- ◆ A stye hurts a lot, grows larger quickly, or does not stop draining.
- ◆ A stye or other eyelid problem blocks your vision.
- ◆ Your eyelids droop suddenly.
- ◆ Your eyes are dry and irritated, or you cannot fully close your eyes.
- ◆ Your eyelashes start to rub on your eyeball.
- ◆ An eyelid problem gets worse even with home treatment or does not improve within 1 week.

Blepharitis

Blepharitis is one of the most common eye problems in older adults. It makes the edges of your eyelids red, irritated, and crusty. The crusty area may be dry or greasy. Eyelashes may fall out as well.

Doctors don't know what causes blepharitis, but it is more common in people who have dandruff, skin allergies, or eczema. The problem is often long-term. If you have blepharitis, you are more likely to get styes.

Styes

A stye is an infection of an eyelash follicle. It looks like a small, red bump or pimple either in the eyelid or on the edge of the lid. Styes come to a head and break open after a few days.

Styes are very common and are not a serious problem. But they can hurt, and they may blur your vision. Most will go away with home treatment.

Drooping Eyelids

As some people get older, their eyelids start to droop. This is the result of reduced muscle tone in the muscles that control the eyelids.

- ◆ If your lower eyelids droop down, away from your eyes, they may no longer be able to protect your eyes. Your eyes may become dry and irritated.
- ◆ If the lower eyelids turn inward so that the lashes touch the eyeball, this may irritate or damage your eyes.
- ◆ If your upper eyelids droop low enough, or if the eyelid skin folds over the edge of the lid, you may not be able to see as well.

Drooping eyelids can also keep tears from draining normally, so tears may run down your cheeks. Tearing can also be a sign of increased sensitivity to light or wind, an eye infection, dry eyes, or a blocked tear duct.

Home Treatment

For blepharitis:

Wash your eyelids, eyebrows, and hair each day with baby shampoo. To wash your eyelids:

- Place a warm, wet washcloth over your eyelid for a few seconds.
- Put a few drops of shampoo in a cup of warm water, and dip a cotton ball, cotton swab, or washcloth in the cup. Close your eyes, and gently wipe each eyelid about 10 times from the inside corner to the outside, across the lashes. Rinse well with clear water before you open your eyes.
- Or, let warm water from the shower run over your closed eyes for a few seconds. Then put a few drops of shampoo on a washcloth, and gently wipe the lashes and eyelids. Rinse the shampoo away.

For a stye:

- Do not rub your eye, and do not squeeze or open the stye.
- Apply a warm, moist cloth for 10 minutes, 3 to 6 times a day, until the stye comes to a head and drains.
- Do not wear eye makeup or contact lenses until the stye heals.

For drooping eyelids:

There is no home treatment for drooping eyelids. Sometimes surgery can help.

Fatigue and Weakness

When to Call a Doctor

- You have sudden muscle weakness, and you don't know why.
- You are so tired that you have to limit your usual activities for longer than 2 weeks.
- You have lost or gained weight for no clear reason.
- You do not feel better after 4 weeks of home treatment.
- Fatigue gets worse even with home treatment.

More

Fatigue is a feeling of being very tired or exhausted or not having any energy. Most fatigue is caused by lack of exercise, stress or overwork, lack of sleep, depression, worry, or boredom. People can usually treat fatigue with self-care.

Fatigue that occurs with muscle pain or stiffness may be a sign of fibromyalgia (see page 152) or polymyalgia rheumatica (see page 212).

Weakness is a lack of physical or muscle strength and the feeling that moving an arm, a leg, or any other part of your body takes a lot of extra effort. Unexplained muscle weakness is usually more serious than fatigue. It may be caused by diabetes, thyroid problems, stroke, or problems related to the brain and spinal cord.

Colds, flu, and other short-term illnesses often cause fatigue and weakness while you are sick.

Low Thyroid

Not having enough thyroid hormone (hypothyroidism) is a common cause of fatigue, especially in middle-aged and older women. A blood test can tell if your thyroid hormone is too low. See page 238.

Are You Depressed?

If you have been feeling very tired for no clear reason, you may want to think about whether you are depressed.

Depression is more than the normal sadness and moodiness that comes with the ups and downs of life. It's an illness. You may be depressed if:

- You feel sad, anxious, or hopeless much of the time, and these feelings do not go away.
- You have lost interest in many of the things you once enjoyed—hobbies, work, time with friends and family.

You may also have changes in your sleep or eating patterns, weight gain or loss, and trouble concentrating and making decisions. You may feel worthless or guilty for no reason and think about death a lot.

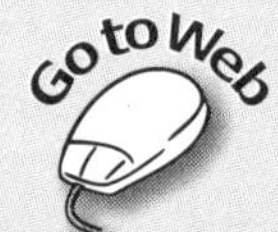

If you think you might be depressed and have felt this way for more than 2 weeks, talk to your doctor or a counselor. If you want to take a self-test for depression, go to the Web site on the back cover and enter **R645** in the search box. If you have already been diagnosed with depression, see Living Better With Depression on page 292.

Treatment can almost always help. If you are just mildly depressed, home treatment may be all you need. Or you may need to try counseling and antidepressant medicines. Without any treatment, depression is likely to get worse.

Anemia

Anemia means that you do not have enough red blood cells, which carry oxygen to your body's tissues. This can make you pale, weak, and tired.

Lack of iron is the most common cause of anemia. You may not be getting enough iron in your diet, or your body may have trouble absorbing it.

To boost your iron:

- Eat foods rich in iron, such as beef, shellfish, chicken, eggs, beans, raisins, whole-grain breads, and leafy green vegetables.
- Use iron pots for cooking.
- Steam vegetables instead of boiling them. They lose iron if you boil them.

Chronic Fatigue Syndrome

Chronic fatigue syndrome can make you so tired and weak that you can't do your normal activities. Even after you rest, you still may not have your usual energy. You may also have memory problems, headaches, a sore throat, painful lymph nodes, muscle and joint pain, and sleep problems.

Chronic fatigue syndrome is hard to diagnose. Depression, thyroid problems, and many other illnesses can cause the same symptoms. You may need tests to rule out some of these other causes. If fatigue and other symptoms go on for at least 6 months and there is no other explanation for them, your doctor may diagnose chronic fatigue syndrome.

Feeling tired and weak may make it hard to get through the day sometimes. But many people do get better over time. Your doctor may be able to help with specific symptoms.

To feel better overall:

- Look for ways to adjust your schedule so that it's easier on you. Schedule rest breaks. Resist the urge to do too much when you have energy. If you overdo it, you may get too tired. Then you may be even more tired the next day.
- If you have problems sleeping, try to improve your sleep habits. See page 233.
- Get light exercise every day. Gentle stretching, light aerobics, swimming, walking, and cycling can help relieve your symptoms.
- Eat a healthy diet. You may feel better if you avoid heavy meals and eat more fruits and vegetables.
- Join a support group with other people who have chronic fatigue syndrome. These groups can be a good source of information and tips on ways to feel better.

More

You can also get anemia from a gradual loss of blood, such as from heavy vaginal bleeding or bleeding in your stomach or colon. If a health problem is causing your anemia, treating that problem may correct your anemia and help you feel better.

Home Treatment

These tips help with most cases of fatigue. If you have anemia or another health problem, talk to your doctor about what other home treatment you should do.

- Get some exercise every day. Daily exercise, balanced with plenty of rest, is often the best treatment for fatigue. If you feel too tired to exercise hard, try a short walk.
- Make sure you get enough sleep. See page 232.
- Eat a healthy diet. This can help you stay at your best.
- Do not ignore emotional problems like depression or anxiety. There are treatments that can help. See Living Better With Depression on page 292 and Anxiety on page 77.
- Try to reduce stress. See page 356.
- Ask your doctor or pharmacist whether any of your medicines can make you tired. Cold and allergy medicines are common causes of fatigue.
- Drink less caffeine and alcohol.
- If you smoke or chew tobacco, quit. See page 351 for help.
- Watch less TV. Spend time with friends instead, or try new activities.
- Be patient. It may take a while to get your energy back.

Female Pelvic Problems

When to Call a Doctor

- You have heavy vaginal bleeding or discharge, especially if it occurs after menopause.
- You have trouble urinating, or it hurts when you urinate.
- You have pain during sex.
- You have pain, cramping, or bloating in your lower belly.
- You have irregular bleeding for 3 months or more while taking hormone therapy.
- You feel very tired or have lost weight, and you don't know why.

For information on vaginitis or yeast infections, see page 245.

Bleeding After Menopause

If you have gone through menopause (see page 201) and are not taking hormones, you should not have any vaginal bleeding. If you do, you may have an abnormal growth in your uterus and should see a doctor.

If you are taking hormones, a little bleeding after menopause may be normal. But be sure to tell your doctor about it.

Pelvic Cancers

The best way to find these cancers early is to have regular pelvic exams and Pap tests. See page 323.

Uterine (endometrial) cancer affects the lining of the uterus. It can be cured if it is found before it spreads beyond the uterus.

Cervical cancer affects the cervix, the lower part of the uterus that opens into the vagina. This form of cancer can be cured most of the time, especially if it is found early. It can usually be found at a very early stage with a Pap test.

Ovarian cancer affects the ovaries, which hold and release a woman's eggs. When found early, ovarian cancer may be successfully treated. But it is often hard to detect until it has grown and spread.

Do You Need a Hysterectomy?

Hysterectomy is surgery to remove the uterus. Most of the time it is done to treat disease. Hysterectomy is often the best treatment for:

- Uterine, cervical, or ovarian cancer.
- Severe endometriosis.
- Severe uterine bleeding.
- Large, noncancerous tumors (fibroids) that cause severe bleeding and pain or press on the bladder.
- Severe uterine prolapse (uterus falls into the opening of the vagina).

For some problems, other treatments may work as well with fewer risks. These include:

- Precancerous changes on the cervix.
- Abnormal uterine bleeding.
- Fibroids that cause mild symptoms.
- Mild to moderate uterine prolapse.

To learn more about hysterectomy, when it is a good idea, and when it isn't, go to the Web site on the back cover and enter **H477** in the search box.

Go to Web

Fever

When to Call a Doctor

- You have a fever of 104 °F or higher.
- You have a fever of 103 °F to 104 °F that does not come down after 12 hours of home treatment.
- You have a long-lasting fever. Many viral illnesses cause fevers of 102 °F or higher for short periods of time (up to 12 to 24 hours). Call a doctor if the fever stays high:
  - 102 °F to 103 °F for 1 full day
  - 101 °F to 102 °F for 3 full days
  - 100.4 °F to 101 °F for 4 full days
- Body temperature rises to 102.3 °F or higher, all sweating stops, and the skin is hot, dry, and red. These are signs of heat stroke. See page 39.
- You have a fever with signs of a skin infection. These may include increased pain, swelling, warmth, or redness; red streaks; or pus.
- You have a fever with a very stiff neck, headache, vomiting, and confusion. These may be signs of a serious illness. See page 151.
- You have a fever with shortness of breath and a cough. See Pneumonia on page 210.
- You have a fever with pain above the eyes or the cheekbones. See Sinusitis on page 227.
- You have a fever with pain or burning when you urinate. See Bladder and Kidney Infections on page 90.
- You have a fever with belly pain, nausea, and vomiting. See Appendicitis on page 67 and Food Poisoning on page 155.
- Fever occurs with confusion, decreased alertness, odd behavior, or other troubling symptoms. Even a small change can be important in a person who is very old or frail.
- You get a fever after you start a new medicine.

A fever is a high body temperature. By itself, a fever is not dangerous unless it gets too high. In fact, it can help your body fight illness and infection. Most healthy adults can handle a fever as high as 103 °F to 104 °F for a short time without problems.

But a high fever can put extra strain on your heart. It may even trigger heart failure in a person who has heart disease. If you have heart disease, use home treatment to bring a fever down. Call your doctor if you have symptoms of heart failure, such as shortness of breath or swelling in your legs.

You can have a severe illness without having a high fever. This is especially true as you age, because as you get older, your body loses some of its ability to produce a fever. An 80-year-old person with a fever of 100 °F may be just as sick as a young person with a fever of 105 °F.

Home Treatment

- Drink plenty of water and other fluids.
- Take acetaminophen (Tylenol), aspirin, or ibuprofen (Advil, Motrin) to lower a fever.
- Take and write down your temperature every 2 hours and whenever symptoms change.
- Take a sponge bath with warm (not hot) water if you feel uncomfortable.
- Watch for dehydration. See page 29.
- Wear lightweight clothing. This will help your body cool down.
- Eat light foods that are easy to digest, such as soup.

What About a Low Temperature?

A low temperature can be a problem. A temperature below normal (especially below 94 °F) may be a sign of a severe infection, a thyroid problem (see page 238), shock (see page 47), or hypothermia (see page 41).

Encephalitis and Meningitis

Encephalitis is swelling (inflammation) of the brain. It can happen after you have a virus like the flu, cold sores, or genital herpes. You can also get it from certain ticks or mosquitoes (see page 16).

Meningitis is swelling (inflammation) in the tissues that surround the brain and spinal cord. It may follow an ear or sinus infection or other illness. But you can get it even if you have not been sick.

Either illness can be very serious. The symptoms are:

- Fever with a bad headache, stiff neck, and vomiting.
- Trouble staying awake, confusion, or seizures.
- A rash that forms quickly and looks like bruises or tiny purple or red blood spots under the skin.

Call your doctor right away if you get these symptoms, especially if you have recently been ill, been exposed to someone with meningitis or encephalitis, or been bitten by mosquitoes.

Fibromyalgia

When to Call a Doctor

- You have severe joint or muscle pain.
- You think you have injured a muscle or joint, and the pain does not go away in a few days.
- You feel sad, helpless, or hopeless; lose interest in things you used to enjoy; or have other symptoms of depression. See Are You Depressed? on page 146.

Fibromyalgia is a painful condition that can make you ache all over and feel tired and weak. It also causes tender spots at specific points of the body that hurt only when you press on them. You may have trouble sleeping. These problems can upset your work and home life.

Symptoms tend to come and go, though they may never go away completely. Fibromyalgia does not harm your muscles, joints, or organs.

Even the experts do not understand fibromyalgia very well. Its cause is unknown. Your doctor may suggest prescription medicines to help with some of your symptoms.

Home Treatment

- Get regular exercise, such as walking, biking, or swimming. This is the best thing you can do for fibromyalgia. It may help with pain and sleep problems and help you feel better.
- Try to get a good night's sleep every night. Go to bed and get up at the same time each day, whether you feel rested or not. Make sure you have a good mattress and pillow. See page 233 for more tips.
- Reduce stress. Avoid things that cause you stress, if you can. If not, work at making them less stressful. Learn to use biofeedback, meditation, or other methods to relax. See page 356.
- Use a heating pad set on low or take warm baths or showers for pain. Using cold packs for up to 15 minutes at a time can also relieve pain. Put a thin cloth between the cold pack and your skin.
- Take acetaminophen (Tylenol), ibuprofen (Advil, Motrin), or naproxen (Aleve) for pain.
- Think about joining a support group with others who have fibromyalgia to learn more and get support.

Some people with fibromyalgia find that other types of treatments help them manage their symptoms. For example, acupuncture or massage may help relieve stress, ease muscle tension, and help you feel better and healthier.

Flu

When to Call a Doctor

It is common for adults with the flu to have a high fever (up to 104°F) for 3 to 4 days. When trying to decide if you need to see a doctor, think about how likely it is that you have the flu rather than some other illness. If it is flu season and lots of people have been getting the flu, chances are good that you have it too.

Call your doctor if:

- You have a fever with a stiff neck, severe headache, and confusion. These may be signs of a serious illness. See page 151.
- You start to get signs of a worse infection, such as fast or shallow breathing; a cough that brings up colored mucus from the lungs; or pain, fever, and fatigue that are getting a lot worse.
- You have a long-term health problem and may have the flu. Antiviral medicine can help prevent problems.
- You have the flu and want to take antiviral medicine to make it less severe.
- You seem to get better and then get worse again.

Flu (influenza) is a viral illness that tends to occur in the winter, and it often affects many people at the same time. If you have the flu, you may feel very tired and have a fever and shaking chills, lots of aches and pains, a headache, and a cough.

The flu is not the same as the common cold.

- Flu symptoms are worse and come on faster.
- The flu lasts for up to 10 days, and you feel pretty bad the whole time.

For most people, the flu does not usually lead to more serious problems. But the flu can be dangerous and even deadly, especially for people older than 65 and those with health problems like diabetes, asthma, or heart disease.

Antiviral medicine is advised for some of these high-risk people. The medicine can make the illness shorter and less severe if you take it before you have symptoms or within 2 days after symptoms appear. Even if you are not at high risk, your doctor may prescribe these medicines to help you feel better faster and help prevent the spread of the flu. For help deciding whether you should take them, go to the Web site on the back cover and enter **H957** in the search box.

Go to Web

Antibiotics will not help you get over the flu. Home treatment will help you feel a little better until the illness ends.

More

Home Treatment

- Stay home from work and avoid public places for several days after you get sick so you don't give the flu to anyone else.
- If you live alone, have a friend or family member call or check in on you every day while you're sick to make sure you're okay.
- Get plenty of rest.
- Drink plenty of water. This helps replace fluids lost from fever and ease a scratchy throat. Other good choices are hot tea with lemon, fruit juice, and soup.
- Take acetaminophen (Tylenol), aspirin, or ibuprofen (Advil, Motrin) to relieve your fever, headache, and muscle aches.
- Do not smoke or let others smoke around you.

Should You Get a Flu Shot?

Flu shots help prevent the flu. They are not foolproof, because there is more than one flu virus and it can change from year to year. But flu shots give you the best chance of avoiding the illness.

All adults over 50 should get a flu shot every fall. No one wants to get the flu, and the older we are, the worse the flu can be.

Flu shots are even more important if you are at high risk for problems from the flu or if you live or work with someone at high risk. Think about whether you would expose a baby, older adult, or other high-risk person to the flu if you got it.

Stay Well During Flu Season

- Wash your hands often!
- Keep your hands away from your nose, eyes, and mouth.
- Keep up your resistance to infection by eating a healthy diet, getting plenty of rest, and getting regular exercise.
- Get a flu shot before flu season starts.

Food Poisoning

When to Call a Doctor

Call 911 if:

- ◆ You have signs of severe dehydration. These include little or no urine for 12 hours; sunken eyes, no tears, and a dry mouth and tongue; skin that sags when you pinch it; feeling very dizzy or lightheaded; fast breathing and heartbeat; and not feeling or acting alert.
- ◆ You think you may have food poisoning from a canned food, and you have blurred or double vision, trouble swallowing or breathing, and muscle weakness. These are symptoms of botulism.

Call a doctor if:

- ◆ You have bloody diarrhea.
- ◆ Severe diarrhea (large, loose bowel movements every 1 to 2 hours) lasts longer than 2 days.
- ◆ Vomiting lasts longer than 1 day.
- ◆ Symptoms of mild dehydration (dry mouth, dark urine, not much urine) get worse even with home treatment.

Food poisoning may occur when you eat food that has bacteria growing in it. Meats, dairy foods, and spreads like mayonnaise are often the source of the problem. Bacteria can grow in these foods if they are not handled right, not cooked well, or not stored below 40°F.

You may start to feel sick as soon as 1 or 2 hours or as late as 2 days after you eat the food. Nausea, diarrhea, and vomiting are the usual symptoms.

You may have food poisoning if:

- ◆ Others who ate the same food now have the same symptoms.
- ◆ Symptoms start after you eat foods that were left sitting out (at a party, picnic, or buffet).

Botulism is a rare but often deadly type of food poisoning. Most people get it from eating contaminated home-canned foods that have a low acid content, like beans and corn. Bacteria that survive the canning process may grow and make poisons in the jar. Symptoms include blurred or double vision and trouble swallowing or breathing.

Home Treatment

- ◆ Symptoms of food poisoning will usually go away in a day or two. Good home care can help you get well faster. See Diarrhea on page 127 and Vomiting on page 253.
- ◆ Watch for and treat early signs of dehydration. See page 29. Older adults can quickly get dehydrated from diarrhea and vomiting.

Food Safety

- ◆ If food looks or smells spoiled, throw it out.
- ◆ Keep hot foods hot and cold foods cold.

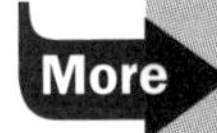

- Follow the 2-40-140 rule. Do not eat meat, dressings, salads, or other foods that have been kept between 40°F and 140°F for more than 2 hours.
- Use a thermometer to check your refrigerator. It should be between 34°F and 40°F.
- Defrost meats in the refrigerator or microwave, not on the counter.
- Keep your hands and your kitchen clean. Wash your hands, cutting boards, and counters with hot, soapy water. After you touch raw meat, especially chicken, wash your hands and utensils very well before you prepare other foods.
- Cook meat until it's well done. Use a meat thermometer to make sure you have cooked meat, chicken, and fish to a safe temperature. This temperature varies depending on the food.
- Never eat undercooked hamburger. It's the main source of *E. coli* infection. All of the pink should be gone, and all of the meat (not just the surface) should have reached a temperature of at least 160°F.
- Do not eat raw eggs, uncooked dough, or sauces made with raw eggs.
- Throw away cans or jars with bulging lids or leaks. Do not eat food from a jar that doesn't make a "pop" sound or have a good seal when you first open it.
- Follow home canning and freezing instructions carefully. Contact your county agricultural extension office for advice.

Hepatitis A

Hepatitis A is a virus that affects the liver. If stool that contains the virus gets into the water or food supply, the virus may infect anyone who drinks the water or eats the food.

The United States does not tend to have this problem with its water and food supply. But sometimes a large group of people who eat at the same restaurant gets infected. This usually happens when an employee with hepatitis A does not wash his or her hands well after using the bathroom and then prepares food.

- Symptoms may not appear for 2 to 7 weeks after you are exposed.
- You may have fatigue, nausea, a fever, sore muscles, headaches, and pain in your upper right belly. Your skin and the white part of your eyes may turn yellow. Symptoms usually last less than 2 months.
- Hepatitis A usually goes away on its own and does not cause long-term liver problems.

If you or someone in your home has hepatitis A, take care not to spread it to others. Always wash your hands well after using the bathroom, after changing a baby's diapers, and before preparing or eating food.

If you live in an area where hepatitis A is common or you are at high risk, you may want to get the hepatitis A vaccine.

Fungal Infections

When to Call a Doctor

- You have signs of a worse infection, such as increased pain, redness, swelling, or warmth; pus; or fever.
- You have diabetes and get athlete's foot.
- You have sudden hair loss, along with flaking, broken hairs, and redness of the scalp, or others in your household start to lose hair.
- Ringworm is severe and spreading or is on the scalp.
- You have white patches inside your mouth that look like cottage cheese but are hard to remove.
- A fungal infection does not improve after 2 weeks or clear up after 1 month, even with home treatment.

Fungal skin infections most often affect the feet, groin, scalp, or nails. Fungi grow best in warm, moist areas, such as between the toes, in the groin, and in the area just beneath the breasts.

You can get a fungal infection by sharing towels, clothing, or sports equipment. You can also get one by touching an infected person. Sometimes people get a fungal infection from working with cats, dogs, or cattle.

Home Treatment

For jock itch or ringworm of the skin:

- Use a nonprescription antifungal powder or lotion, such as Micatin, Lamisil, or Lotrimin AF. Do not use hydrocortisone cream on a fungal infection.
- Wash and dry the area well before you apply the powder or lotion.
- Use the medicine for 1 to 2 weeks after the symptoms clear up so the infection doesn't come back.
- Keep your groin area clean and dry. Shower or bathe soon after you exercise, or at least change out of sweaty clothes. Wear cotton underwear, and avoid tight pants and panty hose.
- To keep from spreading a fungal infection, do not share hats, combs, brushes, or towels.

For a fungal nail infection or athlete's foot:

- For a nail infection, try an antifungal medicine you put on your skin or nail, such as Lamisil or Penlac. For athlete's foot, use an antifungal powder or lotion, such as Micatin, Lamisil, or Lotrimin AF.

More

Common Fungal Infections	Symptoms	Comments
Athlete's foot	Itching and cracked, blistered, peeling areas between the toes and on the soles of the feet	Often comes back; needs to be treated each time
Jock itch	Severe itching and moistness in groin and on upper thighs; red, scaly raised areas that may ooze pus or fluid	Often comes back; needs to be treated each time
Ringworm of the skin	Patches that are clear in the center and red, peeling, or bumpy on the edges; itching	Can spread quickly to other areas
Ringworm of the scalp and beard	Bald patches that are scaly, red, crusty, or swollen with small bumps	Hair or beard may have flakes that look like dandruff; treated with prescription pills
Nail infections	Discolored (often yellow), cracking, thickened, or softened nails	Hard to treat
Thrush of the mouth (yeast infection)	White patches inside the mouth that look like cottage cheese but is hard to remove	May occur after taking antibiotics; may need prescription medicine

- Keep your feet clean, cool, and dry. Dry well between your toes after you swim or shower. Use antifungal powder such as Desitin or Zeasorb in your shoes and socks and on your feet to prevent reinfection.
- Wear leather shoes or sandals that let your feet "breathe," and wear cotton socks to absorb sweat. Give shoes 24 hours to dry before you wear them again.
- Wear flip-flops or shower sandals in public pools and showers.
- When you get dressed, put on your socks before your underwear. This can keep a fungal infection from spreading from your feet to your groin.

For thrush:

If you have thrush, see your doctor. You may need prescription medicine. These steps can help you feel better during treatment:

- Drink cold liquids or eat flavored ice treats or frozen juices.
- Eat foods that are easy to swallow, such as Jell-O and ice cream.
- If the patches are painful, try drinking from a straw.
- Rinse your mouth several times a day with warm saltwater. Mix 1 teaspoon of salt in 8 ounces of warm water.

Gallstones

When to Call a Doctor

If you have not been diagnosed with gallstones, see When to Call a Doctor on page 66 in Abdominal Pain.

Call your doctor if you know you have gallstones and:

- ◆ You have sudden, severe belly pain. Severe belly pain can be a sign of a serious or even life-threatening problem.
- ◆ Your skin and the white part of your eyes look yellow, or you have dark yellow-brown urine or light-colored stools.
- ◆ You have belly pain along with fever and chills.
- ◆ You have another attack of gallstone symptoms.

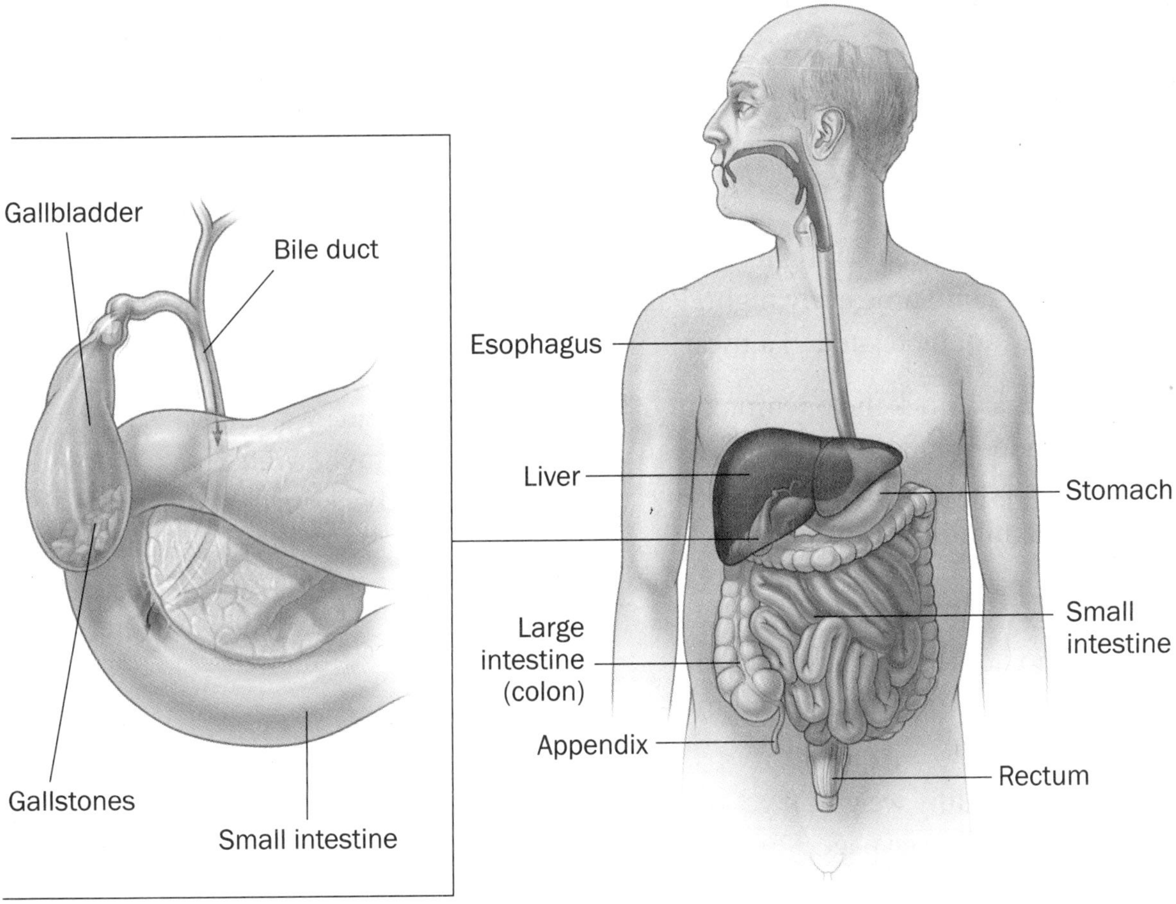

Gallbladder
Bile duct
Gallstones
Small intestine
Esophagus
Liver
Stomach
Small intestine
Large intestine (colon)
Appendix
Rectum

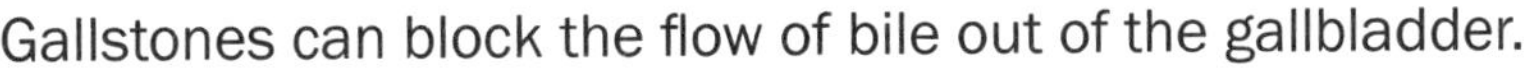

Gallstones can block the flow of bile out of the gallbladder.

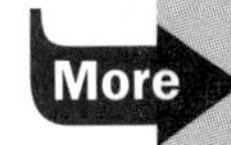

Gallstones are stones made of cholesterol and other substances that form in the gallbladder or bile duct. The gallbladder stores bile, which helps you digest fats. Gallstones may be as small as a grain of sand or as large as a golf ball.

Most people who have gallstones don't have any symptoms. But sometimes stones can irritate the gallbladder. When this happens, you may have:

- A sudden aching or cramping pain that starts in the upper right or upper middle of your belly, just below your breastbone (see the picture on page 67). It may spread to your right upper back or shoulder blade.
- Sudden, severe pain that lasts several hours and then quickly fades.
- Fever and vomiting.

Symptoms often occur at night, usually at about the same time every night. Pain may or may not be related to a meal.

Gallstones can block the opening out of the gallbladder, and the gallbladder can then get infected. If this happens, you will need antibiotics and surgery.

Home Treatment

There is no home treatment for gallstones. You may be able to avoid more gallstones if you:

- Stay at a healthy weight. If you need to lose weight, see page 326 to learn how to do it safely. Crash diets may increase your risk of gallstones.
- Eat a healthy, low-fat diet. Avoid foods that cause symptoms, especially fatty foods.
- Get regular exercise.

Do You Need Gallbladder Surgery?

People who have frequent or severe pain from gallstones often have surgery to remove the gallbladder.

- If your first attack of gallstone pain is mild, it is often safe to wait and see if you have another attack before you get treatment. You may not need surgery if gallstones do not cause problems for you.
- Besides the pain of gallstones, there may be other medical reasons why you need the surgery.
- Surgery costs a lot and has some risks. If you don't need it, don't have it.

For help deciding if surgery is right for you, go to the Web site on the

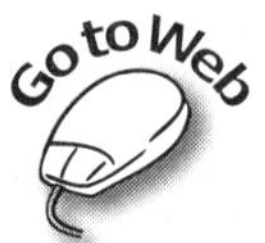

back cover and enter **Q327** in the search box. Then talk to your doctor.

Gas

When to Call a Doctor

Call 911 if you have gas that occurs with chest pain or any other symptoms of a heart attack. See page 38.

Call your doctor if:

- You have gas and severe belly pain for several hours or more. See page 66.
- You have problems with burping, hiccups, swallowing, or bloating that don't get better with a week or so of home treatment.
- You think a medicine is causing gas. Don't stop taking the medicine without talking to your doctor first.
- You have gas, and you have lost your appetite or lost weight for no known reason.

Gas is made in the stomach and intestines as your body breaks down food. Everyone passes gas, but some people have more gas than others. It is normal to pass gas from 6 to 20 times a day. Gas is usually not a cause for concern, but it can be embarrassing.

Home Treatment

There are things you can do to help cut down on gas:

- Avoid foods that cause gas. These vary from person to person, but common problem foods include beans, broccoli, cabbage, and bran. Dairy products can cause gas in people who are lactose-intolerant. See page 128.
- Drink more fluids, especially water. Avoid carbonated drinks and alcohol.
- Try not to swallow air when you eat. Eat more slowly, and chew your food well before you swallow.
- Try a nonprescription treatment for gas. Some that may help include:
  - Activated charcoal tablets, such as CharcoCaps. These may decrease the odor from gas.
  - Antacids, such as Di-Gel, Maalox Anti-Gas, and Mylanta Gas. These help you belch gas instead of passing it.
  - Food enzymes, such as Beano. You can add these to certain foods to help break down the sugars that cause gas.

Glaucoma

When to Call a Doctor

Call 911 if:

- ◆ You have sudden vision loss or blurring that does not clear.
- ◆ You have sudden, severe eye pain.

Call your doctor if:

- ◆ You have blind spots in your side vision.
- ◆ Your vision has gotten worse.
- ◆ You have a family history of open-angle glaucoma, and you have not had an eye exam in the past year.

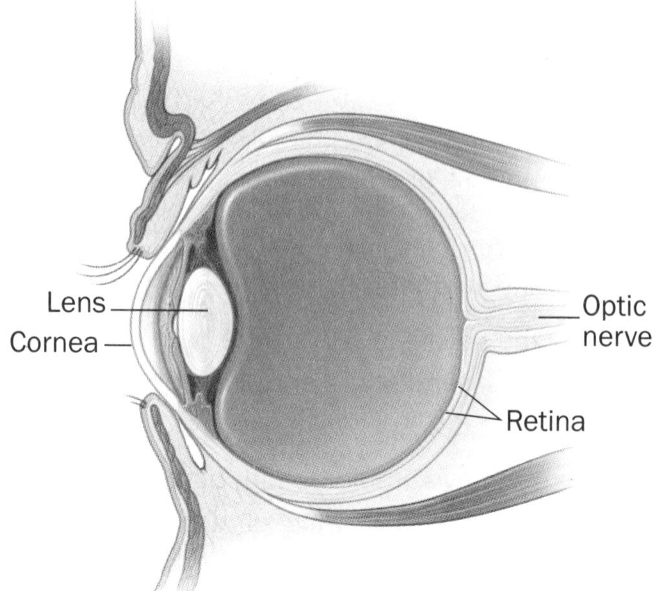

Glaucoma damages the optic nerve at the back of the eye.

Glaucoma is an eye disease that damages the optic nerve at the back of the eye. (The optic nerve carries signals from the eye to the brain, which turns them into images that you see.) The damage is often related to increased pressure in the eye.

Open-angle glaucoma is the most common form. It tends to affect side (peripheral) vision. It's usually painless and can develop slowly over several years without your knowing. You may not notice any vision changes until a lot of damage has occurred.

Closed-angle glaucoma is not common but can be very serious. It occurs when the flow of fluid in the eye gets blocked. This can cause a quick rise in eye pressure that causes sudden vision changes and severe pain. You can lose vision within just a few hours.

Home Treatment

- ◆ Use eyedrops and medicines for glaucoma as directed.
- ◆ Make sure your other doctors know that you have glaucoma. You may need to avoid certain medicines, such as antihistamines. Check with your doctor before you take any medicines, including ones you buy without a prescription.

If glaucoma has already affected your sight, see Tips for Living With Reduced Vision on page 251. Some of the ideas there may help you adapt.

Finding Glaucoma Early

Untreated glaucoma is a leading cause of blindness in adults. But the disease is easy to find in an eye exam. It usually can be controlled if you find it early.

Talk to your doctor about how often to have a glaucoma test. It's especially important for people at higher risk to be tested. You may be at higher risk for glaucoma if:

- You are over 65.
- There is a history of glaucoma in your family.
- You have diabetes or high blood pressure.
- You have had an eye injury or eye surgery, including cataract surgery.
- You are African American or East Asian.

Gout

When to Call a Doctor

- You have joint pain and a fever.
- A joint hurts so much that you can't use it.
- You have sudden swelling, redness, warmth, or severe pain in one or more joints, and it is different from your usual gout attacks or you have not been diagnosed with gout.
- Your symptoms get worse or are not improving after 2 to 3 days.
- You have any problems with your gout medicine.

Gout is a type of arthritis caused by a buildup of uric acid crystals in a joint. It causes sudden pain, swelling, redness, and stiffness in the joint. Gout usually affects the big toe, but it can also affect the ankles, knees, wrists, or elbows.

Gout can seem to strike without a cause. Or it can be brought on by eating meats and seafood that are high in chemicals called purines. Taking certain medicines or drinking alcohol also can bring on an attack of gout.

Home Treatment

- Put ice or a cold pack on the joint for 10 to 15 minutes at a time. Always put a thin cloth between the ice and your skin. See Ice and Cold Packs on page 51.
- Rest the sore joint. Avoid activities that put weight or strain on the joint for a few days.
- Take ibuprofen (Advil, Motrin) or naproxen (Aleve) for pain and swelling. Or if the doctor gave you a prescription pain medicine, take it as prescribed.
- Do not take aspirin. It can make gout worse.

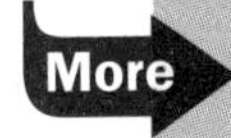

- Avoid alcohol, especially beer, during an attack.
- Do not eat a lot of red meat, seafood, or organ meats such as liver.
- Drink plenty of water and other fluids. This can help your body get rid of uric acid.
- Lose some weight if you are overweight. This may reduce your attacks. But avoid crash diets and low-carbohydrate diets. They can make gout worse.

Gum Disease

When to Call a Dentist

- You have teeth that are loose or have moved.
- Your teeth are sore or sensitive to touch.
- You have pus coming from your gums.
- Your gums have pulled away from your teeth.
- You have bad breath that doesn't go away when you brush and floss.
- Your gums are red, swollen, or tender.
- Your gums bleed easily when brushed.

Gum disease is an infection of the tissues that surround and support the teeth. It is the main cause of tooth loss in older adults. It's very common.

Early gum disease is called **gingivitis**. It causes red, swollen gums that bleed easily when brushed.

If gingivitis is not treated, it can become advanced gum disease, called **periodontitis**. Over time, it can damage the bones that support the teeth.

You are more likely to get gum disease if you have diabetes, you have a dry mouth (see page 133), or you smoke or chew tobacco.

Home Treatment

You may be able to stop and even reverse early gum disease:

- Brush your teeth in the morning and before bed. Use a tartar-control toothpaste that contains fluoride.
- Floss once a day. Any type of floss works, so choose a type you like.
- Use an antiseptic mouthwash, such as Listerine, or an anti-plaque mouthwash.
- Do not smoke or chew tobacco. If you need help quitting, see page 351.

Hair Loss

When to Call a Doctor

- Hair loss is sudden or severe.
- You have patchy hair loss, or hair falls out in clumps.
- You have hair loss after starting a new medicine.
- Hair loss occurs with a scalp rash or any other skin change on your scalp.
- You are losing your hair bit by bit and want to talk about treatment.

Many people lose hair as they age. While men tend to lose hair from the hairline and crown of the head, women's hair gets thinner all over. This hair loss is natural and tends to run in families. It increases your risk of sunburn and skin cancer of the scalp, but you can avoid both of these by wearing sunscreen and a hat.

Bald spots are not the same as baldness.

- Wearing tight braids or having a habit of tugging or twisting your hair may cause bald spots.
- Ringworm of the scalp is a fungal infection that causes scaly bald spots. See page 157.
- Alopecia areata causes patchy hair loss that may need treatment with medicines. Alopecia totalis can cause total hair loss, including the eyelashes and eyebrows.

Thinning hair can be a sign of a problem such as thyroid disease or lupus. Mental or physical stress can cause short-term hair loss all over the head. So can hormone changes or menopause.

Treatment for Hair Loss

If you are thinking about medicine (such as minoxidil) or surgery for hair loss, make sure you understand the risks of treatment, how many treatments you will need, what it costs, and how long the results will last. For help deciding about medicine, go to the Web site on the back cover and enter **Q958** in the search box.

Go to Web

Headaches

When to Call a Doctor

Call 911 if:

- ◆ You have a sudden, severe headache unlike any you have had before. The headache may seem to "explode" out of nowhere.
- ◆ You have a headache with signs of a stroke. These may include sudden weakness, numbness, inability to move, loss of vision, slurred speech, confusion, behavior changes, or a seizure. See page 54.

Call a doctor if:

- ◆ You have a headache with a stiff neck, a fever, vomiting, drowsiness, or confusion. You may have a serious illness. See page 151.
- ◆ You have had a recent head injury, and your headaches are getting a lot worse.
- ◆ You have a headache with severe eye pain or vision changes. These may be signs of a serious problem. See pages 162 and 169.
- ◆ You have a headache with dizziness and vomiting, and others in your household have the same symptoms. These may be signs of **carbon monoxide poisoning**.
- ◆ You often have severe headaches with no clear cause.
- ◆ You think your headaches are migraines, but you have not talked to your doctor about it. There may be medicine that can help prevent them.
- ◆ You have a lot more headaches than you used to, or they are worse than they used to be.
- ◆ You often get headaches during or after exercise, sex, coughing, or sneezing.
- ◆ Headaches wake you from a sound sleep or are worse first thing in the morning.
- ◆ You are using pain medicine to control headaches more than once a week, or you need help dealing with your headaches.

If your headache seems unusual or occurs with other symptoms, you may also want to check the chart on page 64.

Most headaches are **tension headaches**, which get worse when you are under stress. You may have tightness or pain in the muscles of your neck, back, and shoulders with the headache. A past neck injury or arthritis in the neck can also cause tension headaches.

A tension headache may cause pain all over your head, pressure inside your head, or a feeling that you have a tight band around your head. Some people feel a dull, pressing, burning sensation above the eyes. With a tension headache, you can rarely point to an exact spot where it hurts.

Your headaches may be **migraines** if:

- The pain is severe, throbbing, or piercing.
- The pain is on one side of your head.
- Headaches occur with nausea and vomiting, or sound seems too loud or light too bright when you get a headache.
- You have an "aura"—flashing lights, blind spots, numbness or tingling, strange smells or sounds—about an hour before you get the headache. (Some people may have less noticeable symptoms like hunger or mood changes a day or two before the headache.)

Tracking Your Headaches

If you have headaches often, keep a record of your symptoms. This record will help your doctor if you need to be checked or treated. It may also help you take control of your headaches, especially if they are migraines.

Write down:

1. The date and time each headache starts and stops.
2. Anything that could have triggered the headache. This might be food, smoke, bright light, stress, or activity.
3. Where the pain is. Is it in one spot or all over your head?
4. What kind of pain you have. Is it throbbing, aching, stabbing, or dull?
5. How bad the pain is. Rate it from 1 to 10 (10 is the worst pain you can imagine).
6. Any other symptoms you have, such as nausea, vomiting, vision changes, or being extra sensitive to light or noise.
7. (Women only) Any link between your headaches and hormone therapy or your menstrual cycle.

More

Preventing Headaches

- Reduce stress. Take time to relax before and after you do something that has caused a headache in the past. Try relaxation techniques such as meditation or progressive muscle relaxation. See page 358.
- Reduce muscle tension. Try to relax your jaw, neck, shoulder, and upper back muscles.
- Use good posture at work. When you sit at a desk, change positions often, and stretch for 30 seconds each hour. See page 205 for other tips.
- Exercise every day. It can help reduce stress and muscle tension.
- Get regular massages. Some people find this very helpful in relieving tension.
- Limit caffeine to 1 or 2 drinks a day. People who drink a lot of caffeine often get a headache several hours after they have their last caffeine drink. Or they may wake up with a headache that does not go away until they drink caffeine. Cut down slowly to avoid caffeine-withdrawal headaches.

If you get migraines

You may find that certain foods, events, medicines, or activities tend to "trigger" your headaches. Learning what your triggers are and finding ways to limit or avoid them can help you prevent headaches. Tracking your headaches is one thing that can help.

For help figuring out what triggers your migraines, go to the Web site on the back cover and enter **E170** in the search box.

Cluster Headaches

Cluster headaches occur in "clusters" over a period of days or months and then disappear for months or even years. During a cluster period, you may have several headaches each day.

These headaches cause sudden, very severe, sharp, stabbing pain on one side, usually in the temple or behind the eye. The eye and nostril on that side may be runny, and the eye may be red. The headaches often start at night and may last from a few minutes to about an hour.

To prevent headaches during a cluster period:

- Avoid alcohol and tobacco.
- Get plenty of sleep.
- Reduce stress.

If you think you are having cluster headaches, talk to your doctor.

Home Treatment

- If you get migraines and your doctor has prescribed medicine for them, take it at the first sign that you're getting a migraine.
- Stop what you're doing, and sit quietly for a moment. Close your eyes, and breathe slowly. If you can, go to a quiet, dark place and relax. If you have a migraine, sleeping may help.
- Some people find that taking a pain medicine such as acetaminophen (Tylenol) or ibuprofen (Advil, Motrin) at the first sign of a headache helps. But using these medicines too often may make headaches worse or more frequent when the medicine wears off. This is called a **rebound headache**.
- Put a cold pack on the painful area or on your forehead.
- Gently massage your neck and shoulder muscles. Try the neck exercises on page 206.
- Put a heating pad on painful or tight muscles, or take a hot shower. But do not use heat if you have a migraine.
- Try a relaxation exercise such as progressive muscle relaxation. See page 358.

Other Causes of Head or Facial Pain

Head and facial pain can have a number of causes. Two problems that occur in older adults, especially women, are temporal arteritis and trigeminal neuralgia.

Temporal arteritis is an inflammation of blood vessels leading to your head and eyes. It causes a dull, throbbing headache on one side of the head around the eye or near the temple. Sometimes the pain feels like stabbing or burning. It may also cause jaw pain and vision loss.

Temporal arteritis needs quick treatment to prevent blindness or stroke.

Trigeminal neuralgia is a problem with the large nerve that brings feeling to the face. It causes a sudden, sharp pain on one side of the face. Just touching your cheek or talking can set off shooting pain toward the ear, eye, or nose.

An attack can last from a few seconds to a couple of minutes. Some people have long periods when they don't have pain, and then it returns. The attacks often get worse and happen more often over time.

This problem is not dangerous, but the pain can be hard to live with. Medicine, surgery, or other treatment can help control the pain. Progressive muscle relaxation may help relieve pain and anxiety. See page 358.

Hearing Problems

This topic covers two common hearing problems:

- Hearing loss
- Ringing in the ears (tinnitus)

Protect Your Hearing

- Avoid harmful noise. The noise from machines, guns, snowmobiles, motorcycles, lawn mowers, power tools, household appliances, loud music, and other sources can damage your hearing.
- Use hearing protectors such as earplugs or earmuffs when you have to be around harmful noise. These can greatly reduce the noise that reaches the ear. Cotton balls or tissues stuffed in the ears do not help much.
- Control the volume when you can. Don't buy noisy appliances or tools if there are quieter choices. Turn down the stereo, TV, car radio, and personal music player.
- Never use cotton swabs, hairpins, or other objects to remove earwax or to scratch your ears. They can damage the ear. See page 137 to learn how to remove earwax safely.
- Ask your pharmacist if any medicines you take can affect your hearing. For example, antibiotics, blood pressure medicines, ibuprofen (Advil, Motrin), and large doses of aspirin can cause hearing loss or ringing in your ears.
- During air travel, swallow and yawn a lot when the plane is coming down. If you have a cold, the flu, or a sinus infection, take a decongestant or use a decongestant nose spray a few hours before the plane lands.
- Control diseases that affect your circulation, such as heart disease, high blood pressure, and diabetes. Some hearing loss may be the result of decreased blood flow to the inner ear.

Check Your Hearing at Home

Age-related hearing loss often occurs so gradually that many people may not even know it has happened. It is important to find out if you have hearing loss, whatever the cause. If not found and treated, hearing loss can make a person feel depressed, isolated, and dependent.

Here are two simple tests you can do to check your hearing:

- The radio test: Have someone adjust the volume on a radio or TV so it is pleasing to that person. Can you hear it well, or do you have to strain to hear it?
- The telephone test: When you talk on the phone, switch the phone from ear to ear to hear if the sound is the same. Hearing loss that is related to aging usually affects both ears, but it is possible for only one ear to be affected.

Hearing Loss

When to Call a Doctor

- Hearing loss develops suddenly (within a matter of days or weeks).
- You have hearing loss in one ear only.
- You develop a hearing problem while taking medicine, including aspirin or ibuprofen (Advil, Motrin).
- Hearing loss occurs with vertigo (you feel like the room is spinning) or loss of movement in your face.
- You think your hearing is slowly getting worse.
- You wonder if you need a hearing aid.

Millions of people cope with reduced hearing. The most common causes are:

- **Noise.** Over time, the noise you are exposed to at work, at play (such as listening to very loud music), or even during common chores (like mowing the lawn) can lead to hearing loss. Hearing usually gets worse over many years.
- **Age.** Changes in the inner ear that occur as you grow older cause a gradual but steady hearing loss. This is called **presbycusis**.

Other causes of hearing loss include earwax buildup, an object in the ear, an injury to the ear or head, an ear infection, and other ear problems. Some common medicines—aspirin, ibuprofen (Advil, Motrin), antibiotics—can affect your hearing. Check with your pharmacist. Sometimes hearing loss can be a sign of a serious health problem.

Home Treatment

Hearing loss can affect your work and home life. It can make you feel lonely, depressed, or helpless. But there are things you can do to hear better and feel connected to others.

- Protect the hearing you have. Always wear hearing protection around loud noises. Avoid loud noise when you can.
- Learn to pay close attention to a speaker's face, posture, gestures, and tone of voice. These clues can help you understand what a person is saying. Face the person you're talking to, and have him or her face you. Make sure the lighting is good so that you can see the other person's face clearly.
- Consider a hearing aid. See an expert who can help you pick one that fits. Be sure to have your hearing tested and the hearing aid adjusted over time. See page 172.

More

- Use other helpful devices, such as:
  - Telephone amplifiers.
  - Hearing aids that can connect to a TV, stereo, radio, or microphone.
  - Devices that use lights or vibrations to alert you to the doorbell or a ringing phone.
  - TV closed-captioning that shows the words at the bottom of the screen. Most new TVs have this option.
  - TTY (text telephone), which lets you type messages back and forth on the phone instead of talking or listening. These devices are also called TDD.

Caring for a Person With Hearing Loss

- Speak to the person at a distance of 3 to 6 feet. Make sure that your face, mouth, and gestures can be seen clearly. Arrange furniture so everyone can see everyone else's face.
- Do not speak directly into the person's ear. Visual clues will be missed.
- Speak slightly louder than normal, but don't shout. Speak slowly.
- Cut down on background noise. Turn down the TV or radio. Ask for quiet sections in restaurants.
- If a certain word or phrase is not understood, find another way of saying it. Do not repeat the same words over and over.
- If the subject of conversation changes, tell the person, "We are talking about _____ now."
- Treat the hearing-impaired person with respect. Involve the person in discussions, especially those about him or her. Do what you can to help the person feel less isolated.

Hearing Aids

A good-quality hearing aid can help you hear better and feel more connected to family and friends. But there are some important things you should know before you get a hearing aid:

- Not all hearing loss can be corrected with hearing aids. Whether hearing aids will help depends on what is causing your hearing loss.
- Hearing aids work by making all sounds, both soft and loud, louder. They do not restore normal hearing. Digital hearing aids may let you choose different settings depending on whether you are in a noisy or quiet place.
- It takes time and practice to get used to hearing aids. You may need to try more than one type to get the best results. Wear your hearing aids every day, and give yourself time to get used to the way they work.

Go to Web

For help deciding if you should get a hearing aid, go to the Web site on the back cover and enter **Q972** in the search box.

Ringing in the Ears

When to Call a Doctor

- Ringing in the ears (tinnitus) starts suddenly and affects only one ear.
- You have new tinnitus with hearing loss, vertigo (you feel like the room is spinning), loss of balance, nausea, or vomiting.
- Ringing in your ears does not stop or change.
- You get tinnitus after an injury to your head or ear.
- Tinnitus lasts longer than 2 weeks, even with home treatment. There may be no cure, but your doctor can help you learn how to live with the problem.

Most people have ringing, roaring, hissing, or buzzing in their ears from time to time. The sound usually lasts only a few minutes. If it does not go away or it happens often, you may have a problem called tinnitus.

Tinnitus is most often caused by being around too much loud noise. But it can have other causes like ear infections, dental problems, and medicines (especially antibiotics and large amounts of aspirin). Be sure to discuss it with your doctor. Drinking alcohol or lots of caffeine can add to the problem.

Home Treatment

- Cut back on alcohol and caffeine.
- Limit your use of aspirin, ibuprofen (Advil, Motrin), and naproxen (Aleve).
- If you have an earwax problem, remove the wax safely. See page 137.

Hearing Specialists

Otologists or **otolaryngologists** are medical doctors (MDs or DOs) who can diagnose and treat hearing problems and do surgery.

Audiologists are hearing specialists who are trained to identify, diagnose, and measure hearing problems. They can recommend the best method to treat hearing loss. Look for an audiologist who is licensed by your state or who is certified by the American Speech-Language-Hearing Association (the letters CCC-A will appear after the audiologist's name).

Hearing aid specialists or dispensers are licensed in nearly all states and may be certified by the National Board for Certification in Hearing Instrument Sciences (NBC-HIS). They can fit you with hearing aids.

If you are thinking about buying hearing aids, first get checked by a medical doctor and an audiologist to find out what type of hearing loss you have and whether it can be treated in other ways.

Heartbeat Changes

When to Call a Doctor

Call 911 if:

- You have chest pain or pressure, especially if it occurs with other symptoms of a heart attack (sweating, shortness of breath, nausea or vomiting, feeling dizzy or lightheaded). See page 38.
- You have signs of a stroke. These may include sudden weakness, numbness, inability to move, loss of vision, slurred speech, confusion, behavior changes, or a seizure. See page 54.
- You have a change in your heartbeat and you faint.

Call your doctor if:

- You have a change in your heartbeat and you feel:
  - Weak or very tired.
  - Confused.
  - Dizzy or lightheaded.
  - Like something bad is going to happen.
- You feel a fast pounding or fluttering in your chest, or it feels like your heart skips beats.
- You have a change in your heartbeat that is new or different than before, and it does not go away with home treatment.

Normally your heart beats in a regular way and at a rate that is just right for the work your body is doing at that moment. An abnormal change in your heartbeat is a heart rhythm problem, or **arrhythmia**. Your heart may beat too fast or too slowly or beat with an uneven or skipping rhythm. A change in the heart's rhythm may feel like a rapid pounding or fluttering in your chest.

Many heartbeat changes are not serious and do not need treatment. For example, they may be caused by:

- Stress or fatigue.
- Too much alcohol, caffeine, or nicotine.
- Medicines, including diet pills, antihistamines, decongestants, and some herbal products.

Looking for the Heart Failure topic? See page 303.

But some heartbeat changes can be serious:

- **Atrial fibrillation** is a common heartbeat problem that starts in the upper parts (atria) of the heart. It is dangerous because it greatly increases your risk of blood clots and stroke. It can also lead to heart failure or heart attack.
- **Ventricular arrhythmias** start in the lower parts (ventricles) of the heart. The ventricles are the heart's main pumps. This type of problem can be life-threatening, because it can keep the body from getting the blood it needs.

Finding and treating a heart problem early is the best way to prevent serious illness. See your doctor for a checkup if you have changes in your heart rate or rhythm and you have heart disease (such as a previous heart attack) or are at higher risk for it (for example, if you smoke or are not very active, or if you have high blood pressure, high cholesterol, or a lot of stress).

Home Treatment

- Take deep breaths, and try to relax.
- If you start to feel like you may faint, lie down so that you don't fall.
- Write down the date and time, your pulse rate, what you were doing when the problem started, how long it went on, and any other symptoms. Having a record can help you and your doctor figure out the cause of the problem.

To prevent further problems:

- Do not smoke. If you need help quitting, see page 351.
- Cut down on caffeine and alcohol.
- Check with your pharmacist or doctor to see whether any of your medicines can cause heartbeat changes.
- Reduce stress. See page 356. If you have problems with anxiety, see page 77.
- Get regular exercise. Talk to your doctor before you start an exercise program.

Preventing Stroke if You Have Atrial Fibrillation

Many people with atrial fibrillation need to take blood-thinning (anticoagulant) medicine to help prevent strokes. People at low risk for stroke may take daily aspirin instead.

The most common blood thinner is warfarin (Coumadin). If you take warfarin, you will need to have regular blood tests. These let your doctor check how long it takes your blood to clot so he or she can adjust your medicine as needed. Blood thinners can increase your risk of bleeding, so you will also need to watch for signs of bleeding.

If you are over 55 and have atrial fibrillation, take a quiz to find out your risk of having a stroke in the next 5 years. Go to Web

5 years. Go to the Web page on the back cover and enter **L143** in the search box.

Heartburn

When to Call a Doctor

Call 911 if:

- ◆ You have pain in your upper belly with chest pain or pressure or other symptoms of a heart attack. See page 38.
- ◆ You vomit a lot of blood or what looks like coffee grounds.

Call your doctor if:

- ◆ There are streaks of blood in your vomit.
- ◆ It often hurts when you swallow, or you have trouble swallowing.
- ◆ You are losing weight, and you don't know why.
- ◆ You think a medicine may be causing heartburn. Drugs that sometimes cause heartburn include antihistamines, medicines for anxiety, and the anti-inflammatory medicines aspirin, ibuprofen (Advil, Motrin), and naproxen (Aleve).
- ◆ Heartburn lasts more than 2 weeks, even with home treatment. Call sooner if your symptoms are severe or do not improve at all with antacids or acid reducers. Also see Ulcers on page 243.

Heartburn occurs when stomach juices flow backward into the esophagus, the tube that leads from the mouth to the stomach. The backflow, called **reflux**, causes a feeling of burning, warmth, or heat under the breastbone. You may feel it spread in waves up into your neck, and you may get a sour taste in your mouth.

Heartburn can last up to 2 hours or longer. It gets worse when you lie down or bend over. It gets better when you sit or stand up.

Don't worry if you have heartburn now and then. Nearly everyone does. Use the home treatment tips to get relief.

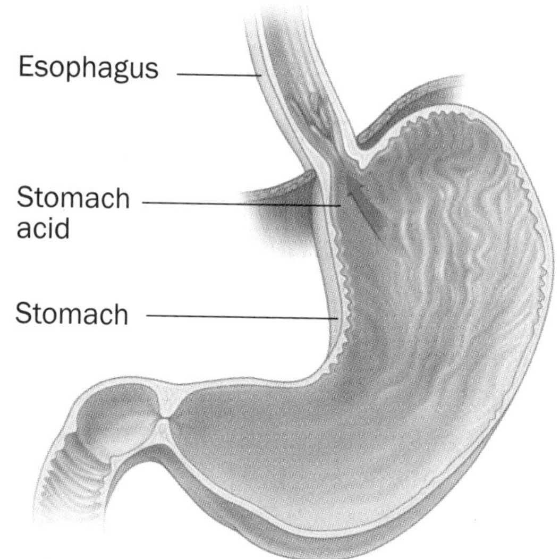

You get heartburn when stomach acid flows up (refluxes) into the esophagus.

If you have heartburn often, you may have **gastroesophageal reflux disease (GERD)**. GERD can lead to other health problems. You need to see a doctor if you have heartburn often and home treatment doesn't help.

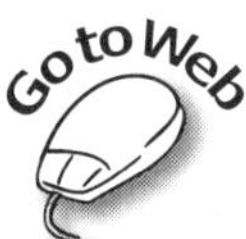

If you have GERD, go to the Web site on the back cover and enter **L498** in the search box to learn what you can do to control your symptoms.

Home Treatment

- Eat smaller meals, and avoid late-night snacks. After eating, wait 2 to 3 hours before you lie down.
- Avoid foods that bring on heartburn. These may include citrus fruits and juices (orange, tomato), chocolate, fatty or fried foods, peppermint- or spearmint-flavored foods, alcohol, carbonated drinks, and coffee and other drinks with caffeine.
- Do not smoke or chew tobacco. If you need help quitting, see page 351.
- If you get heartburn at night, raise the head of your bed 6 to 8 inches. Put the head of the frame on blocks, or place a foam wedge under the head of your mattress. Adding extra pillows doesn't work well.
- Take a nonprescription product for heartburn. For mild heartburn, an antacid, such as Maalox, Mylanta, or Tums, may help. Or try an acid reducer, such as Pepcid AC, Tagamet HB, or Zantac. You can also buy an acid blocker called Prilosec OTC. Ask your pharmacist to help you choose one of these medicines.
- Do not wear tight clothing around your middle.
- Lose weight if you need to. Losing just 5 to 10 pounds can help. See page 326 to get started.
- Do not take aspirin, ibuprofen (Advil, Motrin), or naproxen (Aleve). These can cause heartburn or make it worse. If you need something for pain, try acetaminophen (Tylenol).

Heel Pain and Plantar Fasciitis

When to Call a Doctor

- Heel pain occurs with redness or heat in your heel or with fever.
- You have numbness or tingling in your heel or foot.
- A heel injury causes pain when you put weight on your heel.
- You have pain when you are not putting any weight on your heel.
- Heel pain lasts more than 1 to 2 weeks, even with home treatment.

Heel pain is often caused by **plantar fasciitis**. The plantar fascia is a band of tissue that connects your heel bone to your toes and supports the arch of your foot. If it gets irritated, it causes pain in your heel.

You are more likely to get plantar fasciitis if:

- You are overweight.
- You stand, walk, or run for long periods of time, especially on hard surfaces.
- Your feet roll inward (pronate) too much when you walk. Wearing shoes that are worn out or have poor arch support, having tight calf muscles, or running downhill or on uneven surfaces can make your foot roll inward even more.

You may get a **heel spur** if calcium builds up where the plantar fascia attaches to the heel bone. Heel spurs usually do not cause pain and do not need to be treated. (Rarely, a painful heel spur may need to be removed.) Many people think their pain is caused by heel spurs, but in most cases it is caused by plantar fasciitis.

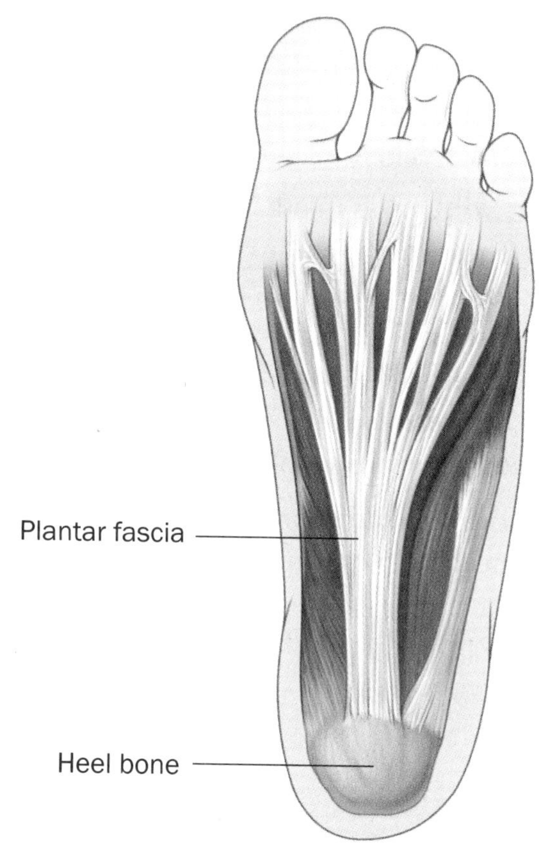

Heel pain is often caused by an irritated plantar fascia.

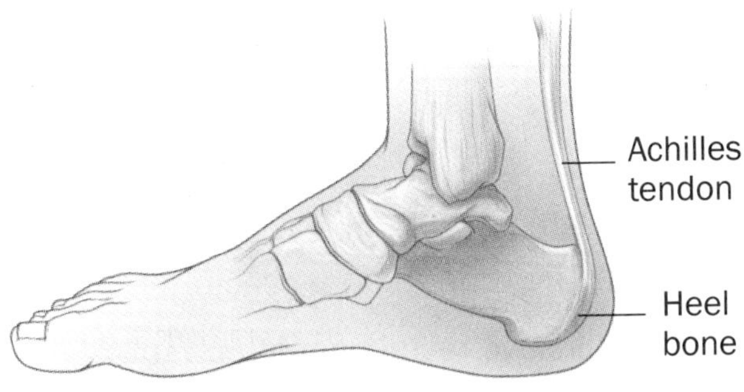

Problems with the Achilles tendon can cause pain in the back of the heel.

Achilles tendinosis can cause pain in the back of the heel. See Bursitis and Tendinosis on page 105. If you think you may have torn your Achilles tendon, see Strains, Sprains, and Broken Bones on page 49.

Home Treatment

- Start treating heel pain as soon as you feel it. If you ignore it until it gets bad, it may take a lot longer to get better.
- Cut back on activities that make your feet hurt. For exercise, try something that gets you off your feet, such as cycling or swimming. You may need to check with your doctor about when you can gradually get back to high-impact activities like running.
- Stretch your Achilles tendon and calf muscles several times a day. See the calf stretch on page 350.
- Put ice on your heel at least once a day. Always put a thin cloth between the ice and your skin. See Ice and Cold Packs on page 51.
- Don't go barefoot. Wear shoes or sandals with good cushioning and good arch support anytime you will be standing up or walking. If you get up at night to go to the bathroom, put on shoes.
- If your shoes are worn out, get a new pair. Pick shoes with good arch support and a cushioned sole. You can also try nonprescription arch supports.
- Take aspirin, ibuprofen (Advil, Motrin), or naproxen (Aleve) to relieve pain.
- For Achilles tendinosis or plantar fasciitis, try heel lifts or heel cups in both shoes. Use them only until the pain is gone.

If you have plantar fascia problems, there are special exercises and stretches that may help. To learn how to do them, Go to Web go to the Web site on the back cover and enter **S301** in the search box.

Your doctor may also suggest other treatments for plantar fasciitis, such as taping, heel splints, shoe inserts, or steroid shots. Surgery is usually done only as a last resort when other treatments have not worked.

Hemorrhoids and Rectal Problems

When to Call a Doctor

Call 911 if you have severe rectal bleeding. Severe means you are passing a lot of stool that is maroon or mostly blood.

Call your doctor if:

- You have severe rectal pain.
- Your stools have blood in them, or they are black or look like tar.
- Stools are narrower than usual (they may be no wider than a pencil).
- You still have rectal pain after a full week of home treatment.
- Any unusual material or tissue seeps or sticks out of the anus.
- A lump near the anus gets bigger or more painful, and you have a fever.

Hemorrhoids

Hemorrhoids are enlarged and inflamed veins that may form inside or outside the anus. Straining to pass hard stools, being overweight or pregnant, and sitting or standing for long periods can all cause hemorrhoids.

Hemorrhoids usually last several days and often come back. You may have:

- Bright red streaks of blood on stools or toilet paper, or blood dripping from the anus.
- Mucus leaking from the anus.
- Irritation or itching.
- The feeling that you cannot complete a bowel movement.
- Tissue or a lump sticking out of the anus.

Pain is not usually a symptom, unless a blood clot forms in a hemorrhoid or the blood flow to a hemorrhoid is cut off (strangulated). A clotted hemorrhoid may be extremely painful, but it is not dangerous. But a strangulated hemorrhoid may need emergency care.

Hemorrhoids may get better with home treatment. But if you have hemorrhoids that bleed a lot, hurt, or make it hard to keep your anal area clean, you may want to talk to your doctor about surgery or other treatments. For help deciding what

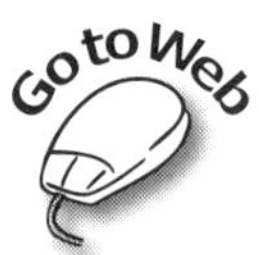

treatment is right for you, go to the Web site on the back cover and enter **V717** in the search box.

Other Rectal Problems

The rectum is the lower part of the large intestine (see the picture on page 159). At the end of the rectum is the anus, where stools pass out of the body.

Most people have rectal itching, pain, or bleeding at some time. These problems are often minor and will go away on their own or with home treatment.

Anal itching can have many causes:

- Skin around the anus may be irritated by stool. But trying to keep the area too clean by rubbing it with dry toilet paper or using harsh soap may damage the skin.
- Itching can be a sign of pinworms, especially in homes with children.
- Caffeine and spicy foods can irritate the rectum.

An **anal fissure** may cause pain during bowel movements and streaks of blood on stools. A fissure is a long, narrow sore that may form when the tissue near the anus is torn during a bowel movement.

Rectal bleeding, recent changes in bowel habits, and rectal pain are also symptoms of **colorectal cancer.** If you have these symptoms, see your doctor to find out if you need tests (see page 121). People over 50 should be tested regularly for colorectal cancer. This is especially important if you have a family history of colon cancer.

Home Treatment

- Take warm baths. They are soothing and cleansing, especially after a bowel movement. Warm baths with just enough water to cover the anal area—called sitz baths—can help with hemorrhoids but may make anal itching worse.
- Wear cotton underwear and loose clothing to decrease moisture in the anal area.
- Put a cool, wet cloth on the anus for 10 minutes, 4 times a day.
- Ease itching and irritation with zinc oxide, petroleum jelly, or hydrocortisone (1%) cream. Use a suppository such as Preparation H to ease pain and moisten the rectum. Ask your doctor before you use any product that has an anesthetic (check the ingredient list for names that end in "-caine," such as lidocaine). These products cause allergic reactions in some people.
- To keep your stool soft, drink plenty of water and eat lots of fresh fruits, vegetables, and whole grains. You may need to use a nonprescription stool softener until you are better. See Constipation on page 125.
- Try not to strain when you pass stools. Never hold your breath.
- Avoid sitting or standing too much. Take short walks to increase blood flow in your pelvic region.
- Keep the anal area clean, but be gentle when you clean it. Use water and a mild soap, such as Ivory. Or use baby wipes or Tucks pads.

Hernia

When to Call a Doctor

- A testicle swells and hurts. This could be very serious.
- You have a known hernia and you have sudden, severe pain in your groin or scrotum, along with nausea, vomiting, and fever.
- Mild groin pain or an unexplained bump or swelling in the groin lasts for more than 1 week.
- The skin over a hernia or bulge in the groin or belly turns red.
- You cannot push a hernia back into place with gentle pressure when you are lying down.

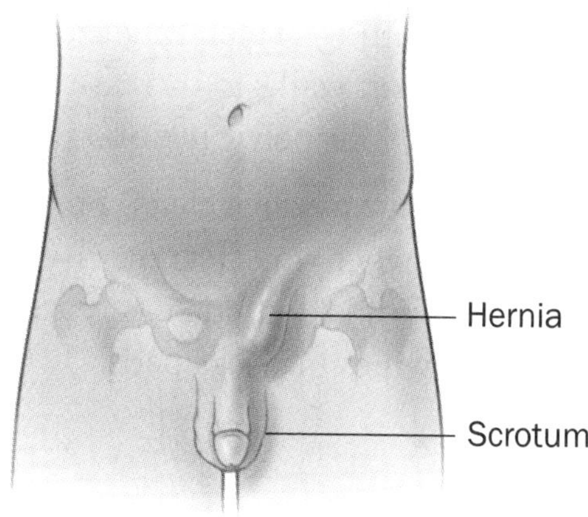

A hernia can cause a bulge or lump in the groin or scrotum.

Most hernias occur when tissue bulges through a weak spot in the belly wall into the groin. These are called inguinal hernias. They are more common in men than in women. In men, inguinal hernias often bulge into the scrotum.

If you have a hernia:

- You may have the sense that something has "given way."
- You may have a tender bulge in your groin or scrotum. The bulge may appear slowly over time, or it may form suddenly after heavy lifting, coughing, or straining. The bulge may flatten when you lie down.
- You may have groin pain that extends into the scrotum. Pain may get worse with bending or lifting. But not all hernias cause pain.

A hernia can form anywhere there is a weakness in the belly wall. Besides the groin, common places for this are the belly button and the site of an incision from a past surgery. Some people are born with a weak spot in the belly wall.

Once in a while, tissue may get trapped in the hernia. If the blood supply to the tissue is cut off, the tissue will swell and die. Then it can get infected. Pain in the

Hiatal Hernias

A hiatal hernia occurs when part of the stomach bulges into the chest cavity. Sometimes this will cause a backflow of stomach acid. This can cause heartburn and a sour taste in the mouth.

See Heartburn on page 176.

groin or scrotum that is quickly getting worse is a sign that this may have happened and that you need medical care now.

Home Treatment

These tips will help prevent hernias:

- Use proper lifting techniques. See page 85. Do not lift weights that are too heavy for you.
- Lose weight if you need to. See page 326.
- Avoid constipation, and don't strain when you pass stools or urinate. See page 125 for tips on avoiding constipation.
- Stop smoking, especially if you have a long-term cough. If you need help quitting, see page 351.

What About Hernia Surgery?

Hernias don't go away on their own, and with time they may get bigger and more painful. Surgery to repair a hernia can relieve the pain and discomfort and make the bulge go away.

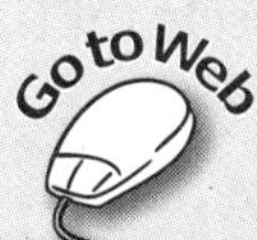

But you may not need surgery right away. Some people are able to wait months or even years. Others need to have surgery sooner. For help deciding if and when to have surgery, go to the Web site on the back cover and enter **U899** in the search box.

High Blood Pressure

When to Call a Doctor

Call 911 if you have high blood pressure and get a sudden, severe headache.

Call your doctor if:

- Your high blood pressure is usually under control, but it suddenly rises much higher than normal.
- You take your blood pressure, and it is 180/110 or higher.
- You have high blood pressure and get new chest pain or discomfort. See Chest Pain on page 114.
- You have high blood pressure and often get short of breath. This could be a sign of heart failure.
- Your blood pressure is higher than 140/90 on two or more occasions.
- You have any problems with your blood pressure medicine.

More

Blood Pressure Level	Systolic (Top Number)	Diastolic (Bottom Number)
Normal for adults	119 or below	79 or below
Borderline-high (prehypertension)	120 to 139	80 to 89
High (hypertension)	140 or above	90 or above

Blood pressure is a measure of the force of blood against the walls of your arteries. (Arteries are the blood vessels that carry oxygen-rich blood throughout your body.) Blood pressure readings include two numbers, such as 130/80. (Say "130 over 80.")

- The first (or top) number in the reading is the systolic pressure. This is the force of blood when the heart beats.
- The second (or bottom) number is the diastolic pressure. This is the force of blood between heartbeats, when the heart is at rest.

If you have high or borderline-high blood pressure, changes in your lifestyle may help lower your blood pressure. Some people also need medicines to get their blood pressure under control.

Despite what a lot of people think, high blood pressure usually does not cause headaches or make you feel dizzy or faint. It is often called the "silent killer" because it usually has no symptoms.

But it does increase your risk for heart attack, stroke, and kidney and eye damage. Your risk goes up as your blood pressure goes up. The longer your blood pressure stays high, the higher your risk.

Home Treatment

If your blood pressure is normal, the steps below will help you keep it that way. If you have borderline-high or high blood pressure, these steps may help you lower your blood pressure or keep it from getting worse:

- Try to reach and stay at a healthy weight. This is especially important if you put on weight around the waist rather than in the hips and thighs. Losing even 10 pounds can help lower your blood pressure. See page 326.
- Exercise for at least 30 minutes on most days of the week. You do not have to do all 30 minutes at once. Try three 10-minute walks. See Exercise for Health on page 340.
- Do not drink much alcohol.
- Limit salt. To learn how to reduce salt in your diet, see page 304.
- Make sure you get enough potassium, calcium, and magnesium. Eat plenty of fruits (such as bananas and oranges), vegetables, dried beans and peas, whole grains, and low-fat dairy products to get these minerals.

- Limit saturated fats. Saturated fat is found in animal products such as milk, cheese, and meat. Limiting these foods will help you lose weight and lower your risk for heart disease. See page 334 for tips on how to cut down on them.
- If you smoke, quit. Smoking increases your risk for heart attack and stroke. If you need help quitting, see page 351.

If you know you have high blood pressure:

- Take any prescribed blood pressure medicines as your doctor tells you. If you stop taking them, your blood pressure may quickly go back up.
- Talk to your doctor about taking an aspirin each day to reduce your risk of a heart attack or stroke. Do not start taking aspirin before you have talked to your doctor about it.
- See your doctor at least once a year.
- If you take blood pressure medicine, talk to your doctor before you take decongestants or anti-inflammatory drugs such as ibuprofen (Advil, Motrin) or naproxen (Aleve). Some of these can raise blood pressure.
- Check your blood pressure at home regularly. Go to Web: To learn how, go to the Web site on the back cover and enter **L311** in the search box.

Are You at Risk for High Blood Pressure?

You are more likely to have high blood pressure if:

- You smoke.
- You are overweight.
- Others in your family have high blood pressure.
- You are African American.
- You don't get regular exercise.
- You drink too much alcohol.
- You have a lot of salt or not enough potassium, calcium, or magnesium in your diet.
- You use decongestants, steroid medicines, or anti-inflammatory drugs such as ibuprofen (Motrin, Advil) or naproxen (Aleve) on a regular basis. Aspirin does not increase your risk for high blood pressure.

High Cholesterol

When to Call a Doctor

- Your cholesterol is over 200, and your doctor does not know about it (for instance, if you had a cholesterol test at a health fair or at work).
- You have never had your cholesterol checked. This is especially important if your family has a history of heart disease, diabetes, or high cholesterol.

Cholesterol is a kind of fat your body makes. You also get it from foods that come from animals, such as meat, milk and dairy foods, eggs, chicken, and fish.

Your body needs some cholesterol. But when you have too much, it can build up in your arteries and make it harder for blood to flow through them. This problem is called **atherosclerosis**. It is the starting point for most heart and blood flow problems, including heart attacks and strokes.

Good and Bad Cholesterol

Your body has a few kinds of cholesterol.

- **LDL** is the "bad" cholesterol. For LDL, a lower number is better. High LDL increases your risk for heart disease, heart attack, and stroke.
- **HDL** is the "good" cholesterol. It helps clear the bad cholesterol from the body. For HDL, a higher number is better. Raising your HDL may reduce your risk for heart disease, stroke, and a blood flow problem called peripheral artery disease.
- **Triglycerides** are another type of fat in the blood. High triglycerides may increase your risk of heart disease and stroke.

What Do the Numbers Mean?

The numbers in the chart below are for people who are at average risk for heart disease. If you have diabetes or heart disease or are at higher risk for heart disease, your doctor may use different numbers for what your cholesterol should be.

Total cholesterol
Normal: Less than 200
Borderline-high: 200 to 239
High: 240 and above
LDL ("bad" cholesterol)
Best: Less than 100
Near-best: 100 to 129
Borderline-high: 130 to 159
High: 160 to 189
Very high: 190 and above
HDL ("good" cholesterol)
Best: Above 60
Too low: Less than 40
Triglycerides
Borderline-high: 150 to 199
High: 200 to 499
Very high: 500 and above

When to Have Cholesterol Tests

You and your doctor can decide how often you should be tested, based on your risk for heart disease.

You may need to have your cholesterol checked more often if:

- Your total cholesterol was over 200 in a previous test.
- Your family has a history of early heart attack. Early means before age 55 in your father or brother or before age 65 in your mother or sister.
- You smoke.
- You have high blood pressure (over 140/90) or take blood pressure medicine.
- You have diabetes.
- Your HDL was below 40 or your triglycerides were over 150 in a previous test.

These all increase your risk for heart disease.

Basic cholesterol tests are easy, quick, and cheap. Call your local health department to find out where you can get a free or low-cost test.

How to Reduce Your Cholesterol

- Eat a heart-healthy diet that is low in saturated fat and cholesterol.
    - Eat less total fat, especially saturated fat. See the tips for eating less fat on page 334. Your total fat intake can be up to 35 percent of total calories, as long as most of it is unsaturated fat.
    - Ask your doctor or a registered dietitian about the TLC (Therapeutic Lifestyle Changes) diet. This diet will help you lower saturated fat to 7 percent or less of your total calories and your cholesterol from food to less than 200 mg a day.
    - Eat at least 2 servings of fruits and 3 servings of vegetables each day.
    - Eat 2 to 3 servings (4 to 6 ounces) of baked or broiled fish each week. Ask your doctor about fish oil supplements.
    - Eat more fiber (fruit, beans and peas, whole grains). See page 336.
- Exercise for at least 30 minutes most days of the week. It increases your HDL level and may lower your LDL level. It can also help you lose weight and lower your blood pressure. For help getting started, see page 340.
- If you smoke, quit. Smoking increases your risk of heart attack and stroke. If you need help quitting, see page 351.
- Lose weight if you need to. Losing even 5 to 10 pounds can lower triglycerides and raise HDL. Your LDL may fall as well. See Reaching a Healthy Weight on page 326.

Start with these changes. Regular exercise and a diet low in saturated fat are often enough to lower cholesterol.

More

Some people also need to take medicines. They may have very high cholesterol or diabetes, be at high risk for heart disease, or have other health problems. For help deciding if you should take medicines for high cholesterol, go to the Web site on the back cover and enter **S781** in the search box.

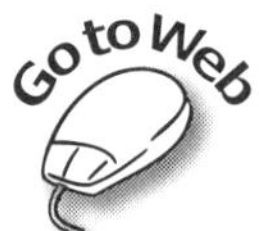

You can do everything right and still have high cholesterol. Although a lot of cholesterol comes from food, your liver makes cholesterol too. Cholesterol goes up as you age, no matter how healthy you are. High cholesterol may run in your family. But healthy habits can help you avoid some of the problems related to high cholesterol, like heart attack, heart disease, and stroke.

Hives

When to Call a Doctor

Call 911 if hives occur with dizziness, wheezing, trouble breathing, tightness in the chest, or swelling of the tongue, lips, or face.

Call a doctor if:

- You get hives soon after you start a new medicine.
- Hives cover all or most of your body.
- You still have hives after a full day of home treatment.

Hives are raised, red, itchy, often fluid-filled patches of skin that may come and go. Some people call them wheals or welts. Hives may last a few minutes or a few days. They can range in size from less than ¼ inch to more than 3 inches across.

An insect sting may cause a single hive. You may get many hives in response to a medicine, food, or infection. Other causes include breathing or touching something (such as a plant) that you are allergic to, stress, makeup, and being exposed to heat, cold, sunlight, or latex. Often you may not know the cause.

Home Treatment

- If you know what caused the hives, avoid it. If it was a food, don't eat it again. If it was makeup, don't wear it again. If it was a medicine, don't take it again. But be sure to tell your doctor if you stop taking a medicine. You may need a different one instead.
- Use cool, moist cloths to help reduce itching. For more tips, see Relief From Itching on page 134.
- Take nonprescription antihistamine pills to treat the hives and relieve itching. Some antihistamines, such as Claritin and Alavert, won't make you sleepy. After the hives go away, slowly lower the dose of the medicine over 5 to 7 days.

Ingrown Toenail

When to Call a Doctor

- You have increasing pain, swelling, warmth, or redness around the nail; red streaks leading from the nail; pus; or fever.
- You have diabetes or blood flow problems and get an ingrown toenail.

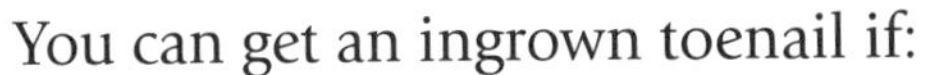

You can get an ingrown toenail if:

- You trim your toenail so that the nail cuts into the skin at the edge of the nail. Always cut your toenails straight across, not curved.
- You wear shoes that are too tight.

Because the nail can easily get infected, an ingrown toenail needs prompt care.

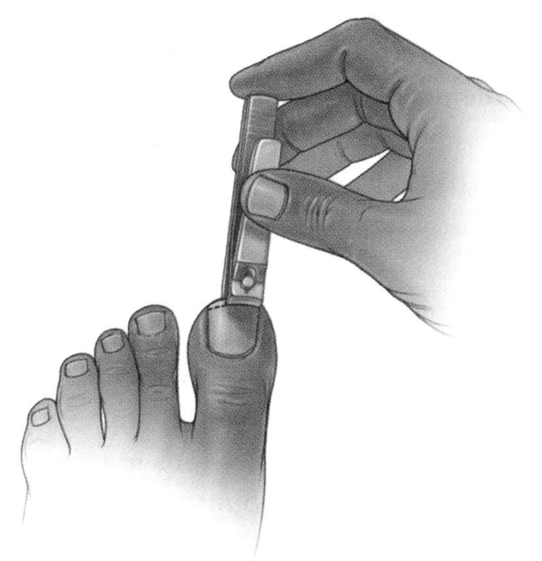

Cut toenails straight across.

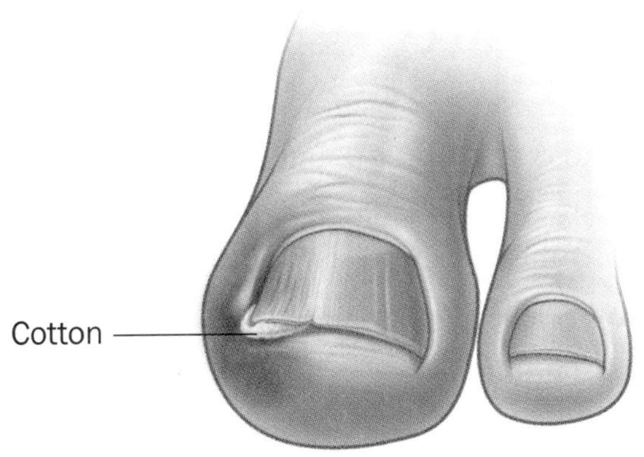

Use a piece of wet cotton to cushion and lift the nail.

Home Treatment

- Soak your foot in warm water for 15 minutes each day to soften the skin around the nail. (This may also relieve swelling and pain while the nail grows out.) You may want to add Epsom salt to the water.
- To keep the nail from cutting the skin, wedge a small piece of wet cotton under the corner of the nail to cushion it and lift it slightly. Repeat each day until the nail has grown out and you can trim it.
- Cut the toenail straight across. Leave it a little longer at the corners so that the sharp ends don't cut into the skin.
- Wear roomy shoes, and keep your feet clean and dry.

Irritable Bowel Syndrome

When to Call a Doctor

- Your symptoms get worse, start to disrupt your usual activities, or do not respond as usual to home treatment.
- You are more and more tired all the time.
- Your symptoms often wake you.
- Your pain gets worse when you move or cough.
- You have belly pain and a fever.
- You have belly pain that does not get better when you pass gas or stools.
- You are losing weight, and you don't know why.
- Your appetite has decreased.
- Your stools have blood in them, or they are black or look like tar.

Irritable bowel syndrome (IBS) is one of the most common problems of the digestive tract. Symptoms often get worse when you are under stress or after you eat. They include:

- Bloating, belly pain, and gas.
- Mucus in the stool.
- The feeling that you cannot complete a bowel movement.
- Changes in bowel movements. You may go back and forth between diarrhea and constipation. Stools may be hard sometimes and loose and watery other times.

People can have IBS for many years. An episode may be worse than the one before it, but IBS does not get worse over time or lead to more serious diseases such as cancer. Symptoms tend to get better over time. Medicines can help control the constipation and diarrhea caused by IBS. Home treatment can help too.

If you often have digestive problems but have not been diagnosed with IBS, try to rule out other reasons for your stomach upset, such as new foods, stress, or the flu. Try home treatment for 1 to 2 weeks. If it does not help, call your doctor.

There are no tests that can diagnose irritable bowel syndrome, but your doctor may want to do tests to rule out other problems. Be sure to think about and discuss how much testing is right for you. This may depend on your age, your symptoms, your response to treatment, and your chances of having a more serious problem.

Tests come with risks and costs, and the results may or may not change your treatment. For questions to think about as you decide about testing, go to Go to Web the Web site on the back cover and enter **Q852** in the search box.

Home Treatment

If constipation is your main symptom:

- Eat more fruits, vegetables, beans, and whole grains. Add these fiber-rich foods to your diet slowly so they don't make gas or cramps worse.
- Add unprocessed wheat bran to your diet. Start by using 1 tablespoon a day, and slowly increase to 4 tablespoons a day. Sprinkle bran on cereal, soup, and casseroles. Drink extra water to avoid bloating.
- Get some exercise every day. Exercise helps the digestive system work better.
- Try a fiber supplement, such as Citrucel, FiberCon, or Metamucil. Start with 1 tablespoon or less each day, and drink extra water to prevent bloating.
- Use a laxative only if your doctor suggests it.

If diarrhea is your main symptom:

- Try the diet tips for relieving constipation. Fiber-rich foods and wheat bran can sometimes help relieve diarrhea.
- Avoid foods that make diarrhea worse. Try cutting out one food at a time; then add it back bit by bit. If a food does not seem to be related to symptoms, you don't need to avoid it. Many people find that the following foods or ingredients make their symptoms worse:
  - Alcohol, caffeine, and nicotine
  - Beans, broccoli, cabbage, and apples
  - Spicy foods
  - Foods high in acid, such as citrus fruit
  - Fatty foods, including bacon, sausage, butter, oils, and anything deep-fried
- Avoid dairy products that have lactose (milk sugar) if they seem to make symptoms worse. But be sure to get enough calcium in your diet from other sources. See Lactose Intolerance on page 128.
- Avoid sorbitol, an artificial sweetener, and olestra, a fat substitute used in some processed foods.
- Add more starchy food (whole-grain breads, rice, potatoes, pasta) to your diet.
- If diarrhea doesn't stop, a nonprescription medicine such as loperamide (in products such as Imodium) may help. Check with your doctor if you are using loperamide more than 3 times a week.

To reduce stress:

- Keep a record of the life events that occur with your symptoms. This may help you see any link between stress and your symptoms.
- Get regular, brisk exercise, such as swimming, cycling, or walking.
- Learn and use a relaxation technique. See page 358.

Look for more tips in Managing Stress on page 356.

Jaw Pain and Temporomandibular Disorder

When to Call a Doctor

Call 911 if you have jaw pain along with chest pain or pressure or other signs of a heart attack. See page 38.

Call your doctor if:

- You have jaw pain with vision loss. This may be sign of a serious problem called temporal arteritis. See page 169.
- Jaw pain is severe.
- You have jaw pain or other problems after an injury to the jaw.
- Your jaw locks.
- A jaw problem has not improved after 2 weeks of home treatment.
- You have noticed a change in the way your teeth fit together when you close your mouth.

The temporomandibular joint connects the lower jawbone to the skull. When you have pain in this joint and in the jaw muscles, you have a problem called **temporomandibular (TM) disorder**. You may also hear it called TMJ, TMD, or TM problems.

- You may feel pain in one or both jaws when you chew or yawn.
- You may have painful clicking, popping, or grating in the jaw joint.
- Your jaw may lock, or you may not be able to open your mouth wide.
- You may often have headaches or pain in your neck, face, or shoulders.

The most common cause of TM disorder is tension in the jaw, neck, and shoulder muscles. Stress or habits such as clenching or grinding your teeth can cause a lot of tension in these muscles. TM disorder can also occur if there is a problem in the jaw joint itself, such as arthritis.

Home treatment can relieve most TM problems. Your doctor may also suggest a plastic mouth plate or physical therapy. Surgery is rarely needed and may make things worse.

Home Treatment

The key to treating TM disorder is to reduce tension in your jaw.

- Try not to clench or grind your teeth. Do not bite your nails or tuck the phone receiver between your shoulder and jaw.

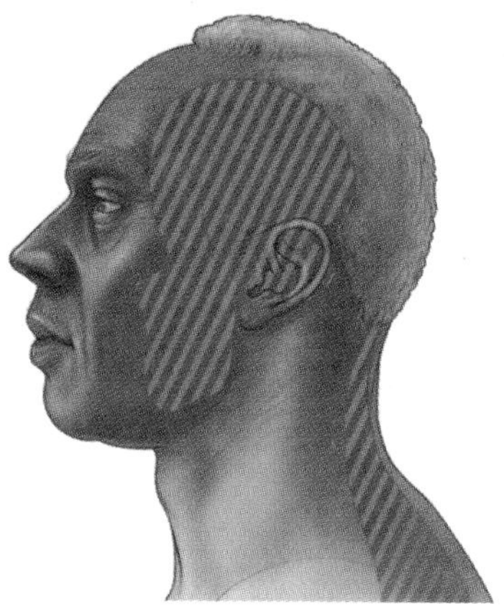

TM disorder causes pain in the shaded areas.

- At the first sign of pain in your jaw muscles, stop chewing gum, ice, hard candy, or tough foods. Eat softer foods, and use both sides of your mouth to chew.
- Use good posture. Poor posture may disturb the way the muscles and bones in your face work together.
- Rest your jaw, keeping your teeth apart and your lips closed. (Keep your tongue on the roof of your mouth, not between your teeth.) Do not open your mouth too wide.
- Put an ice pack on the joint for 10 minutes, 3 times a day. (Always put a thin cloth between the ice and your skin.) Gently open and close your mouth while the ice pack is on. If the jaw muscle is swollen, use ice 6 times a day. See Ice and Cold Packs on page 51.
- Take ibuprofen (Advil, Motrin) or naproxen (Aleve) to reduce pain and swelling.
- If there is no swelling, you can put moist heat on your jaw for 10 to 15 minutes, 3 times a day. Gently open and close your mouth while the heat is on. You can also alternate heat with cold.
- Relax. If you have a lot of stress in your life, try a relaxation technique. See page 358. Get help if you are under severe stress or suffer from anxiety or depression.

Looking for the Kidney Disease topic? See page 308.

Kidney Stones

When to Call a Doctor

- You think you have a kidney stone. Symptoms include:
  - Sudden pain in your side, groin, or genital area that gets worse over 15 to 60 minutes until it is steady and severe.
  - Nausea and vomiting.
  - Blood in the urine.
  - Feeling like you need to urinate often or having pain when you urinate.
  - Diarrhea, constipation, or loss of appetite.
  - Not being able to find a comfortable position.
- You have fever or chills and increasing pain in your back, just below your rib cage.
- You have blood in your urine.
- You pass a stone, even if there was little or no pain. Save the stone, and ask your doctor if it needs to be tested.

More

Kidney stones can form from the minerals in urine. The most common cause is not drinking enough water.

As long as they stay in the kidneys, kidney stones usually cause no problems. But a stone may block the flow of urine and cause severe pain if it moves into the ureter, which is the tube that leads to the bladder (see the picture on page 91). In fact, it may be the worst pain you have ever had.

When the stone moves into the bladder, the pain may vanish suddenly. But it can hurt again when the stone passes out of the body.

Most small kidney stones pass without your needing treatment other than pain medicine. In rare cases, you may need surgery or a procedure called lithotripsy that uses sound waves to break the stones into small pieces.

Home Treatment

- Drink enough water to keep your urine clear—about 8 to 10 glasses a day. This will help the stone pass and can help prevent future stones.
- Take aspirin, acetaminophen (Tylenol), or ibuprofen (Advil, Motrin) to relieve pain.
- Use heat on sore areas on your back or belly for 20 minutes at a time. Moist heat works better than dry heat. Use a hot pack, or take a hot bath or shower.

Knee Problems

When to Call a Doctor

- Your knee gives out or will not bear weight.
- You felt or heard a "pop" in your knee at the time of an injury.
- Your knee swells a lot within 30 minutes of an injury.
- You have signs of damage to the nerves or blood vessels, such as numbness, tingling, a pins-and-needles feeling, or pale or blue skin below the injury.
- Your knee looks deformed.
- You cannot straighten or bend your knee, or the joint locks.
- Your knee is red, hot, swollen, or painful to touch.
- The pain is bad enough that you are limping, or it does not improve with 2 days of home treatment.

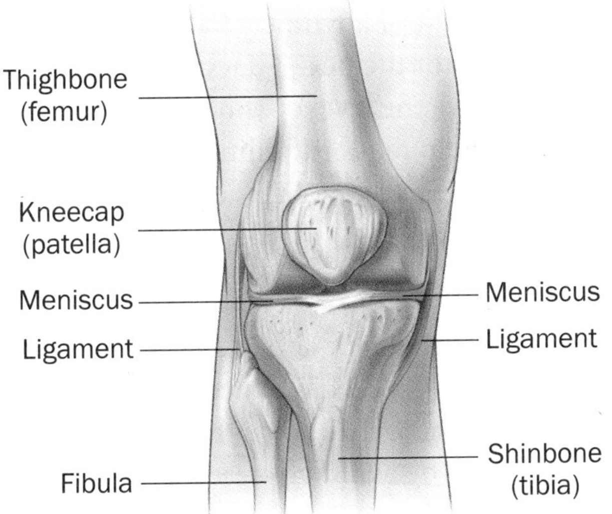

You can have knee problems when the structures that support the joint are injured or inflamed.

The knee is a joint that can get hurt easily. It is the place where three long leg bones meet and are held together with ligaments and muscles. Problems can occur when you overstress or injure your knee. Four common problems are:

- **Sprained knee ligaments**. (Ligaments connect bone to bone.) Sprains are usually the result of the knee bending or twisting too far in a direction that it's not supposed to go. Sometimes a ligament may tear.
- **Cartilage tear**. Cartilage is tissue that cushions the joint. If you tear cartilage in your knee, you will have pain and may have a sense of your knee locking.
- **Kneecap pain**, also known as patellofemoral pain. This is pain around or behind the kneecap. You may have it when you go up or down stairs, when you run downhill, or after you sit for long periods of time.
- **Jumper's knee**, also known as patellar tendinosis. This affects the tendon that attaches your kneecap to your shinbone and causes pain right below your knee. It is common in people who play basketball or volleyball.

Preventing Knee Problems

- Strengthen and stretch the leg muscles evenly, especially those in the front of the thigh (called the quadriceps) and the back of the thigh (called the hamstrings). See page 350. This is the best way to prevent knee problems.
- Do not do deep knee bends. Imagine a line that starts at the tip of your toes and goes straight up. When you do knee bends, your knees should not jut past that line.
- Do not wear high-heeled shoes.
- Wear shoes with good arch supports. Replace running or walking shoes every 300 to 500 miles.
- Do not run downhill unless your muscles are well trained and strong enough for it.
- Do not wear shoes with cleats if you play contact sports.

More

Also see Strains, Sprains, and Broken Bones on page 49 and Bursitis and Tendinosis on page 105.

If knee pain is not related to exercise or a recent or past injury, it could be arthritis. See page 266.

Home Treatment

- Rest and protect your knee. Take a break from anything that causes pain. After several days of rest, you can start gentle exercises and stretching.
- Put ice or a cold pack on your knee for 10 to 15 minutes at a time. Always put a thin cloth beneath the ice and your skin. See Ice and Cold Packs on page 51.
- Prop up your knee on a pillow when you ice it or anytime you sit or lie down for the next 3 days. Try to keep it above the level of your heart. This will help reduce swelling.
- Take ibuprofen (Advil, Motrin) or naproxen (Aleve) for pain and swelling.
- Ask your doctor about wearing a brace or an elastic or neoprene sleeve with a hole that holds the kneecap in place. This will help ease pain during activity. You can buy one at a pharmacy or sporting goods store.

Laryngitis

When to Call a Doctor

- You are hoarse or have lost your voice and have a high fever. See the fever guidelines on page 150.
- You have symptoms of a worse infection, such as fast or shallow breathing; a cough that brings up colored mucus from the lungs; or pain, fever, and fatigue that are getting a lot worse.
- You are hoarse for more than 2 to 3 weeks.

Laryngitis is an infection or irritation of the voice box (larynx). If you have laryngitis, you may be hoarse, lose your voice, and feel like you need to clear your throat a lot. You may also have fever, throat pain, and a cough and feel more tired than usual.

You can get laryngitis because of:

- A virus, such as a cold.
- Allergies.
- Lots of talking, singing, or yelling.
- Cigarette smoke.
- Backflow (reflux) of stomach acid into the throat.

Your voice box will usually heal in 5 to 10 days. Medicine does not help much.

If you drink a lot of alcohol or you smoke, you may reach a point where your throat and voice box are irritated all the time.

Home Treatment

- If a cold makes you hoarse, treat the cold. See page 119. You may be hoarse for up to a week after a cold goes away.
- Rest your voice. Try not to talk much or clear your throat.
- Do not smoke, and avoid other people's smoke. If you need help quitting, see page 351.
- Use a humidifier in your bedroom or your whole house. Or try standing in the steam from a hot shower.
- Drink extra water and other fluids.
- To soothe your throat, gargle with warm salt water (1 teaspoon of salt in 8 ounces of water). Or drink weak tea or hot water with honey or lemon juice in it.
- If you think that acid reflux may be the cause, reducing heartburn may help. See page 177.

Leg Pain and Muscle Cramps

When to Call a Doctor

- You have sudden leg pain, and the skin of your lower leg, foot, or toes is cold, pale, or blue-black. This could be a serious problem.
- You have swelling, redness, and pain in the leg or calf. (You may also have a fever.) These are signs of phlebitis or infection (cellulitis). See the chart on page 198.
- Leg pain always starts after you walk a certain distance and then goes away when you stop walking. This is a sign of a blood flow problem. See Peripheral Artery Disease on page 208.
- Home treatment does not relieve your muscle cramps.

Leg pain and muscle cramps are common. They often occur at night or during exercise, especially if the weather is hot or humid. Dehydration, low levels of potassium, or using a muscle that is not stretched well may cause cramps.

These aches and pains become even more common as we age. There are a number of things that can help.

Home Treatment

If you have pain, swelling, or a heavy feeling in the calf of only one of your legs, or if you have other symptoms that cause you to suspect phlebitis or infection (cellulitis), call your doctor before you try home treatment.

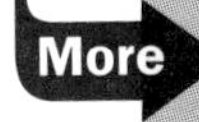

Common Causes of Leg Pain	Symptoms	Comments
Muscle cramps	Sudden cramping pain, usually in lower leg; leg may feel like it is in "knots"	Often happens at night or during exercise
Shin splints	Pain in front of lower leg	Often caused by overuse or high-impact exercise (such as running on a hard surface), especially if you are not used to it
Arthritis	Pain in leg joints (knees, ankles, toes)	See Living Better With Arthritis, p. 266.
Sciatica (a back problem)	Leg pain that extends from buttocks down back of leg and into foot	See Sciatica, p. 80.
Phlebitis (an inflamed vein)	Pain and swelling in one leg (but it can occur anywhere); common after surgery, bed rest, and extended air travel	Can be serious if blood clot forms, breaks loose, and travels to lungs. See Blood Clots in the Leg, p. 96.
Decreased blood flow (intermittent claudication)	Cramping pain, usually in calf, that starts after you walk a certain distance and goes away when you rest; leg pain and cold, pale skin	See Peripheral Artery Disease, p. 208.
Cellulitis (skin infection)	Warm, red, swollen, and tender area on the leg; may include fever, chills, and swollen lymph nodes	Needs to be treated right away to keep infection from spreading through the body. See Cellulitis, p. 220.

- Warm up well and stretch before exercise. Also stretch after you exercise. If a muscle cramps, gently stretch and massage it.
- Drink plenty of fluids. Drink extra fluids before and during exercise, especially if the weather is hot or humid.
- Get plenty of potassium in your diet (unless your doctor has told you to limit potassium). Bananas, orange juice, and potatoes are good sources.
- If leg cramps wake you at night, take a warm bath and do some stretches before you go to bed. Keep your legs warm while you sleep.
- For shin splints:
  - Put a cold pack on your leg for 10 to 15 minutes at a time. Put a thin cloth between the ice and your skin.
  - Take acetaminophen (Tylenol) or ibuprofen (Advil, Motrin) for pain.
  - Take 1 to 2 weeks of rest from high-impact activities like running. Return to exercise slowly.

Restless Legs Syndrome

Restless legs syndrome is an unpleasant feeling in your legs when you lie down to sleep. Most people also have a very strong urge to move their legs, and moving the legs sometimes makes them feel better. But all this moving can make it hard to sleep. You may start to have problems during the day because you are so tired.

Tell your doctor if you have restless legs. Sometimes it is caused by a problem that can be treated, such as not getting enough iron. Some medicines, such as antidepressants and cold and sinus medicines, can make your symptoms worse.

If your symptoms are mild, you may just need to make a few lifestyle changes. Here are some things to try:

- Get regular exercise.
- Stretch or massage your legs before bed or when symptoms begin.
- Use heat or ice packs, or take hot or cold baths.
- Avoid tobacco, alcohol, and caffeine.
- Keep your bedroom cool, quiet, and comfortable, and use it only for sleeping and sex.

If these changes don't help, you may need to take medicine to control your leg movements and help you sleep.

Lung Cancer

When to Call a Doctor

If you already know you have lung cancer, you may want to read Living Better With Cancer on page 276.

Lung cancer may not cause symptoms early on. **Call your doctor if:**

- You have a cough that doesn't go away.
- You have chest pain that gets worse when you breathe deeply, cough, or laugh.
- Your voice is hoarse a lot of the time.
- You cough up bloody or rust-colored mucus.
- You are often short of breath.
- You have started wheezing.
- You have bronchitis or pneumonia that keeps coming back.
- You have lost weight and don't feel like eating.

Lung cancer is the most deadly type of cancer in both men and women. It happens when the lungs are damaged by breathing smoke (including secondhand smoke) or other harmful substances, such as asbestos, radioactive dust, or radon.

Lung cancer occurs most often in people over 40 who have smoked for many years. The longer you smoke and the more you smoke, the higher your risk.

Lung cancer may not cause symptoms early on, or the symptoms may be like those caused by other lung problems: coughing, wheezing, or shortness of breath. As a result, lung cancer is often not found early, when treatment works best. If it is not found early, it may spread to the lymph nodes and other organs.

If your doctor thinks you might have cancer, you will need tests to diagnose it and find out if it has spread. Then you can have surgery to remove the cancer or have radiation or take medicines (chemotherapy) to kill the cancer. A combination of treatments may be used.

Smoking and Lung Cancer

Smoking is the biggest risk factor for lung cancer. So the best thing you can do for yourself is to stop smoking. Over time, this will reduce your risk.

If you already have lung cancer, quitting smoking can help your treatment work better and may help you live longer.

See page 351 for help with quitting.

Menopause

When to Call a Doctor

- Your periods are longer, heavier, or harder to predict than usual.
- You have bleeding between periods.
- You have bleeding after your periods have stopped for 6 months.
- You have vaginal dryness, and a lubricant does not help. Your doctor may prescribe an estrogen cream or suppository.
- You have started leaking urine.
- Your symptoms are disrupting your life, even with home treatment.
- You have unexplained vaginal bleeding (different from what your doctor told you to expect) while you are taking hormones.
- You have been on hormone therapy for a long time. Ask your doctor if it is still a good idea for you.

Menopause occurs when the body starts making less of the female hormones estrogen and progesterone. This happens between ages 45 and 55 for most women, and it may take several years to complete.

Having both ovaries removed (oophorectomy) also causes menopause, though you can take hormones to help with the symptoms.

Hormone changes may cause:

- **Irregular periods**. Your flow may be lighter or heavier than usual. The time between periods may get shorter or longer. You may have spotting. Some women have regular periods until their periods stop suddenly. Others have irregular periods for a long time.
- **Hot flashes**. These cause intense heat, sweating, and flushing that can last from a few minutes to an hour. A hot flash usually starts in the chest and spreads out to the neck, face, and arms. If hot flashes often wake you up at night, you may feel tired and distracted because you're not sleeping enough.
- **Vaginal dryness**. Your vagina may become drier, thinner, and less stretchy. These changes can make sex hurt. And they may increase your risk for infections (see page 245) and bladder control problems (see page 92).
- **Mood changes**. Some women feel nervous, moody, or depressed as they go through menopause. You may have less energy or have trouble sleeping.

More

Hormone Therapy

Your doctor may prescribe hormone therapy to treat symptoms of menopause. There are two types:

- Estrogen replacement therapy (ERT). ERT is estrogen alone. Because ERT may increase the risk of uterine cancer, it is usually used only for women who have had their uterus removed (hysterectomy).
- Hormone replacement therapy (HRT). HRT is estrogen and progesterone, another female hormone. Progesterone helps protect against uterine cancer.

Hormone therapy comes as a pill that you take every day. You can get some forms of hormone therapy as skin patches, vaginal creams, or vaginal rings.

Benefits of therapy

- Reduces hot flashes and vaginal dryness.
- Helps keep bones strong and lowers your risk of osteoporosis. But there are other medicines that can help with this too. See page 207.

Risks of therapy

- Increases the risk of blood clots in your legs or lungs.
- May increase your risk of breast cancer, stroke, and heart problems.
- May cause bloating, sore breasts, vaginal bleeding, and other side effects.
- Not advised for women who have had breast cancer, uterine cancer, blood clots, heart attack, stroke, liver disease, undiagnosed uterine bleeding, or a family history of breast cancer.

For some women, the short-term benefit of reducing menopause symptoms may outweigh the risks. Using hormone therapy for 1 to 2 years may help with symptoms while they are at their worst with less chance of causing the long-term side effects.

Talk with your doctor about whether hormone therapy is a good idea for you. For help with your decision, go to

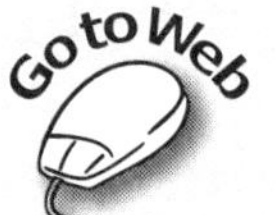

the Web site on the back cover and enter **V655** in the search box.

If you already take hormones, talk with your doctor each year about whether it is still the right thing for you.

You may also need to think about some other issues, including:

- **Osteoporosis**. Having lower estrogen levels weakens your bones and makes them more likely to break. Hormone therapy can help prevent this, but it has risks. There are also other medicines you can take for your bones. To learn more, see page 207. Be sure to get plenty of calcium and vitamin D.
- **Birth control**. Until you have finished menopause, your body will continue to release eggs (ovulate). This means you could get pregnant. If you don't want to get pregnant, use birth control until your doctor confirms that you have finished menopause or until you have not had a period for 12 months.
- **Heart disease**. Women who are at the age to start menopause are more likely to get heart disease. Work with your doctor to learn what you can do to prevent it.

Home Treatment

- For hot flashes:
  - Keep your home and workplace cool, or use a fan.
  - Dress in layers that are easy to take off. Wear natural fibers like cotton and silk.
  - Drink cold drinks, not hot ones.
  - Limit caffeine and alcohol, and do not smoke.
  - Get regular exercise. Women who exercise regularly have fewer problems with hot flashes.
  - Try a relaxation technique. See page 358.
- For vaginal dryness and pain during sex, use a water-soluble lubricant, such as Astroglide or Replens. Do not use Vaseline or other oil-based products.
- Make exercise part of your life. Regular exercise can ease stress, keep your bones strong, and reduce your risk of heart disease and other health problems.
- Get support if you need it. Talking with other women may help.
- Try to stay relaxed about menopause. Being tense may make you feel worse.
- Keep a written record of your periods. You may need to discuss them with your doctor.

Neck Pain

When to Call a Doctor

Call 911 if:

- Neck pain occurs with chest pain or other symptoms of a heart attack. See page 38.
- A person has signs of damage to the spine after an injury (such as a car accident, fall, or direct blow to the spine). Signs may include:
  - Being unable to move part of the body.
  - Severe back or neck pain.
  - Weakness, tingling, or numbness in the arms or legs.
  - Loss of bowel or bladder control.

Call your doctor if:

- You have a stiff neck with a fever and a severe headache. You may have a serious illness. See page 151.
- You suddenly lose bowel or bladder control. This could be a sign of a serious problem.
- You have new weakness or constant numbness in your arms or legs.
- Neck pain goes down one arm, or you have numbness or tingling in your hands.
- A blow or injury to your neck (whiplash) causes new pain.
- You cannot control your pain with home treatment.
- Pain has not gotten better after 2 weeks of home treatment.

Most people have pain, stiffness, or a kink in the neck from time to time. Neck pain is most often caused by tension, strain, or spasm in the neck muscles or a problem with the ligaments, tendons, or joints in the neck. This can happen when:

- You stay too long in a position that stresses the neck. Some examples are cradling the phone between your ear and shoulder, sleeping on your stomach or with your neck twisted, or looking up or down at a computer screen all day.
- You repeat movements that stress the neck. You might do this during exercise or sports, on the job, or at home.

Arthritis or damage to the discs in the neck can cause a pinched nerve. With this problem, the pain usually spreads down one arm. Your arm or hand may tingle or feel numb or weak. If you have symptoms of a pinched nerve, you need to see your doctor.

Home Treatment

Much of the home treatment for back pain also works for neck pain. See page 81. These tips may also help:

- Put ice or a cold pack on your neck for 10 to 15 minutes several times a day for the next 2 to 3 days. This will reduce pain and speed healing. If the problem is near your shoulder or upper back, icing the back of your neck may work best. Put a thin cloth between the ice and your skin.
- After the first 3 full days (or if you have chronic neck pain), you may put heat on the sore area for 20 minutes at a time.
- Take aspirin, ibuprofen (Advil, Motrin), or acetaminophen (Tylenol) to help relieve pain.
- Take some easy walks. The gentle swinging motion of your arms often relieves pain. Start with short walks of 5 to 10 minutes, 3 or 4 times a day.
- After the pain starts to get better, try the neck exercises on page 206.

If neck pain occurs with a headache, see page 166.

Preventing Neck Pain

You can prevent most neck pain by using good posture, getting regular exercise, and not stressing your neck too much or too often. You can strengthen and protect your neck by doing neck exercises. See page 206.

Reducing stress may help too. Try the relaxation exercise on page 358.

To avoid pain at the end of the day, be careful how you sit, stand, and move during the day.

- Sit straight in your chair with your lower back supported. Do not sit for long periods without getting up or changing positions. Take short breaks several times each hour to stretch your neck.
- If you work at a computer, have the top of the screen at eye level. Use a document holder that puts the copy at the same level as the screen.
- If you use the phone a lot, use a headset or speakerphone.

To avoid neck stiffness in the morning, you may need better neck support when you sleep. (Morning neck pain may also be the result of things you did the day before.)

- Fold a towel lengthwise into a 4-inch-wide pad and wrap it around your neck. Pin the ends together for good support.
- You may need a special neck support pillow. Look for a pillow that supports your neck comfortably when you lie on your back and on your side (try before buying). Do not use pillows that push your head forward when you are on your back.
- Do not sleep on your stomach with your neck twisted or bent.

More

Neck Exercises

These exercises make your neck stronger and more flexible, so they can help you avoid neck problems. You do not need to do every exercise. Do the ones that help the most. Go slow, and stop any exercise that hurts. Do the exercises 2 times a day.

Dorsal glide

Sit or stand tall, looking straight ahead (a "palace guard" posture). Slowly tuck your chin as you glide your head backward over your body. Hold for a count of 5; then relax. Repeat 6 to 10 times. This stretches the back of the neck. If you feel pain, do not glide so far back.

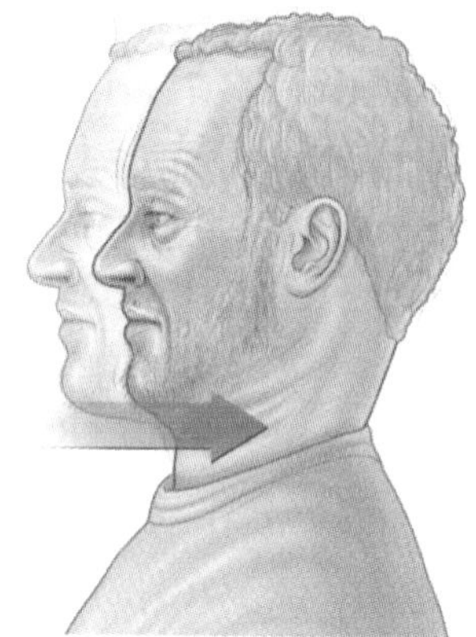

Dorsal glide

Shoulder lifts

Lie facedown with your arms beside your body. Lift your shoulders straight up from the floor as high as you can without pain. Keep your chin down, and face the floor. Keep your belly and hips pressed to the floor. Repeat 6 to 10 times. See the picture on page 87.

Chest and shoulder stretch

Sit or stand tall, and glide your head backward as in the dorsal glide. Raise both arms so that your hands are next to your ears. As you exhale, lower your elbows down and back. Feel your shoulder blades slide down and together. Hold for a few seconds and then relax. Repeat 6 to 10 times.

Hands on head

Move your head backward, forward, and side to side against gentle pressure from your hands. Hold each position for several seconds. Repeat 6 to 10 times.

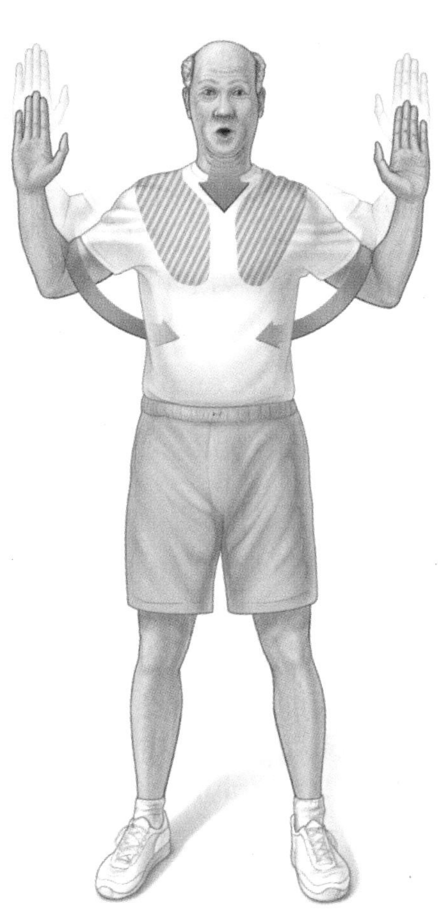

Chest and shoulder stretch

Osteoporosis

When to Call a Doctor

- You think you have a broken bone, or you cannot move a part of your body.
- You have sudden, severe pain or cannot bear weight on a body part.
- One of your arms or legs is not its normal shape. This may mean you have a broken bone.
- You are concerned about your risk for osteoporosis.

Also see Strains, Sprains, and Broken Bones on page 49.

Osteoporosis means that your bones are thin and weak and can break easily. The problem affects millions of older adults, especially older women.

Osteoporosis is more common after menopause, when the body makes less estrogen. Having rheumatoid arthritis or too much thyroid hormone also can weaken your bones.

You are at highest risk for osteoporosis if:

- Other people in your family have had it.
- You do not get much exercise and have not gotten much in the past.
- You have a slender body frame.
- You smoke, or you drink a lot of alcohol.
- You are of Asian or European heritage.

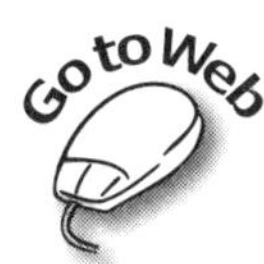

To find out your risk for osteoporosis, go to the Web site on the back cover and enter **T409** in the search box.

Osteoporosis usually develops over many years without symptoms. The first sign may be a broken bone, loss of height, back pain, or a slowly forming curve or hump in the upper back.

A special X-ray called a **DEXA scan** measures bone thickness (density) and can tell you how much bone loss you have. If you are at high risk for osteoporosis, or if you are a woman over age 65, a bone density test may give you and your doctor information that can help you decide whether you need treatment. For help deciding if you need this test, go to the Web site on the back cover and enter **W380** in the search box.

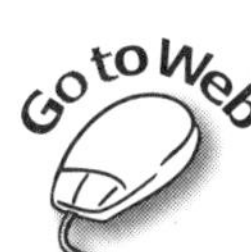

What You Can Do

Weakening bones are a natural part of growing older. But if you started healthy habits early in life, you may delay the problem. If you already have osteoporosis, these same habits can help slow the disease process and may reduce your risk of broken bones.

- Get plenty of exercise. Walking, jogging, dancing, lifting weights, and other exercises make bones stronger.

More

- Eat a healthy diet with lots of calcium and vitamin D. You need both of these for strong, healthy bones.
  - Get calcium from yogurt, cheese, milk, and dark green vegetables.
  - Get vitamin D from eggs, fatty fish, and fortified cereal and milk.
  - Talk to your doctor about taking a calcium and vitamin D supplement if you think you might need one. Most people don't get enough calcium.
- If you smoke, quit. If you need help quitting, see page 351.
- Limit alcohol to 1 drink a day or less.
- Cut down on cola soft drinks (including the diet versions). They may make your bones thinner.

There are medicines that can help prevent osteoporosis. Hormone therapy is one choice, but it has risks. Talk with your doctor about what's right for you. Also see Hormone Therapy on page 202.

If you have osteoporosis, medicines can help slow bone loss and build bone strength. Bisphosphonates (such as Fosamax) are the medicines used most often.

If you know your bones are weak, be extra careful to avoid falls. See page 364 for tips on how to make your home safer.

Peripheral Artery Disease

When to Call a Doctor

- You have sudden leg pain or numbness, or pale, blue-black skin on your legs or feet.
- You have leg pain that always starts after you walk a certain distance and goes away when you rest.
- You have foot or toe pain when resting.
- You have peripheral artery disease and have an open sore on your foot or leg.

Peripheral artery disease is narrowing of the blood vessels in the arms, legs, or belly. This reduces blood flow to that area. The legs are affected most often.

Plaque usually is the cause of narrow blood vessels. Plaque is a buildup of cholesterol and other substances. This buildup is called "hardening" of the arteries, or **atherosclerosis**.

You are more likely to have peripheral artery disease if you smoke or have high cholesterol, high blood pressure, diabetes, or a family history of peripheral artery disease.

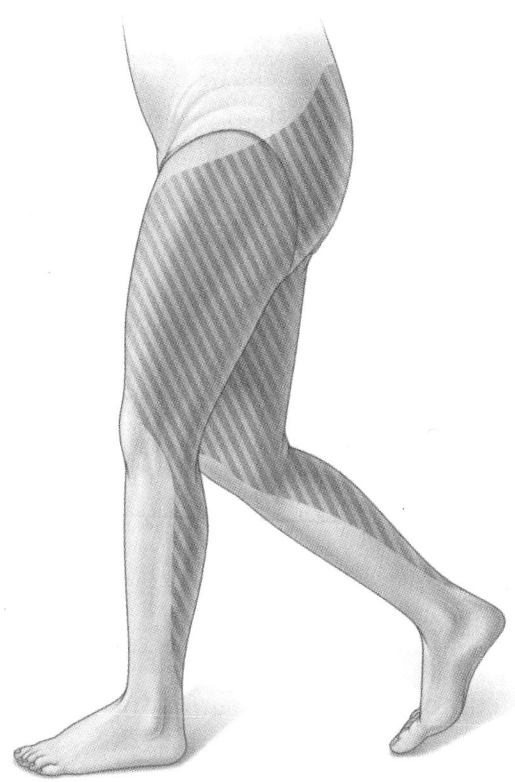

Peripheral artery disease of the legs most often causes pain in the shaded area.

The main symptom of peripheral artery disease is a tight aching or squeezing pain in the calf, foot, thigh, or buttock that you get when you exercise. This is called **intermittent claudication**. The pain usually goes away when you rest. As the disease gets worse, your leg may hurt even at rest. But not everyone has this symptom. Some people have numb or cold feet or toes, or sores that are slow to heal.

You may need to take medicines or have surgery to treat peripheral artery disease. There are things you can do at home to help with your symptoms.

Foot Care

Take good care of your feet and legs. If you have a blood flow problem, even a minor injury could lead to a serious infection. Good foot care is even more important if you also have diabetes or another problem that decreases feeling in your feet.

- Inspect your feet at least once a day. If you can't see well, have someone else check them for you. This will help you find problems early so they can be treated.
- Wash your feet every day, and use lotion on your feet to keep the skin from drying and cracking. Place cotton or lamb's wool between your toes to prevent rubbing and to absorb extra moisture. Before you put on shoes and socks, be sure to dry your feet well.
- Treat cuts and scrapes on your legs right away.
- Don't wear shoes that are too tight or that rub your feet. Shoes should feel good and fit well.
- Don't wear tight socks or stockings. These can make blood flow problems worse.
- If you have a sore on your leg or foot, keep it dry and cover it with a nonstick bandage until you can see your doctor.

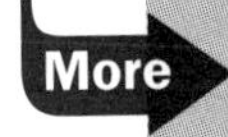

Home Treatment

- If you smoke, quit. This is the single most important step you can take. If you need help quitting, see page 351.
- Keep your blood pressure in a normal range. See page 183.
- Lower your cholesterol. See page 186.
- If you have diabetes, keep your blood sugar in a normal range. See page 296.
- Try to get some exercise every day. If your doctor approves, start a walking program. Each day, walk until the pain starts, then rest until it goes away. Try to walk a little farther each day. Don't try to walk through the pain. The goal is to increase the amount of time you can walk before the pain starts.
- Eat a heart-healthy diet. See page 289.
- Take good care of your feet. See Foot Care on page 209.

Pneumonia

When to Call a Doctor

- You have fever and a cough that brings up yellow, green, rust-colored, or bloody mucus from your lungs.
- You have new pain in your chest that gets worse when you take a deep breath or cough.
- You have had the flu or bronchitis, and you get worse instead of better (such as getting more short of breath).

Pneumonia is an infection of the lungs. It sometimes follows the flu or bronchitis. Having a lung disease, such as COPD, may make you more likely to get pneumonia.

Pneumonia is usually caused by bacteria, but it can be caused by viruses and other things too. A person who has bacterial pneumonia is usually very sick and may have:

- A bad cough that brings up yellow, green, rust-colored, or bloody mucus (sputum) from the lungs.
- A fever and shaking chills.
- Fast, shallow breathing.
- Pain in the chest muscles (chest-wall pain) that is worse when you cough or take a deep breath.
- A fast heartbeat.
- Tiredness that is worse than you would get from a cold.

Home Treatment

Pneumonia can be a very serious problem for older adults and people who have long-term health problems. They may need to be treated in the hospital.

If you are at home with pneumonia:

- Take any medicines your doctor prescribes.
- Drink extra fluids.
- Take acetaminophen (Tylenol), aspirin, or ibuprofen (Advil, Motrin) to reduce fever and pain.
- Get lots of rest. It takes time to get well.
- Have a family member or friend stop by or call you every day while you're sick to make sure you aren't getting worse.

Preventing Pneumonia

Pneumonia can be very serious, even deadly. Anyone can get it, but it is most common in older adults and people who have other health problems. Here's what you can do to reduce your risk:

- Get the pneumococcal vaccine if your doctor recommends it. This may help prevent severe illness. See page 320.
- Get a flu shot every year. Flu can lead to pneumonia. Ask those you live or work with to do the same, so they don't get the flu and pass it to you. See page 154.
- Wash your hands often, especially during cold and flu season.
- If you smoke, quit. This can help make your lungs healthier. If you need help quitting, see page 351.

Polymyalgia Rheumatica

When to Call a Doctor

- You have polymyalgia rheumatica, and you have a headache, jaw pain, or vision problems. These may be signs of a serious problem called temporal arteritis. See page 169.
- You take steroid medicines, and you have trouble with the side effects.

Polymyalgia rheumatica causes pain and stiffness in your joints and muscles, mainly in the hips, neck, and shoulders. The symptoms may be worse in the morning. It may also cause fever, weight loss, and fatigue. Polymyalgia rheumatica almost always affect people over 50, and most of them are women.

Some people who have polymyalgia rheumatica also get **temporal arteritis** (see page 169). Temporal arteritis is the more serious problem. It can cause severe headaches and lead to blindness or stroke if it is not treated.

Doctors prescribe steroid medicines to treat polymyalgia rheumatica. Most people need to take these medicines for 1 or 2 years to keep the problem from coming back.

Home Treatment

Long-term treatment with steroids can cause serious problems, such as high blood pressure and bone thinning (osteoporosis). You can take steps to prevent these problems.

- Take your medicine just the way your doctor tells you to. Do not stop or change your medicine without talking to your doctor first.
- Get some exercise every day. This will help keep your bones strong and can also lift your mood.
- Eat a healthy diet with lots of fresh fruits and vegetables, whole grains, and lean protein, such as fish. Limit salt, sugar, and alcohol. See page 333.
- Get plenty of calcium and vitamin D to keep your bones strong. Ask your doctor if you need to take supplements.
- Don't smoke, and avoid secondhand smoke. If you need help quitting, see page 351.

Pressure Sores

When to Call a Doctor

- There are signs of a pressure sore. Skin may be painful or tender and look red or dark like a bruise. Later, the skin may tear or break open and form an ulcer.
- There are signs of infection. These may include increased pain, swelling, redness, or warmth; red streaks leading from the sore; pus; or fever.

Pressure sores can happen if you lie in bed or sit for a long time. They are also called bedsores. They are caused by constant pressure against your skin. The pressure blocks the blood supply to your skin. This kills skin cells and creates a sore.

Pressure sores usually form over bony areas, such as the tailbone, hips, lower back, elbows, heels, and shoulders. They may also form on the back of the head, the backs of the ears, and between the knees.

The sores can become very deep and take a long time to heal. If a sore gets infected, you will need antibiotics to treat it.

Home Treatment

- Keep the sore clean and covered. Use lotion to keep the skin from drying and cracking. Ask your doctor what kind of cleanser and lotion to use.
- Keep the skin around the sore clean and dry.
- Change positions often to take weight off the area.
- Eat healthy foods, and make sure you get enough protein, which helps healing.

More

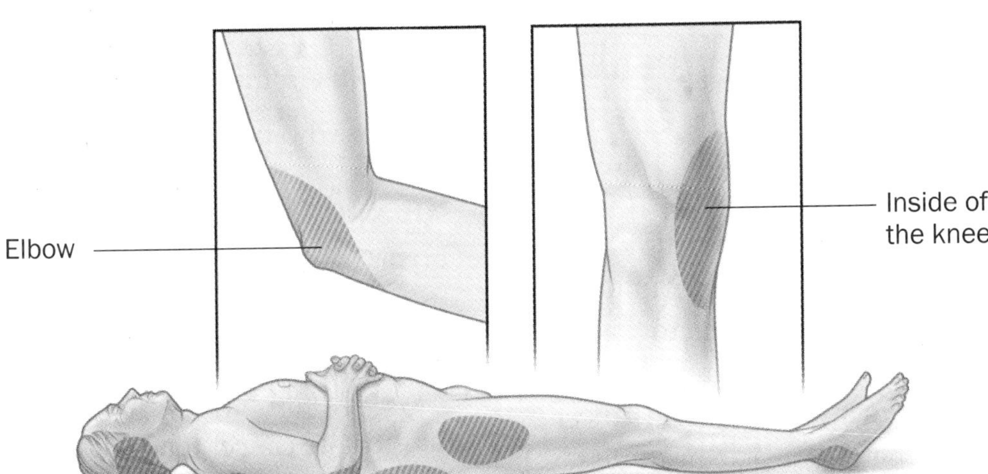

Shading shows areas where pressure sores often form.

Caregiver Tips for Preventing Pressure Sores

If you care for someone who has trouble moving:

- Help the person change positions every 1 to 2 hours.
- Put pillows or foam pads under bony areas when the person is sitting or lying down. Using a special mattress made to spread body weight evenly can also help.
- Check the person's skin every day for signs of pressure sores. They often start as red or dark spots that are tender or painful. Pay special attention to bony areas, such as the tailbone, hips, lower back, elbows, heels, shoulders, and the back of the head.

Prostate Cancer

When to Call a Doctor

- You have blood or pus in your urine.
- You have urinary problems that come on quickly, bother you enough that you want help, or last longer than 2 months. (Also see Prostate Enlargement on page 215.)
- You already have prostate problems, and you develop back or bone pain.

Prostate cancer is the second leading cause of cancer deaths in men. (See a picture of the prostate on page 218.) But it can often be cured if it is found early, before it has spread to other organs. Prostate cancer tends to grow slowly. Many older men with prostate cancer die of another cause (like heart disease) before the cancer has grown enough to cause problems.

Most men with prostate cancer have no symptoms. In a few cases, the cancer can cause urinary problems like those of prostate enlargement. See page 215. If it spreads to bones or other organs, it can cause pain and other symptoms.

Any man can get prostate cancer. But the risk is highest for:

- Older men. Most men who get prostate cancer are over 65.
- Black men.
- Men who have a family history of prostate cancer.
- Men who eat a high-fat diet.

Should You Be Treated?

If you have prostate cancer, here are a few things you should know:

- You may not die any sooner than you would have without the cancer. Prostate cancer tends to occur later in life and usually grows slowly.

- If the cancer does not cause symptoms, it may not affect your quality of life.
- The younger you are and the larger or more advanced the cancer is, the more serious the disease may be.
- Treatment can be painful and can cause lasting problems with bladder control or erections.

Learn all you can about your treatment options—which may include not treating the cancer. You need to consider your age, your health, and the nature of the cancer itself when you make treatment decisions. For example, if you are older and the cancer is not growing much, it may make sense to take a wait-and-see approach.

To help decide what approach you want to take, go to the Web site on the back cover and enter **X212** in the search box. Your doctor can help you with the decision.

Should You Be Tested?

Doctors can use one of two simple tests to look for prostate cancer:

- Digital rectal exam, in which the doctor puts a gloved finger in your rectum and feels the prostate
- PSA blood test

Many experts are not sure that routine testing is right for men without symptoms. Finding prostate cancer early can save lives in some cases. But for men who are older and do not have symptoms, knowing they have prostate cancer may not extend or improve their lives.

Think about whether testing is right for you. For help, go to the Web site on the back cover and enter **T530** in the search box. Then talk to your doctor.

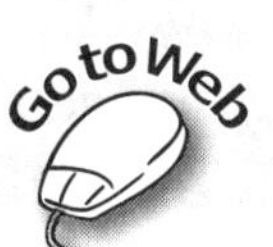

Prostate Enlargement

When to Call a Doctor

- You cannot urinate at all.
- You feel like you cannot empty your bladder completely.
- You have urinary problems along with a fever, chills, vomiting, or pain in your back or belly.
- It hurts or burns when you urinate.
- There is blood or pus in your urine.
- You have new or worse urinary problems after you start a new medicine.

More

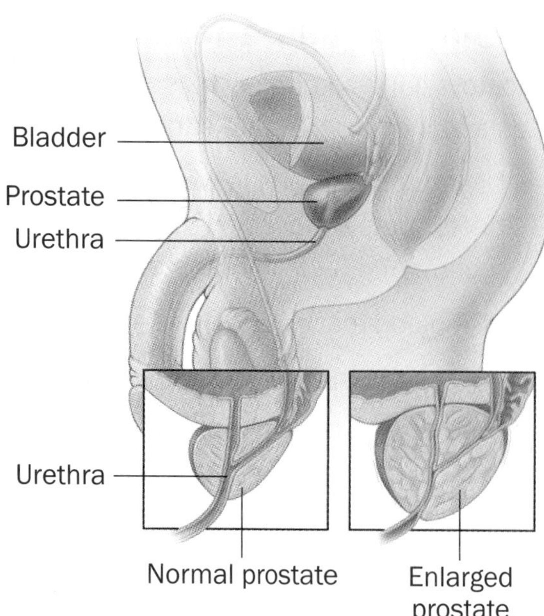

As the prostate gets bigger, it may squeeze the urethra.

As a man ages, his prostate gland may get bigger. This is called **benign prostatic hyperplasia**, or **BPH**. As the gland gets bigger, it may squeeze or partly block the urethra (the tube that carries urine out of the body). This can cause problems with urine flow, such as:

- Trouble getting the urine stream started or fully stopped. This may cause dribbling. (But dribbling is very common. It may not mean you have BPH.)
- Needing to urinate more often, especially at night.
- A weak urine stream.
- Feeling like you can't empty your bladder all the way.

BPH is not serious unless you have a lot of trouble urinating or unless backed-up urine causes bladder or kidney problems.

Many men find that they can manage their symptoms with self-care. Sometimes symptoms clear up on their own. In these cases, the best treatment may be no treatment at all.

The main factor in deciding if and how to treat your symptoms is how much the symptoms bother you. To take a quiz that scores your symptoms for you, go to the Web site on the back cover and enter **C155** in the search box.

Some men decide to try medicine that can help with symptoms. For help deciding whether medicine is right for you, go to the Web site on the back cover and enter **K106** in the search box. Then talk to your doctor.

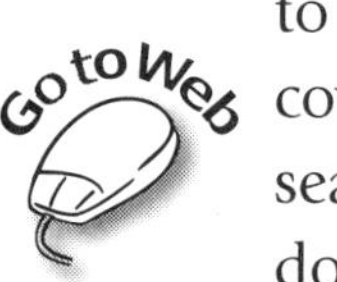

Surgery may also be an option. To help you decide if surgery is a good choice for you, go to the Web site on the back cover and enter **N852** in the search box.

Home Treatment

- Avoid allergy and cold medicines (antihistamines, decongestants, and nasal sprays). They can make urinary problems worse.
- If having to get up at night to urinate bothers you, cut down on fluids before bed, especially those with alcohol or caffeine. But drink plenty of water and other fluids during the day.
- Take plenty of time to urinate. Turn on a faucet, or picture running water. Some men find this helps. Read or think of other things while you wait.

- Sit on the toilet to urinate.
- Try "double voiding." Urinate as much as you can, relax for a few moments, and then try again.
- Herbal products such as saw palmetto help some men with BPH. Talk to your doctor before you take this or any herbal product. See Vitamins, Herbs, and Other Supplements on page 370.

The tips in Bladder Control on page 93 may also help.

Prostatitis

When to Call a Doctor

- You have urinary problems along with fever, chills, vomiting, or pain in your back or belly.
- Your urine is bloody, red, or pink for no clear reason (see page 65).
- Pelvic pain or urinary problems last more than 5 days, even with home treatment.
- Pelvic pain or urinary problems suddenly change or get worse.
- It hurts when you urinate, ejaculate, or pass stool.
- There is an unusual discharge from your penis. Also see Sexually Transmitted Diseases on page 222.

Prostatitis is any painful infection or inflammation of the prostate. If you have this problem:

- You may often feel the urge to urinate but can pass only a little urine each time.
- It may burn when you urinate.
- You may feel like you can't empty your bladder all the way.
- You may have trouble starting to urinate or have a weak urine flow.
- You may have to urinate often at night.
- You may have pelvic pain. You may feel it in your lower back or belly, your scrotum, the area between your scrotum and anus, your upper thighs, or the pubic area.
- It may hurt when you ejaculate.

A prostate infection caused by bacteria usually gets better with home treatment and antibiotics. If the infection comes back, you may need to take more antibiotics.

But most men with prostatitis do not have a bacterial infection. In these cases, home treatment tends to be the best approach.

More

Home Treatment

- Avoid alcohol, caffeine, and spicy foods. They may make your symptoms worse.
- Take hot baths to help soothe pain and reduce stress.
- Eat plenty of high-fiber foods, and drink plenty of water. This will help you avoid constipation. Straining to have a bowel movement can hurt a lot when you have prostatitis.
- Take ibuprofen (Advil, Motrin), naproxen (Aleve), or acetaminophen (Tylenol) for pain.
- If your doctor gives you antibiotics for a prostate infection, take them as you are told.

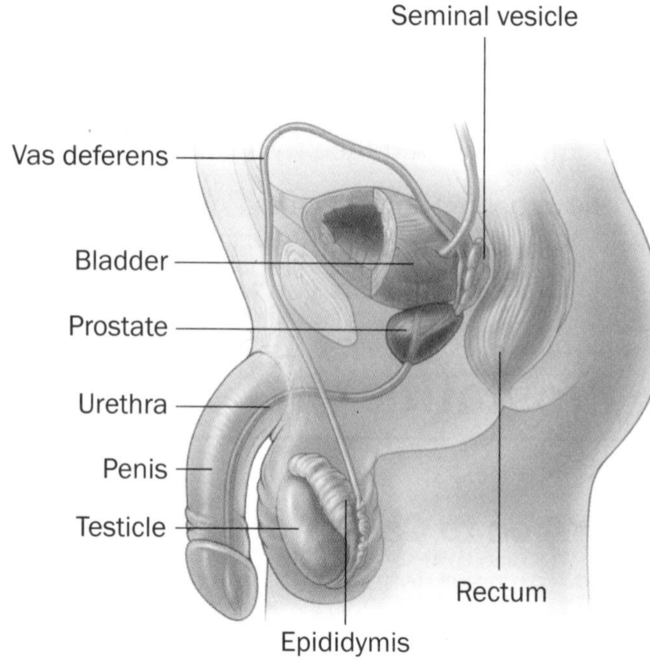

Male pelvic organs
(the prostate is just under the bladder)

Rashes

When to Call a Doctor

- You have a rash that develops quickly and looks like bruises or tiny purple or red blood spots under the skin. You may have a serious illness. See page 151.
- You have a rash with signs of infection. These may include increased pain, redness, swelling, or warmth; red streaks leading from the rash; pus; or fever.
- You get a rash after being bitten by a tick. See page 14.
- You get a rash after you start a new medicine.
- You have a rash with fever and joint pain.
- A rash occurs with a sore throat. Scarlet fever is a rash you may get because of strep throat. Like strep throat, scarlet fever is treated with antibiotics.
- You are not sure what's causing a rash.
- A rash does not clear up after 2 to 3 weeks of home treatment.

Rashes can be caused by lots of things—illness, allergy, bacteria, heat, and stress, to name a few.

When you first get a rash, ask yourself these questions to help find the cause:

- Do you have a rash in an area that came in contact with something new? This could be a plant, soap, detergent, shampoo, perfume, makeup, lotion, jewelry, fabric, a new tool, an appliance, or latex gloves. Any of these could irritate your skin.
- Have you eaten anything new that you may be allergic to?
- Are you taking any new medicines?
- Have you been more stressed or upset than usual?
- Have you been sick?
- Is the rash spreading?
- Does it itch?

Also see the Skin Problems chart on page 61.

Intertrigo (Chafing)

Intertrigo is a rash that occurs in skin folds because of rubbing, warmth, and moisture. It is important to treat the rash so it doesn't get infected.

It may help to lose weight or change positions often. Keep the area clean and dry, and leave the rash open to the air.

Seborrheic Dermatitis

Seborrheic dermatitis is a common type of rash in older adults. It causes reddish yellow, scaly patches on oily areas, such as the scalp, forehead, sides of the nose, eyebrows, behind the ears, or center of the chest.

Dandruff shampoo may work well for seborrheic dermatitis on your scalp. For other areas, try a nonprescription hydrocortisone cream.

Poison Ivy, Oak, and Sumac

The leaves of poison ivy, oak, and sumac have an oil that many people are allergic to. If you touch the leaves or the oil, you may get a red, blistered, and very itchy rash. The rash often appears in lines where the leaves brushed against the skin.

You may be able to prevent or reduce the rash if you act fast.

- Wash your skin with rubbing alcohol or lots of water within 10 to 15 minutes to get the oil off your skin.
- Use soap only after using lots of water.
- Wash your clothes, your dog, or anything else that may have touched the plant.

If you get a rash anyway, follow the tips in Home Treatment.

More

Home Treatment

- Wash the area with water. Soap may irritate the rash. Pat dry.
- Use cold, wet cloths to reduce itching. Also see Relief From Itching on page 134.
- Keep cool, and stay out of the sun.
- Leave the rash open to the air. Baby powder can help keep it dry.
- If you have a plant rash, calamine lotion may help. Use it 3 or 4 times a day. A mild lotion like Cetaphil may soothe some rashes.
- For itching, try nonprescription antihistamine pills. Some types, such as Claritin and Alavert, won't make you sleepy.
- Use hydrocortisone cream to provide short-term relief from itching. Do not use it on the face or the genital area.
- Do not use products that have caused a rash in the past, such as detergents, skin-care products, makeup, clothing, or jewelry.
- Use fragrance-free or hypoallergenic soaps, detergents, lotions, and makeup if you often have rashes.

Cellulitis

Cellulitis is a skin infection that happens when bacteria enter a break in the skin and spread to deeper tissues. At first, the infected area will be warm, red, swollen, and tender. As the infection spreads, you may have a fever, chills, and swollen lymph nodes.

If you have any of the symptoms of cellulitis, you need to see a doctor right away. If it is not treated with antibiotics, the infection can spread to the blood or lymph nodes. This can be deadly.

Some people get cellulitis without having a break in the skin. These include older adults and people who have diabetes or a weak immune system. These people are also more likely to have dangerous problems from cellulitis, such as blood poisoning. And they are more likely to get cellulitis again.

If you are at risk for cellulitis, you can take steps to help prevent it.

- Take good care of your skin. Keep it clean, and use lotion to prevent drying and cracking.
- Check your feet and legs often. This is especially important if you have diabetes.
- Treat any skin infection, such as athlete's foot, right away.
- Ask your doctor if you need to take antibiotics on a regular basis to prevent cellulitis.

Rosacea

When to Call a Doctor

- You think you may have rosacea because you often have red patches or tiny red lines on your face or other symptoms.
- You have rosacea, and the redness, pimples, and eye irritation get worse even with treatment.

Rosacea is a long-term skin problem that causes:

- Red patches, tiny red lines, and small pimples on the face. You may think you have acne.
- Burning and soreness in the eyes or eyelids. Rosacea can lead to more serious eye problems if you do not treat it.
- Large bumps on the nose and face in severe cases.

You are more likely to get rosacea if you have fair skin and blush easily or if your face stays red and flushed longer than most people's. The problem tends to run in families.

The sooner you start to treat rosacea, the better. If it stays mild, you may be able to control it well. Prescription medicines may help if home treatment is not enough.

Home Treatment

- Find out what makes your redness and pimples worse, and try to avoid those things. They may include:
  - Very cold or hot weather. In winter, wear a hat and scarf to shield your face from cold and wind. Use a face moisturizer.
  - Stress. Eat a healthy diet, and get plenty of exercise and sleep.
  - Alcohol, spicy foods, or very hot drinks.
  - Getting too hot when you exercise. Try working out for a shorter time. In the summer, exercise during the cool morning hours or in an air-conditioned gym.
  - Hot showers. Take warm or cool ones instead. Don't use hot tubs or saunas.
- Always wear sunscreen on exposed skin.
- Use soaps, lotions, and makeup made for sensitive skin that don't contain alcohol, are not abrasive, and won't clog pores.
- If you have rosacea on your eyelids, gently wash your eyelids with a product made for the eyes. Use artificial tears if your eyes feel dry.
- Talk to your doctor about antibiotic creams and other medicines that can help with pimples and redness. In advanced cases, laser treatment can reduce redness.

Sexually Transmitted Diseases (STDs)

When to Call a Doctor

All sexually transmitted diseases (STDs) need to be diagnosed and treated. Your doctor or a health professional at your local health department can help with testing and treatment.

Call your doctor if:

- You think you may have been exposed to an STD. Your sex partner(s) may also need to be treated, even if they have no symptoms. Without treatment, you and your partner(s) may reinfect each other or have serious problems.
- You have any unusual discharge from your vagina or penis, burning when you urinate, or any sores, redness, or growths on your genitals.
- You or your partner(s) have done things that put you at risk for HIV. See page 224.
- You have symptoms such as fatigue, weight loss, fever, diarrhea, cough, or swollen lymph nodes that do not go away after a short time and do not seem to be related to any illness.

Sexually transmitted diseases, also called STDs, are infections passed from person to person through sex, genital contact, and contact with body fluids such as semen, vaginal fluids, and blood (including menstrual blood). Some of these infections can also be spread by sharing drug needles, razors, and other items that may have infected blood or fluids on them.

You can get an STD from any kind of sexual contact. This includes:

- Vaginal sex.
- Anal sex.
- Oral sex.

Preventing STDs is a lot easier than treating them or living with them. To learn how to protect yourself, see Safe Sex on page 363.

Some of the most common STDs are described in the chart on page 223. If you think you may have been exposed to any of them, use the chart to check your symptoms and learn more.

HIV: Should You Get Tested?

HIV (human immunodeficiency virus) is a virus that attacks your immune system. This makes it hard for your body to fight infection and disease. AIDS is the last and most severe stage of HIV infection.

Sexually Transmitted Diseases			
Symptoms	**Disease**	**Treatment**	**Other Concerns**
Discharge from vagina or penis; pain or burning when you urinate; for women, pain and bleeding during or after sex	**Chlamydia, gonorrhea, or trichomoniasis**	Antibiotics for all partners. Do not have sex until you and your partner(s) have finished treatment and have no symptoms.	If not treated, can lead to pelvic inflammatory disease. Gonorrhea can spread to joints, causing arthritis.
Red, painless sore in genital or rectal area or on mouth about 3 weeks after exposure Two months later: Rash, patchy hair loss, fever, flu-like symptoms	**Syphilis**	Antibiotics for all partners. Do not have sex until you and your partner(s) have finished treatment and have no symptoms.	If not treated, can cause serious health problems and death.
Painful sores or blisters in genital or anal area 2 to 7 days after exposure; fever, swollen lymph nodes, headache, and muscle aches	**Genital herpes**	No cure. Medicine can reduce pain and speed healing during an outbreak.	Those with frequent or severe outbreaks may take medicine daily to help prevent them. Couples should avoid sex during an outbreak.
Small, fleshy bumps or flat, white patches in genital or anal area	**Genital warts caused by HPV (human papillomavirus)**	No cure for HPV. Warts can be removed but may return. Infection may go away on its own.	HPV can increase a woman's risk for cervical cancer.
Yellowing of skin and whites of eyes; flu-like symptoms; steady pain in upper right belly, under rib cage; diarrhea or constipation; muscle aches and joint pain; skin rash	**Hepatitis B virus**	No treatment for short-term (acute) hepatitis; most people get better in 6 to 8 weeks. Medicine for long-term (chronic) hepatitis, but no cure.	Can become chronic and lead to liver damage or cancer. If you are at risk for hepatitis B, get the vaccine.

More

Sexually Transmitted Diseases			
Symptoms	**Disease**	**Treatment**	**Other Concerns**
Flu-like symptoms soon after infection; then no symptoms for years until disease progresses	**HIV (human immunodeficiency virus)**	No cure, but medicine can slow the disease and prolong life.	Weakens immune system. Without treatment, can lead to AIDS and death.

But having HIV does not mean you have AIDS. If HIV is found before it becomes AIDS, medicines can slow or stop the damage to your immune system. So if you could be infected, it is very important to find out.

Are You at Risk?

All kinds of people get HIV—all ages, men and women, gay and straight, all races. HIV spreads through contact with body fluids such as semen, vaginal fluids, and blood (including menstrual blood). Acts that increase your risk include:

- Having more than one sex partner.
- Having unprotected sex. Unprotected sex means having sex without properly using a condom. This is especially risky if you are a man who has sex with men, but it is a risk for everyone. Sex without condoms is not safe unless both you and your partner are sure that neither of you has HIV and that neither of you is having sex with anyone else.
- Sharing needles or other drug supplies with someone who is HIV-positive.
- Having sex with someone who does any of the above.

You will not get HIV from touching, hugging, or lightly kissing someone who is HIV-positive. HIV is *not* spread by mosquitoes, toilet seats, donating blood, or being touched or coughed on by someone who is HIV-positive or who has AIDS.

Getting Tested

If you do things that put you at risk for HIV infection, be sure to have an HIV test every 6 months. Here's why:

- Medicine for HIV can help delay or prevent AIDS and helps you live longer and better. If you have HIV, the sooner you find out and start getting checked, the better your chances of staying healthy. Regular checks of your immune system will help you and your doctor know when you need to start medicine.
- A blood test is the only way to know if you have HIV. You may not feel sick or notice any symptoms for years. But inside your body, the virus is growing.
- If you have HIV and don't know it, you may spread the disease to others.

All it takes is a simple, cheap blood test. The test checks for HIV antibodies in your blood. If HIV antibodies are found, you are considered HIV-positive. If HIV antibodies are not found, you may need to be tested again. This is to make sure that HIV antibodies don't appear at a later time. It can take up to 6 months after you are first exposed to HIV for antibodies to appear.

You can have the test in your doctor's office or at your local health department.

If you find out you are HIV-positive, work with your doctor to get the right treatment and stay as healthy as you can. Many people with HIV are able to live long and active lives.

If you need help dealing with HIV or AIDS, or if you just want to learn more, call the CDC-INFO hotline at 1-800-232-4636.

Shingles

When to Call a Doctor

If you think you have shingles, call your doctor. There is medicine that can limit the pain and rash and help prevent serious problems. It works best if you start it as soon as symptoms appear.

Also call your doctor if you have shingles and:

- You have a headache, stiff neck, or hearing loss, or you feel weak, dizzy, or confused. These may be signs of a serious illness. See page 151.
- Pain, rash, or other symptoms of shingles affect your forehead, nose, or eyes, or your vision is affected.
- You have pain or loss of movement in your face.
- Sores have spread beyond the area where the rash started.
- You have signs of infection. These may include increased pain, redness, swelling, or warmth; red streaks leading from the rash; pus; or fever.
- You can't control itching.
- The rash has not healed after 2 to 4 weeks.

More

Shingles is caused by the same virus that causes chickenpox. If you have ever had chickenpox, you still have the virus in your body. If the virus becomes active again, years after the original illness, it is called shingles.

Shingles usually affects one or two of the large nerves that spread outward from the spine. This causes pain and usually a rash in a band around one side of the chest, belly, or face. The rash will blister and scab, then clear up over the course of a few weeks.

You can't get shingles from someone who has it. But a person who has not had chickenpox can get chickenpox from being exposed to someone with shingles.

About half of people over 60 who get shingles have pain in the affected nerve for months or sometimes years. This is called post-herpetic neuralgia. Taking medicine for shingles within 2 days of getting the rash may help prevent this problem.

Preventing Shingles

Anyone who has had chickenpox can get shingles. If you are 60 or older, ask your doctor about the shingles vaccine. One shot can help prevent shingles or reduce the pain it causes.

Home Treatment

- Try not to pick at or scratch the blisters. This will cause scars. The blisters will crust over and fall off on their own if you leave them alone.
- Use cool, wet cloths to relieve pain and itching. You can also use calamine lotion. Try not to use so much lotion that it cakes and is hard to remove.
- Put cornstarch or baking soda on the sores to help dry them out so they heal faster. Do not use thick ointment, such as petroleum jelly, on the sores. Ointment will keep them from drying and healing.
- After the sores have formed crusts, soak them with tap water or Burow's solution. This can help decrease oozing and dry and soothe the skin. (You can buy Burow's solution in most drugstores and supermarkets.)
- Take acetaminophen (Tylenol), ibuprofen (Advil, Motrin), or naproxen (Aleve) to relieve pain.
- Avoid close contact with people until the blisters have healed. It is very important to avoid contact with those who have not had chickenpox, especially pregnant women, young babies, and anyone who has a hard time fighting infection (such as people with HIV, diabetes, or cancer).

Sinusitis

When to Call a Doctor

- Cold symptoms last longer than 10 to 14 days or get worse after the first 7 days.
- You have a severe headache that is different from a "normal" headache, and nonprescription medicines don't help.
- You have swelling or redness in your face, or your vision changes or gets blurry.
- Nasal discharge changes from clear to yellow or green after 5 to 7 days of a cold, and pain and fever get worse. If nasal discharge is colored from the start of a cold, call if it lasts longer than 7 to 10 days.
- You have face pain (especially in one sinus area or along the ridge between the nose and lower eyelid) or pain in your teeth after 2 days of home treatment.
- You have finished your antibiotics and still have symptoms.

Sinusitis is an inflammation or infection of the sinuses and nasal passages. The sinuses become blocked, which causes pain and pressure in the face.

Sinusitis most often follows a cold. Sinus problems can also be related to allergies, an infected tooth, air pollution, and other things.

Is It Sinusitis or a Cold?

Colds and sinusitis have some of the same symptoms, like a stuffy nose and cough.

But if you have a sinus problem, you may also have:

- Pain over your cheekbones and upper teeth.
- Pain in your forehead over your eyebrows.
- Pain around or behind your eyes.

Along with the pain, you may have a headache, swelling around your eyes, a fever, or mucus draining down your throat. Face pain and these other symptoms are not likely with just a cold.

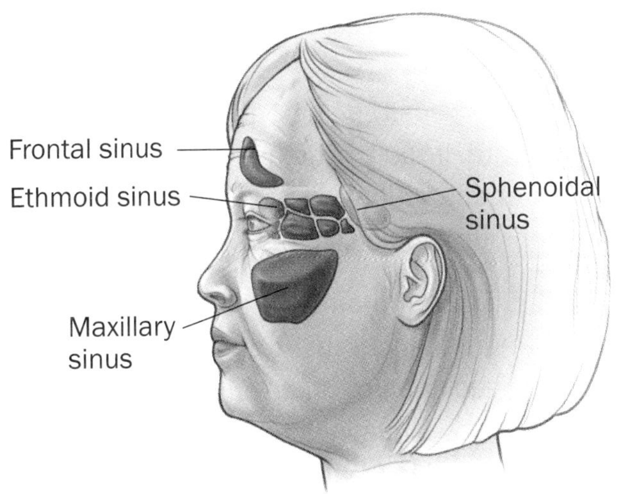

The sinuses are hollow spaces in the head.

More

What About Antibiotics?

There are good reasons not to use antibiotics unless you really need them:

- Antibiotics can cost a lot.
- You will probably have to see the doctor to get a prescription. This costs you time and money.
- Antibiotics can have harmful side effects, such as diarrhea, vomiting, and skin rashes.
- The most important reason of all: If you take antibiotics when you don't need them, they may not work when you do need them. Each time you take antibiotics, you are more likely to carry some bacteria that were not killed by the medicine. Over time, these bacteria get tougher and can cause longer and more serious infections. To treat them, you may need different, stronger, and more costly antibiotics.

Do you need antibiotics for sinusitis?

Sinusitis usually gets better with good self-care. If you try the tips in Home Treatment, you may be able to avoid antibiotics and a trip to the doctor.

But if your symptoms are severe or last more than 10 to 14 days, you may need antibiotics. If you do not treat a bad sinus infection or it does not respond to treatment, it can lead to long-term sinus problems that are harder to treat.

Home Treatment

- Drink plenty of water and other fluids.
- Put a warm, damp towel or gel pack on your face several times a day for 5 to 10 minutes at a time.
- Breathe warm, moist air from a steamy shower, a hot bath, or a sink filled with hot water.
- Use a humidifier in your home, or at least in your bedroom. Avoid cold, dry air.
- Take aspirin, acetaminophen (Tylenol), or ibuprofen (Advil, Motrin) to relieve face pain and headache.
- Use decongestant pills or a decongestant nasal spray. Do not use a nasal decongestant spray for more than 3 days in a row.
- Do not take antihistamines unless your symptoms may also be caused by allergies.
- Do not smoke, and avoid other people's smoke.
- If you see streaks of mucus in the back of your throat, gargle with warm water.
- Blow your nose gently. Do not block one nostril when you blow your nose.
- Use a saltwater (saline) wash to help clear out mucus and bacteria. You can use nonprescription saline nose drops or a homemade saltwater mix. Try the recipe in Saline Nose Drops on page 229.

- Use a bulb syringe to gently squirt the liquid into your nose. Or snuff it from the palm of your hand, one nostril at a time.
- Blow your nose gently when you are done.
- Repeat 2 to 4 times a day.

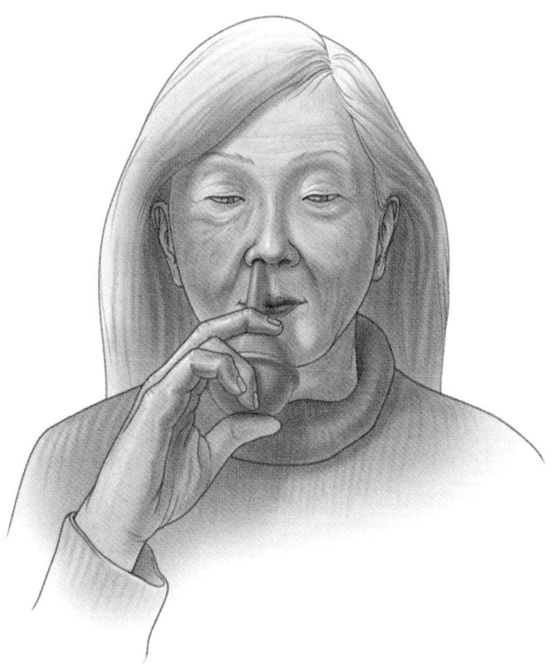

Using a bulb syringe

Saline Nose Drops

Nonprescription saline nasal sprays, such as NaSal and Ocean, are cheap and easy to use. They will keep nasal tissues moist and help clean out mucus and bacteria. Unlike other kinds of nasal sprays, they don't cause swelling inside the nose.

You can also make saline nose drops at home. Mix 1/4 teaspoon of salt with 1 cup of warm water. Store it in a clean bottle with a dropper. After 3 days, throw out the mix and make a fresh one.

Skin Cancer

When to Call a Doctor

- A mole is itchy, tender, or painful.
- A mole starts to get bigger or changes color or shape.
- A mole scales, oozes, or bleeds, or its color spreads into nearby skin.
- You find a new bump or nodule on a mole or any change in how the mole looks.
- You have a sore that does not heal.
- A skin growth looks odd or irritated.

If your moles do not change over time, you probably don't need to worry about them.

If a family member has had melanoma skin cancer, let your doctor know. You are at greater risk.

Skin cancer is the most common type of cancer. Most skin cancer is caused by sun damage, so it tends to occur on areas that get the most sun, such as the face, neck, and arms. People with light skin and blue eyes are more likely to get skin cancer. People with dark skin have less risk.

You are more likely to get skin cancer if you spend a lot of time in the sun or under sunlamps or you have had severe sunburns. Sun damage from earlier years is often the cause of skin cancer later in life.

Most skin cancers are **nonmelanoma** skin cancers. These include basal cell and squamous cell carcinomas. Nonmelanoma skin cancer is rarely life-threatening. But it is still best to find and treat it promptly. It is usually easy to treat.

Melanoma is a more serious type of skin cancer. It may affect only the skin, or it may spread to other organs and bones. Melanoma can be deadly if it is not found and treated early. In most cases it can be cured if the cancer is removed while it is still in the top layer of skin.

Watch for Skin Changes

Once a month, check all areas of your skin with a mirror (or have someone help you). Look for odd moles, spots, bumps, or sores that will not heal. Pay extra attention to areas that get a lot of sun, like your hands, arms, back, chest, back of the neck, face, and ears. Report any changes to your doctor.

Skin cancers differ from other skin growths in these ways:

- They tend to bleed more and are often open sores that do not heal.
- They tend to grow slowly. But melanoma may appear suddenly and grow quickly.

Also watch for any of these **ABCD changes** in a mole or other growth:

- **A**symmetry: One half does not match the other half.
- **B**order: The edges are ragged, notched, or blurred.
- **C**olor: The mole changes color, has shades of red and black, or has a red, white, and blue blotchy appearance.
- **D**iameter (size): A mole grows larger than a pencil eraser.

NCI Visuals Online. Skin Cancer Foundation.

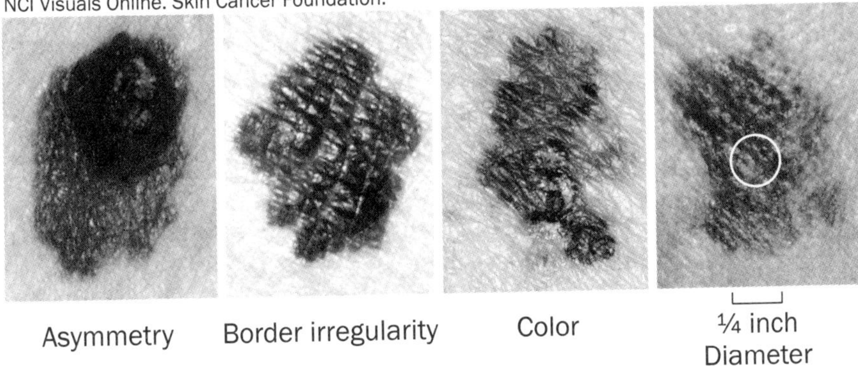

Watch for these "ABCD" mole changes.

Skin Growths and Spots

When to Call a Doctor

- A skin growth changes in size, shape, texture, or color.
- A sore lasts 4 weeks or longer without healing.
- A skin growth bleeds or breaks off.
- A skin growth gets irritated over and over when you shave or when clothing rubs on it.
- You have any signs of skin cancer. See page 230.

Most skin growths and spots are harmless. They often stay the same or even go away on their own. You can have them removed if they bother you.

Seborrheic keratoses are flat-topped, waxy-looking growths that appear on the scalp, face, neck, and body. They may look as if you could easily pick them off the skin. They are usually light brown at first and may get darker over time.

Age spots are dark spots that appear on skin that has been exposed to the sun for many years. They are sometimes called liver spots, but they have nothing to do with your liver.

Cherry angiomas, or ruby spots, are small, reddish purple spots most often found on the body and upper legs. They may also be on the face, neck, scalp, and arms.

More

Skin tags are small, fleshy growths of skin that appear on the face, neck, chest, underarms, and groin.

Sebaceous gland growths are small, yellowish bumps that appear on the forehead and face.

Actinic Keratoses

This type of growth should be watched. Actinic keratoses are small red or yellow-brown patches with a crusted, scaly surface. They are caused by spending too much time in the sun. If you protect them from the sun, the patches may grow smaller and disappear.

Actinic keratoses are not cancer, but if they continue to get sun, they can turn into skin cancer. If you find these spots on your skin, have your doctor check them. They can be treated to keep them from turning into cancer.

Home Treatment

- Wear a long-sleeved shirt, long pants, and a hat with a wide brim when you are outdoors.
- Use a sunscreen that has an SPF of 30 or higher.

Sleep Problems

When to Call a Doctor

- You regularly take sleeping pills and cannot stop taking them.
- You think a medicine or a health problem is causing sleep problems.
- You or your partner snores loudly and often feels extremely sleepy during the day.
- You or your partner often stops breathing, gasps, and chokes during sleep.
- You often wake up because your legs move or get cramps.
- A full month of self-care does not solve your sleep problem.

Insomnia can mean:

- Having trouble getting to sleep (taking more than 45 minutes to fall asleep).
- Waking up often and not being able to fall back asleep.
- Waking up too early in the morning when you don't want to.

None of these are problems unless you feel tired a lot of the time or you fall asleep at the wrong times, like when you're eating or driving. If you are less sleepy at night, or if you wake up early in the morning but still feel rested and alert, there is little need to worry.

Short-term insomnia, lasting from a few nights to a few weeks, is usually caused by worry or stress. Long-term insomnia, which can last months or even years, is often caused by frequent or constant anxiety, medicines, long-term pain, depression, or other health problems.

Sleep apnea is a problem usually caused by a blockage in your airways. When airflow through your nose and mouth is blocked, you repeatedly stop breathing for 10 to 15 seconds or longer while you sleep. People who have sleep apnea often snore loudly and are very tired during the day. They are not aware of waking up at night, but they do have very restless sleep.

Changing some of your pre-bedtime habits may help cure mild insomnia or sleep apnea. More severe insomnia or sleep apnea may need medical treatment.

Sleep patterns change as you get older, and many older adults sleep less than or not as deeply as younger adults. But not sleeping well is not normal, no matter what your age. If you are having trouble sleeping and it is a problem for you, tell your doctor at your next checkup.

Tips for Better Sleep

Try this seven-step approach for 2 weeks:

1. Do relaxing activities in the evening. Read (but not in bed). Take a warm bath. Or do some slow, easy stretches.
2. Use your bed for sleeping and sex only. Do not eat, watch TV, read, or work in bed.
3. Sleep only at bedtime. Do not take naps, especially in the late afternoon or evening.
4. Go to bed only when you feel sleepy.
5. If you lie awake for more than 15 minutes, get up, leave the room, and do something relaxing.
6. Repeat steps 4 and 5 until it is time to get up.
7. Get up at the same time every day, even on weekends.

These tips also may help:

- Review all your prescription and nonprescription medicines with a pharmacist to rule out side effects that upset your sleep.
- Keep your bedroom dark, quiet, and cool. Try using a sleep mask and earplugs. Or try a noise machine that makes relaxing sounds like waterfalls or the ocean.
- Get regular exercise. But don't do a hard workout within 2 hours of going to bed.
- Avoid alcohol and smoking before bedtime. Limit caffeine, and don't have it at all after noon.
- Avoid foods that upset your stomach.
- Drink a glass of warm milk at bedtime. But don't drink more than one glass of fluid before you go to bed, or you may have to get up in the night to go to the bathroom.

You may want to read about anxiety on page 77 or depression on page 146. Either problem can upset your sleep.

More

Snoring

Lots of adults snore. Snoring is caused by blockage of the airways in the back of the mouth and nose. The airways can be blocked for many reasons, such as excess neck tissue or a stuffy nose caused by allergies or a cold. Some people who snore have sleep apnea.

Snoring can disrupt your sleep patterns, which may leave you sleepy and less alert during the day. It can also disrupt the sleep of family members or roommates.

Tips for people who snore

- Exercise each day to stay at a healthy weight and improve muscle tone. But don't exercise within 2 hours of bedtime (it may make it harder to fall asleep).
- Avoid heavy meals, alcohol, sleeping pills, and antihistamines before bedtime.
- Try to sleep on your side instead of your back. (Sew a pocket onto the back of your pajama top, and put a tennis ball in the pocket. This will keep you off your back.)
- Go to bed at the same time every night, even on weekends.
- Let a bedmate or roommate who does not snore fall asleep first.

If snoring is a problem for you or affects your household, see a doctor. You may need an exam of your nose, mouth, and neck.

Treatment will depend on what is making you snore. Your doctor may want to do a sleep study to see if sleep apnea is one of the reasons why you snore. For help deciding if you want

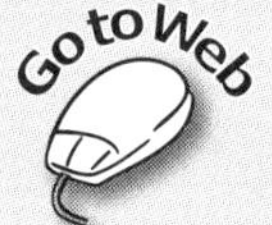

this kind of testing, go to the Web site on the back cover and enter **J109** in the search box.

What About Sleeping Pills?

Prescription and nonprescription sleep medicines may give you fast relief from insomnia. But it's best to use these only for a short time and to stop taking them as soon as you can. Here's why:

- They can cause daytime confusion, memory loss, and dizziness.
- You can get addicted to some of them.
- They may not mix well with other medicines you take.

Continued use of sleeping pills actually makes sleep problems worse in many people. If you want to try sleeping pills, check with your doctor first, and don't take them for long. For help deciding if sleeping pills might help you, go to

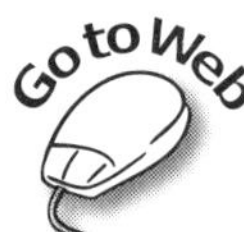

the Web site on the back cover and enter **B686** in the search box.

Sore Throat

When to Call a Doctor

- You have trouble breathing or swallowing because of a sore throat, or you drool a lot because you cannot swallow.
- You have a sore throat with at least 2 of these 3 symptoms of strep throat:
  - Fever of 101 °F or higher
  - White or yellow coating on the tonsils
  - Swollen lymph nodes in the neck, armpits, or groin (see the picture on page 237)
- You get a severe sore throat after being exposed to someone with strep throat.
- A rash occurs with a sore throat. Scarlet fever is a rash you may get because of strep throat. Like strep throat, scarlet fever is treated with antibiotics.
- You have a sore throat that's not related to a cold, allergies, smoking, overuse of your voice, or any other clear reason.
- Any sore throat lasts longer than 2 weeks.

Most sore throats are minor and go away with home treatment. You may get a sore throat because of:

- A cold or other virus.
- Smoking, air pollution, or dry air.
- Yelling.
- Breathing through your mouth when you sleep. People who have stuffy noses from allergies or colds often do this.
- Backflow (reflux) of stomach acid into the throat. If you think this may be the cause of your throat pain, see Heartburn on page 176.

Strep Throat

Strep throat is a sore throat caused by streptococcal bacteria. It is much more common in children than in adults, but anyone can get it. You can get strep throat even if you have had your tonsils taken out.

Most sore throats are not strep throat. The more you feel like you have a cold, the less likely it is that you have strep. Strep throat causes some or all of these symptoms:

- Severe and sudden sore throat
- Fever of 101 °F or higher
- Swollen lymph nodes in your neck
- White or yellow coating on the tonsils

More

Antibiotics are used to treat strep throat and prevent rheumatic fever, a rare but serious problem that can occur if strep is not treated.

Home Treatment

- Gargle with warm salt water several times a day to reduce throat swelling and pain. Mix 1 teaspoon of salt in 8 ounces of water.
- Drink extra fluids to soothe your throat. Honey and lemon in hot water or in weak tea may help.
- Do not smoke, and avoid other people's smoke. If you need help quitting, see page 351.
- Take acetaminophen (Tylenol), aspirin, or ibuprofen (Advil, Motrin) to relieve pain and reduce fever.
- Try nonprescription throat lozenges that have a painkiller to numb your throat, such as Sucrets Maximum Strength. Cough drops or hard candy may also help. If you have diabetes, look for ones that are sugar-free.
- If you have strep throat, stay home from work until 24 hours after you have started antibiotics.

Looking for the Stroke topic? See page 54 if you think someone is having a stroke. See page 314 for help on adapting to life after a stroke.

Swollen Lymph Nodes

When to Call a Doctor

- Your lymph nodes are large, very firm, red, and painful.
- You have swollen lymph nodes and signs of infection in a nearby cut or sore. Signs may include increased pain, redness, swelling, or warmth; red streaks leading from the cut; pus; or fever.
- You have swollen lymph nodes after traveling outside the United States or in wilderness areas.
- Your lymph nodes swell for no clear cause, they keep getting bigger, and the swelling has not gone away after 2 weeks.
- You have swollen lymph nodes in areas other than your neck, armpits, or groin.

The lymph nodes are small glands found all through the body. They swell as the body fights minor infections from colds, insect bites, or small cuts. More serious infections and some types of cancer can make lymph nodes hard, sore, and quite large.

The lymph nodes in the neck are the ones people most often notice. They may swell when you have a cold or sore throat. The lymph nodes in the groin may swell if you have a vaginal or other pelvic infection or if you have a cut or sore on your leg or foot.

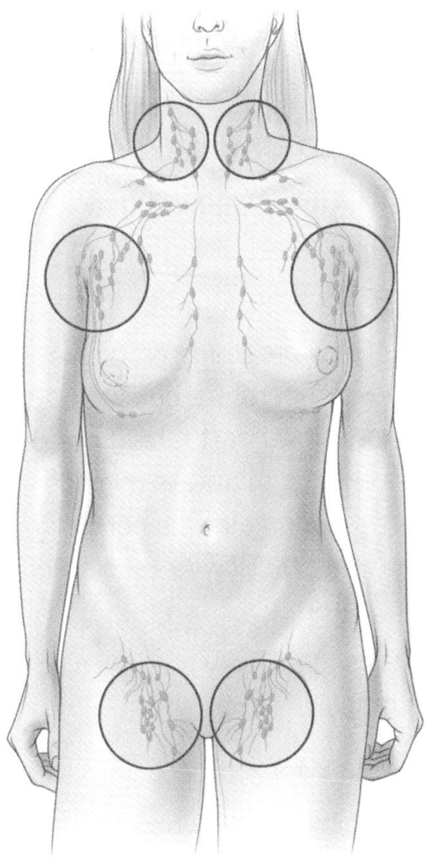

Swollen lymph nodes in the neck, armpits, and groin are usually easy to feel.

Home Treatment

Treat the cold or other infection that is making the lymph nodes large. Use the index in the back of the book or the symptom charts on pages 59 to 65 to find what you need.

Lumps That Aren't Lymph Nodes

Most lumps under the skin are nothing to worry about. A lump that is not a lymph node may be a noncancerous growth such as a lipoma, ganglion or sebaceous cyst, or thyroid nodule; a pocket of pus from an infection under the skin; or a blood vessel pushing against the skin. In rare cases, a lump is cancer.

Call your doctor if:

- You have a lump in your belly, groin, or behind your knee that has a pulse like a heartbeat.
- You have a painful lump that doesn't get better after 2 weeks.
- You have a new, hard lump that doesn't move when you press on it and that changes or grows over a few weeks.
- You are worried about a lump.

See page 99 for information about breast lumps.

Thyroid, Low (Hypothyroidism)

When to Call a Doctor

Call 911 if someone who has hypothyroidism:

- Faints.
- Has new breathing problems, a body temperature below 95 °F, or a very slow heart rate. (Less than 60 beats a minute is considered very slow unless it is normal for that person. See How to Take a Pulse on page 48.)
- Starts to act very confused or behave strangely.

Call your doctor if:

- You think you may have a thyroid problem because you have symptoms that won't go away, such as:
  - Not being able to stand cold temperatures.
  - Feeling weak and tired all the time.
  - Dry skin, brittle nails, or hair loss.
  - Constipation.
  - Steady weight gain.
  - Depression, memory problems, or trouble concentrating.
- You have been taking your thyroid medicine for at least 4 weeks, but do not feel any better.
- Your symptoms went away after you started taking thyroid medicine, but now they have come back.

If you are at risk for thyroid problems and have not had your thyroid level checked, you may want to ask your doctor about it. See Should You Have Your Thyroid Checked? on page 239.

The thyroid is a gland in the front of your neck. It makes a hormone that helps your body use energy. As the thyroid makes more hormone, the body "runs" faster. As it makes less, the body slows down.

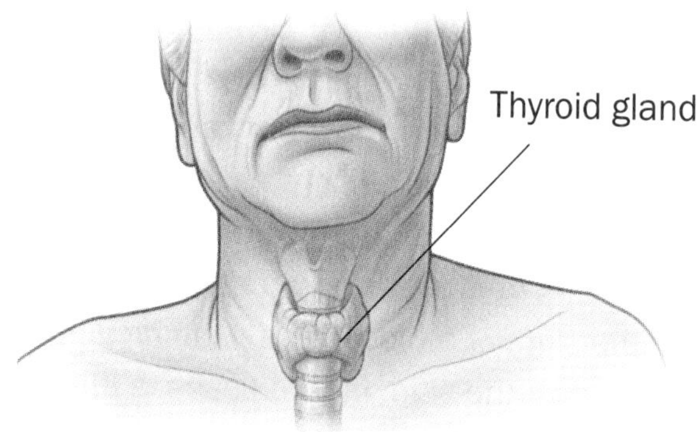

Hormones made by the thyroid gland help your body use energy.

Hypothyroidism means that your thyroid is not making enough thyroid hormone. This is common in women and older people. But the symptoms may develop so slowly that you don't notice them, or you may assume they are part of "normal" aging. When your thyroid level is low, you may feel tired and sluggish, have trouble concentrating or remembering things, and slowly gain weight. You may get cold easily, even when it is warm.

Talk to your doctor if you have symptoms like these. Having these symptoms does not always mean you have a thyroid problem, but a simple blood test can tell for sure.

Low thyroid is easy to treat with medicine. You will probably need to take the medicine for the rest of your life. You will also need blood tests about once a year (or more often if you are having symptoms) to make sure your medicine does not need to be changed.

Home Treatment

- Take your thyroid medicine as directed. Most people do not have side effects if they take the right amount of medicine every time. Do not take extra doses of the medicine. It will not help you get better any faster, and it may cause side effects.
- Make sure your doctor or pharmacist knows about any other medicines you are taking. They can affect your thyroid level.
- Take care of yourself. Eat a healthy diet, get enough sleep, and get regular exercise.

Should You Have Your Thyroid Checked?

Simple blood tests can find changes in the amount of thyroid hormone in your body, sometimes before you notice any symptoms. But experts do not agree on whether adults who don't have symptoms should have their thyroid checked. If you don't have symptoms and your thyroid level is just a little low, you may not need treatment right now. But you will need to see your doctor for regular follow-up testing.

Talk to your doctor about whether you need to be tested. People who are at high risk for thyroid problems may want to get checked. You are at higher risk if:

- You are a woman older than 60.
- You or your family has a history of thyroid problems.
- Your neck has been exposed to radiation either at work or as part of medical treatment.
- You have diabetes, an autoimmune disease (such as rheumatoid arthritis), or certain other health problems.

Toothache

When to Call a Dentist

- You have signs of a tooth or gum infection, such as:
  - Increased pain, swelling, warmth, or redness.
  - Red streaks on the skin over the area.
  - Pus or blood that drains into your mouth.
  - Swollen lymph nodes in your neck.
- You have a severe toothache that does not improve after 2 hours of home treatment.
- Your face is swollen or painful.
- You have a painful bump near the sore tooth.
- A toothache keeps you from sleeping or doing your usual activities.
- You have had a toothache on and off for 2 weeks or longer.

You may have teeth that ache or tingle when you touch them or when you eat or drink something hot, cold, sweet, or sour. The pain may come from a worn-down tooth or from gums that have pulled away from the teeth and exposed the roots and inner parts of the teeth.

If you have sharp pain, you may have tooth decay or infection, have lost a filling, or have a crack in the tooth. Another cause is damage from nervous grinding of your teeth (this can even happen at night while you're sleeping).

A dentist can help find the cause of your toothache and keep your tooth healthy.

Home Treatment

- Put ice or a cold pack on the outside of your cheek for 10 to 15 minutes at a time. Put a thin cloth between the ice and your skin. Do not use heat.
- Take aspirin, ibuprofen (Advil, Motrin), or naproxen (Aleve) to relieve pain and swelling.
- Avoid very hot, cold, or sweet foods and drinks if they make the pain worse.
- Talk to your dentist about special toothpaste for sensitive teeth. Brush with this toothpaste regularly. Or rub a small amount of it on the sensitive area with a clean finger 2 or 3 times a day. Floss gently.
- Do not smoke or chew tobacco. It can make gum problems worse. It also makes you less able to fight infection in your gums. If you need help to quit using tobacco, see page 351.

Tooth Injury

When to Call a Dentist

- You knock out a tooth. The dentist may be able to put it back. This works best within 30 minutes of the injury. (After 2 hours, it probably won't work.)
  - Pick up the tooth by the top, not by the root.
  - Place the tooth in a small cup or jar of milk to take to your dentist. Use tap water if you don't have milk.
- You chip a tooth. A blow that was hard enough to chip a tooth may have moved other teeth out of place or broken the bone that holds the tooth in place. Also, a dentist can fix a chipped tooth.

Tremor (Shaking)

When to Call a Doctor

- You have new shaking (called tremor) in any part of your body.
- A tremor you've had for a while gets worse.
- Shaking keeps you from doing what you want or need to do.
- You develop tremor soon after you start a new medicine.

Tremor is a shaking movement that you can't control. It most often affects the hands and head. It can also affect the voice, torso, or legs.

Essential tremor is one of the most common types. This type of shaking is worse when you are doing something like lifting a cup or pointing at an object. You don't shake when you're not moving. The problem sometimes runs in families, but it's not clear why people get it.

Tremors can also be caused by health problems or medicines that affect the nervous system, such as:

- Parkinson's disease.
- Liver failure.
- Alcoholism.
- Mercury or arsenic poisoning.
- Some antidepressants.
- A thyroid problem.

Sometimes, treating the cause will stop the tremor. Medicine or surgery can help in other cases.

More

Home Treatment

- Reduce stress.
- If your hand shakes, add some weight to it. Wear a heavy bracelet or watch, or hold something in your hand.
- Drink from half-filled cups or glasses, and use a straw.
- Get enough sleep. Tremor may be worse when you are tired.
- Cut down on alcohol, caffeine, and nicotine.

Parkinson's Disease

Parkinson's disease occurs when some of the nerve cells in the brain break down and stop making a chemical called dopamine. Dopamine helps your brain control movement. When you don't have enough dopamine, your muscles don't move as well. It's harder for you to make them do what you want them to.

Symptoms of Parkinson's disease usually start slowly and get worse over time. The most common problems are:

- Tremor (shaking).
- Stiffness.
- Slow movement.
- Problems with walking and balance.

Parkinson's affects muscles all through your body, so it can also lead to problems like constipation and trouble swallowing or speaking. Some people have problems with memory and thinking as the disease gets worse.

Treatment does not stop the disease, but it may help you control some of the symptoms. Your doctor may wait to prescribe medicines until your symptoms start to get in the way of your daily life. Regular exercise and other changes in your lifestyle can help you stay healthy and adapt.

Ulcers

When to Call a Doctor

Call 911 if:

- You have pain in your upper belly with chest pain or pressure or other symptoms of a heart attack. See page 38.
- You have been diagnosed with an ulcer and:
  - You have severe, nonstop belly pain.
  - You have severe vomiting.
  - You vomit a lot of blood or what looks like coffee grounds.
  - You have severe rectal bleeding. Severe means you are passing a lot of stool that is maroon or mostly blood.
  - Your belly is hard and swollen.
  - You faint.

Call your doctor if:

- Belly pain wakes you from sleep.
- Your stools have blood in them, or they are black or look like tar.
- You vomit and there are streaks of blood in your vomit.
- It often hurts to swallow, or you have trouble swallowing.
- You often vomit or feel nauseated right after you eat.
- You often feel full right after you start eating.
- Mild symptoms of an ulcer do not improve after 10 to 14 days of home treatment.
- You are losing weight, and you don't know why.

A peptic ulcer is a sore in the lining of the digestive tract. Without treatment, ulcers can cause dangerous health problems, such as bleeding in the stomach and small intestine.

The two most common causes of ulcers are:

- Infection with *H. pylori* bacteria. Most people who have *H. pylori* in their stomachs don't get ulcers. But it does increase your risk.
- Frequent or long-term use of aspirin, ibuprofen (Advil, Motrin), naproxen (Aleve), and other pain medicines that reduce swelling (anti-inflammatories). This can damage the digestive tract.

Your risk of an ulcer is higher if you smoke or drink a lot of alcohol.

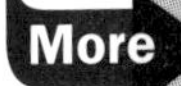

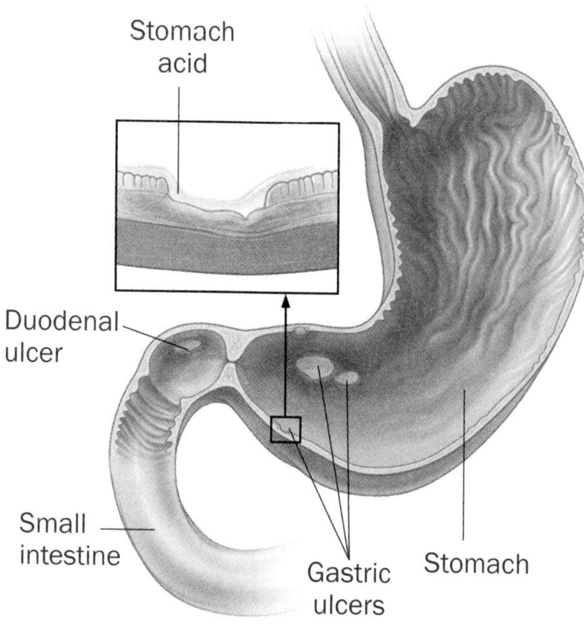

Most ulcers form in the stomach (gastric ulcers) or in the opening to the small intestine (duodenal ulcers).

Symptoms of an ulcer may include a burning or gnawing pain between your belly button and breastbone. The pain often occurs between meals and may wake you during the night. Eating something or taking an antacid usually relieves the pain. Ulcers may also cause bloating, nausea, or vomiting after meals.

In rare cases, stomach ulcers can lead to stomach cancer. So it is important to go to your follow-up visits about your ulcer.

Home Treatment

- Avoid foods that seem to bring on symptoms. Spicy or greasy foods are a problem for many people with ulcers. You don't need to avoid a food if it doesn't cause problems.
- Avoid coffee, tea, cola, and other sources of caffeine. Many people find that caffeine makes their pain worse.
- Try eating smaller, more frequent meals.
- If you smoke, quit. Smoking slows healing of ulcers and increases the chance that they will come back. If you need help quitting, see page 351.
- Limit alcohol. Large amounts may slow healing and make symptoms worse.
- Do not take aspirin, ibuprofen (Advil, Motrin), or naproxen (Aleve). Try acetaminophen (Tylenol) if you need something for pain.
- Try a nonprescription antacid, such as Tums, Maalox, or Mylanta, or an acid reducer, such as Pepcid AC, Tagamet HB, or Zantac 75. You can also buy an acid blocker called Prilosec OTC without a prescription.
    - If you take antacids, you may need frequent, large doses to do the job. Talk with your doctor about the best dose.
    - Your doctor may suggest that you take a prescription medicine such as Prevacid, Prilosec, or Nexium. These drugs greatly reduce the production of stomach acid and can help your ulcer heal.
- Learn to relax and cope better with stress. See page 356.

Vaginitis

When to Call a Doctor

- You have pain in your lower belly or pelvis, a fever, and unusual vaginal discharge.
- You have pain or bleeding during or after sex.
- Your vaginal discharge smells bad or doesn't look normal.
- You think you have a yeast infection but are not sure.
- You know you have a yeast infection, and nonprescription medicine does not clear it up in 3 or 4 days.
- Your vagina is dry and irritated, and a lubricant doesn't help.
- You think you may have a sexually transmitted disease. See page 223. Your sex partner(s) may need to be treated too.
- You get yeast infections often and are not taking antibiotics. This can be a sign of diabetes or other problems.
- You have symptoms of a urinary tract infection (pain or burning, frequent urge to urinate). See page 90.

If you plan to see a doctor, do not douche, use vaginal creams, or have sex for 48 hours before your appointment.

Vaginitis is any infection or irritation of the vagina that changes your normal vaginal discharge. **Yeast infections** are the most common cause of vaginitis in older women.

Atrophic vaginitis is also common in older women. Women get it because of changes in the vagina caused by the drop in estrogen that happens with menopause.

See the chart on page 246 to learn more about the common causes of vaginitis and what to do about them.

If it hurts or burns when you urinate and you feel the need to urinate often, you may have a bladder infection. See page 90.

Home Treatment

- Do not have sex until your symptoms have gone away.
- Do not scratch. Relieve itching with a cold pack or cool bath.
- Make sure the cause of vaginitis is not a forgotten tampon, diaphragm, or other object.
- If you know that you have a yeast infection, try a nonprescription medicine such as Monistat or Gyne-Lotrimin.
- Also follow the tips in Preventing Vaginitis on page 246.

Vaginitis may clear up in a few days. If it doesn't, be sure to call your doctor.

More

Vaginal Problems		
Common Causes	**Symptoms**	**What to Do**
Yeast infection	Itching and redness; white, odor-free discharge that looks like cottage cheese; burning when you urinate or have sex	Infection may clear on its own. Try nonprescription medicine for yeast infection (Monistat, Gyne-Lotrimin). Call your doctor if this doesn't help.
Atrophic vaginitis (happens after menopause)	Burning, pain, and dryness when you have sex	Try a vaginal lubricant (Replens, Astroglide). Ask your doctor about estrogen cream.
Bacterial vaginosis	Thin gray or yellow discharge that smells fishy; pain when you urinate or have sex	You may need treatment. Call your doctor.
Trichomoniasis and other sexually transmitted diseases (see page 223)	Redness and irritation; bad odor; a lot of foamy, white or colored discharge; pain during sex	You need treatment. Call your doctor. Any partner(s) will need treatment too.

Preventing Vaginitis

- Do not take antibiotics unless you really need to.
- Wash your vaginal area once a day with plain water or a mild, unscented soap. Rinse and dry well.
- Do not douche or use feminine deodorant sprays and other perfumed products. They irritate and dry tender skin.
- Limit how many sex partners you have. Use condoms.
- Do not wear panty hose or tight nylon underwear.
- Try a vaginal lubricant during sex if you have a problem with dryness.
- If you have diabetes, keep your blood sugar under control. This can help prevent yeast infections.

Varicose Veins

When to Call a Doctor

- You have sudden pain or swelling in your leg. You may have a clot in a deep vein, which could be serious. See page 96.
- The skin over a varicose vein bleeds heavily on its own or after an injury, and you cannot stop the bleeding. See page 17.
- You have an open sore on your leg or foot.
- A tender lump appears on your leg for no clear reason (you have not bumped or bruised your leg).

Varicose veins are large, twisted veins near the surface of the skin. They are most common in the legs and ankles.

You get a varicose vein when a vein becomes weak and stretched and can no longer help move blood back up to the heart. (This is not harmful, because there are so many other veins in the body.) Blood pools in the weak vein, causing it to swell.

Obesity, pregnancy, or standing for long periods of time can cause varicose veins. They also tend to run in families.

- Varicose veins may not cause any symptoms. The blue color of the veins may be the only reason you notice them.
- Your legs, feet, or ankles may ache, swell a little, and feel tired.
- If the veins get worse, they can cause dry, itchy skin and may break open and bleed, causing open sores.

Some people have tiny varicose veins on the surface of the skin. These are called spider veins. They are not a health problem, but you may not like the way they look.

Varicose veins usually do not need treatment other than self-care. If they bother you or cause bleeding or skin problems, you may want to think about treatments such as sclerotherapy or surgery. For help deciding whether you want or need treatment, go to the Web site on the back cover and enter **M013** in the search box.

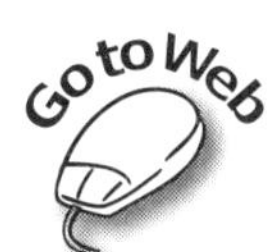

Home Treatment

- Wear supportive, full-length elastic stockings. Do not wear knee-highs. For mild symptoms, regular support panty hose may work. Or your doctor can give you a prescription for compression stockings, which you can buy at a drugstore or medical supply store.
- Do not wear socks or stockings that leave red marks around your legs. Do not wear tight belts or pants that are tight in the waist or thighs.

More

- Put your feet up when you sit. If you cannot put your feet up, then sit with your feet flat on the floor or crossed at the ankles. Do not cross your legs at the knee. At the end of the day, lie down and prop your legs above the level of your heart.
- If you have to sit a lot (at work, for example), get up and walk around often. If you have to stand a lot, move around often. Sit down and put your feet up when you can.
- Get regular exercise, such as walking, cycling, swimming, or dancing. Working your leg muscles keeps blood from pooling in the legs.
- Lose weight if you need to. See page 326.

Vision Changes

By age 50, most people notice changes in their vision:

- You may not be able to see small print or focus on close objects as well as you used to.
- Your vision may get less sharp.
- You may need more light for reading, driving, sewing, and other activities.
- You may have more trouble seeing subtle color differences (blue may look gray, for example).

Problems caused by diseases like diabetes or high blood pressure also become more common as you get older. Some of these can be serious.

Use the When to Call a Doctor list on page 249 and the information that follows it to learn what's normal and what needs to be checked out. If your vision is already poor, you may want to read Tips for Living With Reduced Vision on page 251.

If you don't find what you're looking for here, be sure to review the Eye and Vision Problems chart on page 62 or any of these topics:

- Cataracts, page 113
- Glaucoma, page 162
- Eye Problems, page 140

When to Call a Doctor

Call 911 if:

- You have a sudden loss of vision or double vision that does not clear.
- You see a sudden shower of dark specks ("floaters") or flashes of light that you have never seen before.
- You suddenly notice a blank or dark spot or a dark shadow across your field of vision that does not go away.

Call your eye doctor if:

- Straight lines look wavy or curved, or objects seem to have changed size or shape.
- You have pain or pressure in your eyes.
- Colors seem faded or less bright than they used to.
- Your vision is getting worse. Age-related vision loss (presbyopia) develops slowly, over months to years. If your vision changes more quickly—for example, over just a few weeks—be sure to call your doctor. This may be an early sign of a more serious problem.

Presbyopia

Presbyopia is the normal change in vision that affects nearly everyone as they get older. As the eyes age, changes in the lenses make it harder for them to focus on close objects or small print. You may find that you have to hold objects at arm's length to see them clearly. (People with presbyopia sometimes say that they don't need glasses; they just need longer arms.)

Glasses or contacts can usually solve the problem.

- If you haven't needed glasses or contacts before, you may want to try nonprescription reading glasses first. They cost a lot less than prescription glasses, and they work well for many people. You can buy reading glasses at most drugstores. Check with your eye doctor first to make sure you know what to get.
- If you already wear glasses or contacts, you may need bifocals. Bifocals let you see objects that are close up and those that are far away with the same pair of glasses or contacts.

What About Surgery?

If you don't want to wear glasses or contacts, surgery may be an option. Laser eye surgery, such as LASIK or photorefractive keratectomy (PRK), can sometimes correct presbyopia. You can also have your aging lens removed and get an artificial one to replace it. This is called a lens implant.

Talk to your eye doctor about whether surgery might be a good choice for you.

More

Macular Degeneration

Macular degeneration is an eye disease that destroys your central vision. The macula is the part of the retina that provides the clear, sharp central vision you use to focus on what is in front of you. The disease does not affect your side vision.

Macular degeneration may affect one or both eyes. Symptoms may include dim or fuzzy vision and a blank or dark spot in the center of your visual field. Colors may look faded or dim. As the disease gets worse, straight lines will start to look wavy.

Many people get along well despite the loss of central vision, although walking, reading, driving, and other activities that rely on central vision are much harder.

There are two types of macular degeneration:

- **Dry macular degeneration** is very common in people over age 50. It causes slow vision loss, usually over many years.
- **Wet macular degeneration** is far less common but much more serious. It occurs when abnormal blood vessels grow beneath the retina. This can cause fast vision loss, sometimes over a period of weeks or months.

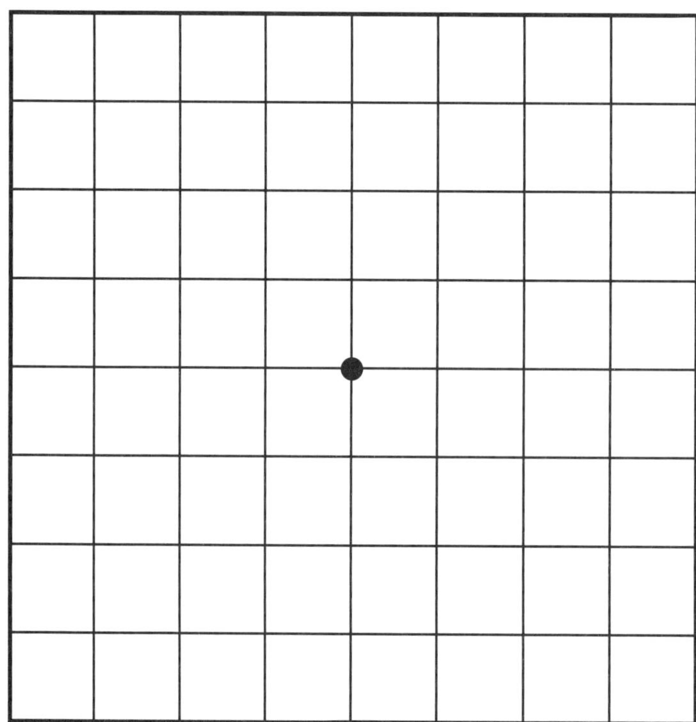

View this Amsler grid from about 10 inches away while wearing your glasses or contacts. Cover one eye and focus on the center dot while noticing the areas around the dot. Repeat with the other eye covered. If the lines around the center dot look wavy or curved, you may have a macular problem. Call your eye doctor if this is the case. In some cases, prompt treatment can help you keep your vision.

Laser surgery and medicines may prevent or delay further loss of vision if macular degeneration is found early. Be sure to see your doctor for regular eye exams as you get older.

Detached Retina

The retina is a layer of nerve cells in the eye that detect light and send signals to the brain about what the eye sees. Problems with the retina can lead to poor vision or blindness.

Retinal detachment happens when the retina separates from the wall of the eye, usually when a hole forms and fluid from inside the eye gets underneath. This causes vision loss in the detached part of the retina.

Diabetic Retinopathy

Diabetic retinopathy is an eye problem caused by diabetes. Diabetes can damage the small blood vessels in the retina, which is the part of the eye that detects light and sends signals to the brain about what the eye sees. Problems with the retina can lead to poor vision and even blindness.

Retinopathy often has no symptoms until it is quite advanced. So if you have diabetes, be sure to have regular eye exams. Eye exams can find the problem early, when it is easier to treat.

Controlling your blood sugar can help prevent eye problems and blindness caused by diabetes. See page 296.

Most retinal detachments are caused by age-related changes in the gel (vitreous) that fills the eye. Getting hit in the head or eye may also cause the retina to detach. Symptoms of a retinal problem may include seeing floaters or flashes of light or seeing a new shadow or "curtain" across your field of vision.

Retinal detachment almost always needs surgery. Surgery can often restore good vision if it is done soon after the detachment occurs.

Tips for Living With Reduced Vision

There are many changes you can make in your home so living with low vision is easier and safer. Here are some suggestions. The tips in Preventing Falls can also help. See page 364.

Change your lighting.

- Aim lighting at what you want to see and away from your eyes.
- Add table and floor lamps in areas where you need extra lighting.
- Use window coverings that let you adjust how much natural light comes in.
- Use nightlights in halls and bathrooms.
- Make sure that doorways, stairs, and other areas that could be dangerous are well-lit.

More

Use contrast.

- Place light objects against dark backgrounds or dark objects against light backgrounds. For example, if you have white or light-colored walls, use dark switch plates for the lights. You can also use switches that glow softly to make them easier to find.
- Use paint in a contrasting color to mark electrical outlets, oven dials, thermostats, and other items.
- Paint door frames in a contrasting color; if the door is light, paint the frame with a dark color. Use dark doorknobs on light-colored doors.
- In your bathroom, use contrasting color for items such as cups, soap dishes, and even the soap.
- Use high contrast, such as bold black letters on a white background, when you make labels, signs, and other markings.

Label and mark things.

- Label your medicines so you know which is which. Use high-contrast labels to "color code" medicines, spices, foods, and other items.
- Mark the settings that you use the most on your stove and oven controls, as well as the "on" and "off" positions. Some appliances come with extra-large, high-contrast markings and dials.
- Mark the faucet settings that provide the right water temperature. In sinks and tubs, mark the water level that you want with a strip of waterproof tape or waterproof marker so that you don't add too much water.
- Mark the areas around stairways and ramps with paint or tape. Use dark tape on light floors, and light tape on dark floors.
- Post signs at eye level.

Here are some other things that might help:

- Ask for large-print books, newspapers, bank checks, medicine labels, and other items.
- Look for household items made to work better for people with low vision. Items include clocks and watches with electronic voices that announce the time, or clocks, phones, and calculators with extra-large buttons and numbers that are easier to see.
- Keep your eyeglasses prescription current.
- Use magnifying lenses. These may range from simple lenses you hold for reading to special eyeglasses or magnifiers much like the lenses that jewelers use. Some have a built-in light, and some are mounted on stands so that your hands are free. For distance vision, try small handheld telescopes or lenses that clip onto your eyeglasses.

Vomiting

When to Call a Doctor

Call 911 if:

- Vomiting occurs with chest pain or pressure or other signs of a heart attack. See page 38.
- You have signs of severe dehydration. These include little or no urine for 12 hours; sunken eyes, no tears, and a dry mouth and tongue; skin that sags when you pinch it; feeling very dizzy or lightheaded; fast breathing and heartbeat; and not feeling or acting alert.
- You vomit a lot of blood or what looks like coffee grounds.

Call a doctor if:

- Vomiting occurs with a stiff neck, severe headache, drowsiness, or confusion. You may have a serious illness. See page 151.
- You vomit after a head injury. See page 36.
- Vomiting occurs with any of these signs of serious illness:
  - Fever and increasing pain in the lower right belly (see page 67)
  - Fever and shaking chills
  - Swelling in the belly
  - Pain in the upper right or upper left belly
- Symptoms of mild dehydration (dry mouth, dark urine, not much urine) get worse, even with home treatment.
- Vomiting and fever last longer than 48 hours.
- There are streaks of blood in your vomit.
- You think that a medicine may be causing the problem.
- Any vomiting lasts longer than 1 week.

Nausea is an unpleasant feeling in the pit of your stomach. You may feel weak and sweaty and produce lots of spit. Intense nausea often leads to vomiting, or "throwing up." Good home treatment will help you feel better and avoid losing too much fluid (dehydration).

Common causes of nausea and vomiting are:

- Viral stomach flu or food poisoning. See page 155.
- Stress or nervousness.
- Medicines, especially antibiotics, aspirin, ibuprofen (Advil, Motrin), and naproxen (Aleve).
- Diabetes.

More

- Migraine headaches. See page 167.
- Head injury. See page 36.

Nausea and vomiting can also be signs of other serious problems. Be sure to check the Digestive Problems chart on page 60 if this topic does not meet your needs.

Home Treatment

- Watch for and treat early signs of dehydration. See page 29. Older adults who are vomiting can quickly get dehydrated.
- After vomiting has stopped for 1 hour, take small sips of a clear liquid every 10 to 15 minutes. Drink more as you feel better and your body can handle it. Clear liquids include apple or grape juice mixed to half-strength with water; rehydration drinks (see page 30); weak tea with sugar; clear broth; and Jell-O. Avoid orange juice and grapefruit juice.
- If vomiting lasts longer than 24 hours, sip a rehydration drink. This can help replace lost fluids and nutrients. See page 30.
- When you feel better, try clear soups and liquids and mild foods. Bananas, rice, applesauce, dry toast, and crackers are good choices. Stick with these mild foods until all symptoms have been gone for 12 to 48 hours.
- Rest until you feel better.

Warts

When to Call a Doctor

- A wart looks infected.
- A plantar wart hurts when you walk, and foam pads do not help.
- You have warts in the anal or genital area. See page 223.
- You have a wart on your face that you want removed.
- You have diabetes or peripheral artery disease, and you get a wart on your foot.

Warts are skin growths caused by a virus. They can appear anywhere on the body. Plantar warts are on the soles of the feet. Most of the wart lies under the skin surface and may make you feel like you are walking on a pebble.

Warts come and go for no clear reason. They can last a week, a month, or even years.

There are several ways to deal with warts:

- Ignore them. If warts don't bother you, there is no reason to spend time and money treating them.

- Use home treatment to remove them. There are three methods for this: salicylic acid, tape, and cryotherapy. See the methods described in Home Treatment. These work a lot of the time but not always.
- Have surgery to remove them. If you have a very painful wart that will not go away, or if your warts bother you, you may want to think about surgery. But you should know that warts may come back after surgery.

Talk with your doctor about your treatment choices and their pros and cons.

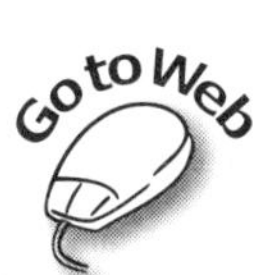

For help deciding what's right for you, go to the Web site on the back cover and enter **V319** in the search box.

Home Treatment

- Do not try to remove genital warts. See page 223.
- Do not pick at a wart. It may spread to the skin under your nails.
- Do not try to cut or burn off a wart.
- Do not try to remove a wart if you have diabetes or peripheral artery disease. Talk to your doctor.
- Wear comfortable shoes and socks. Don't wear high heels or shoes that put pressure on your foot.
- Cushion the wart with a doughnut-shaped pad or a moleskin patch you can buy at a drugstore. Place the pad around the plantar wart. You may also want to place pads or cushions in your shoes.

To Remove Warts

If you are sure that your skin growth is a wart, you can try one of three methods.

- **Method 1:** Use a nonprescription product that contains salicylic acid. Over time, this will soften the wart so that you can rub or file it off. Follow the instructions on the label. Salicylic acid works as well as or better than any other treatment for warts. It may take 2 to 3 months to work.
- **Method 2:** Cover the wart with a piece of waterproof tape (such as duct tape), and leave it on for 6 days. After 6 days, remove the tape and soak the wart in water. Then gently rub it with a nail file or pumice stone. (You will need to clean or replace the nail file or pumice stone often.) Leave the tape off overnight. Repeat the process until the wart is gone, but not longer than 2 months. This method is cheap and works for most people who do it right.
- **Method 3:** Use a nonprescription cryotherapy product. You spray medicine into a foam applicator and then hold the applicator to the wart for a few seconds. This "freezes" the wart off.

If any treatment irritates the area, take a break from it for 2 or 3 days.

If you rub the wart with a pumice stone or file to remove dead tissue, do not use the item for any other purpose. It can spread the wart-causing virus. Wash your hands with soap after you touch the debris from the wart or the pumice stone or file.

Living Better With Chronic Disease

Mastering Chronic Disease: The Basics 258

Living Better With Alzheimer's Disease. 261

Living Better With Arthritis 266

Living Better With Asthma 271

Living Better With Cancer. 276

Living Better With COPD 282

Living Better With Coronary Artery Disease 287

Living Better With Depression . . . 292

Living Better With Diabetes. 296

Living Better With Heart Failure . . 303

Living Better With Chronic Kidney Disease. 308

Living Better After a Stroke 314

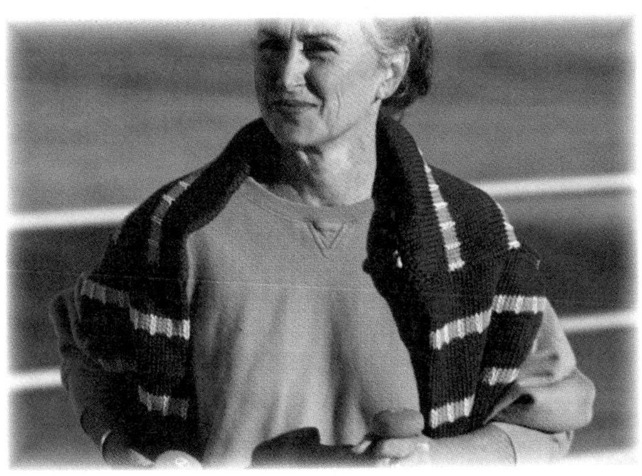

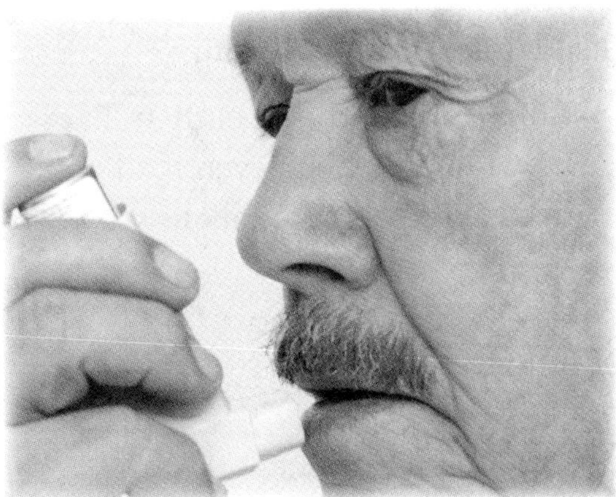

Mastering Chronic Disease: The Basics

Chronic diseases are long-term health problems. They can last for months or years. Most older adults live with at least one chronic disease, and many live with more than one.

If you have a chronic disease, coping with it is probably part of your daily life. But it doesn't have to be the only part. No matter what your health problem is, there are things you can do to help control your disease and live better.

1. Get informed. Learn as much as you can about your health problem. Good information can help you make good decisions.

Don't be afraid to use your doctor as a teacher. See page 2 for tips on how to get the most out of your partnership with your doctor.

2. Keep your health care team informed. Make sure that all your health care providers know what health problems you have, how they are being treated, and what medicines you take.

3. Get support. For major health problems, support can make a big difference in how well you do and how good you feel. Look for support from:

- Family and friends. Let them know how they can help, even if all you need is someone to talk to.
- Support groups in your area or online. People who have the same disease you do can be a great source of emotional and practical help. (Be careful with what you learn, and talk to your doctor before you change your treatment or try any new medicines, vitamins, or herbal products.)
- Large organizations like the American Diabetes Association or the American Heart Association.
- Counselors and therapists. Living with chronic diseases can be overwhelming at times. If you're feeling depressed or not coping well, talking with an expert might help.

A Good-Health Attitude

Good health requires a positive attitude. But this good-health mindset doesn't just happen. It takes work, every day.

- Focus on what you can do instead of what you can't do.
- Focus on your strengths instead of your weaknesses.
- Break down activities into small tasks that you can manage.
- Work fitness and healthy eating into your daily routine.
- Find ways to reduce your stress.
- Balance rest with activity.
- Build a support system of family, friends, and health care workers.

4. Follow your treatment plan. Your doctor can guide your treatment, but whether you stick to the plan is up to you. Depending on what health problems you have, treatment may include things like:

- Taking medicines every day, on time and in the right amount.
- Changing your diet. (Maybe you need to eat a low-sodium diet or avoid certain foods.)
- Making changes in your lifestyle, like being more active, quitting smoking, or getting more rest. For some health problems, changes like these are not just healthy habits. They're vital to treating the disease.
- Doing physical therapy.
- Having treatments like radiation, dialysis, or chemotherapy.

Following your treatment plan may be hard sometimes, but it can make a big difference. Talk with your doctor if you have problems with your treatment. There may be ways to make it easier.

5. Avoid "triggers" when you can. Triggers are things that make your symptoms or disease worse. For example, smoke, dust, and pollution are common triggers for people with breathing problems. For someone with kidney disease, a high-protein meal or certain nonprescription medicines might trigger symptoms. Stress and lack of sleep are triggers for some health problems.

If you're not sure what your triggers are, keep a record of your symptoms. Write down when you have them, how bad they are, and what seems to make them worse or better. With time, you may start to see patterns that can help you recognize your triggers. Then you can try to avoid them.

6. Monitor your health. Part of your self-care job may be to regularly test and keep track of some aspect of your disease. For example, people with diabetes need to check their blood sugar every day. If you have heart failure, you may need to weigh yourself regularly to make sure fluid is not building up in your body.

Doing these "self-tests" can help you:

- Know when there's a problem and, in some cases, stop the problem before it gets worse.
- Know when to call your doctor right away rather than wait for your next visit.
- Know how well your treatment is working. Your records can help your doctor track your health over time.

7. Know what problems to watch for. Sometimes there may be warning signs that your disease is about to flare up. Or you may need to watch for early signs of complications.

Talk to your doctor about what symptoms you should watch for, and have a plan for how to handle them. Should you go to the hospital? Is there medicine you can take? Get instructions for what to do if you suddenly get worse.

More

8. Get regular check-ups. Regular visits and tests let you and your doctor check in on your health and know if your treatment needs to be changed. They can also help your doctor find problems early, when they may be easier to correct.

Agree on a schedule for visits and tests. Once a year? Every 3 months? Work with your doctor to decide what's best for you.

9. Stay as healthy as you can. Chronic diseases can become harder to manage if you start to have other health problems too. Do everything you can to stay well and avoid new problems. For most people, healthy lifestyle choices—eating right, not smoking, being active, reducing stress—can make a big difference.

10. Remember to take care of your whole self. You may want to try palliative care, especially if your health is getting worse.

Palliative Care: Caring for the Whole Person

Palliative care is a kind of care for people who have illnesses that don't go away and often get worse over time. It is different than care to cure your illness. It focuses on improving your quality of life—not just your body, but also your mind and spirit. Sometimes people call it compassionate care.

Although palliative care is often used at the end of life, it is not just for people who are near death. You can have palliative care at the same time that you are getting treatment for a health problem.

Palliative care can help reduce pain or treatment side effects. The doctors, nurses, and others on a palliative care team can help you and your loved ones talk more openly about your feelings and make future plans. They can also make sure the rest of your health care team and your family and friends understand your goals.

Many people value palliative care because it focuses on what's most important to them. If you think it could help you, talk to your doctor.

If you are nearing the end of your life, you may want to consider **hospice care**. See page 387 to learn more about your choices.

Living Better With Alzheimer's Disease

Alzheimer's disease damages the part of the brain involved in memory, problem solving, judgment, language, and behavior. It is the most common type of **dementia** in older adults.

Alzheimer's usually starts with mild memory loss and gets worse over a few years. Medicines may for a short time improve some of the thinking and memory problems, but they do not stop the disease.

Over time, Alzheimer's robs people of the ability to take care of themselves. They may forget how to perform basic tasks such as eating, dressing, bathing, using the toilet, or getting up from a bed or chair and walking. They may become confused and easily frightened and may strike out at others.

More and more people are living with Alzheimer's—whether they have it themselves or take care of a spouse or parent who has it. This section offers a few ways to approach the many challenges of living with Alzheimer's disease.

If You Have Alzheimer's

For most people, finding out that they have Alzheimer's is a shock. You may be afraid and worried about how it will change your life.

Your life is not over. Alzheimer's disease is different for everyone. In some cases, people can function well for a long time. Others get worse more quickly. Whatever turns out to be true for you, you can find ways to get the most out of life now.

Stay Active and Healthy

- Keep doing your hobbies and other activities as long as they don't put you or others at risk.
- Spend time with friends and family.
- Get some exercise every day.
- Eat healthy foods.
- Get enough rest. If you have trouble sleeping, see page 262 for help on how to sleep better.
- Take care of any other health problems, and see your doctor for checkups.

Look for Ways to Adapt

Things you have done for a long time will start to be harder for you. That doesn't mean you have to give them up right away.

- Change tasks to fit your abilities. A task may take longer than it used to, but if you want to keep doing it, give it a try. For example, if you don't want to give up cooking but don't feel as comfortable with it as you used to, try making easier recipes. Or do some of the other related tasks, such as planning meals or setting the table.
- Schedule things for times of day when you are best able to handle them. It may help to have a routine that doesn't change much from day to day.
- Be creative in dealing with memory problems.
  - Use labels, lists, and sticky notes as reminders.

More

- Write your activities on a calendar or daily planner, and keep it where you can check it often.
- Keep calendars and clocks where you can see them.

- Ask for help. Let your friends and family know how they can support you.

Be Safe

- **When you go out:** Tell someone where you are going and when you will be back. Before you go out alone, write down where you are going, how to get there, and how to get back home, and take these notes with you. Do this even if you have gone there many times before. Take someone with you when you can.
- **At home:** Make your home safe. Tack down rugs, put no-slip tape in the tub, and put safety switches on stoves and appliances. Put night-lights in bedrooms, hallways, and bathrooms. Lower the hot water setting to 120°F or lower to avoid burns.
- **If you still drive:** Have a family member or other caregiver tell you if you are driving badly. Go to the driver's license office for a test if there is any question. Deciding to stop driving can be very hard. Driving helps you feel independent. But it can also put you and others at risk. Plan for other means of getting around when you can't drive anymore. See Driving: Are You Safe? on page 365.

Sleep Problems and Alzheimer's

Some people with Alzheimer's may have trouble sleeping at night. It may help to:

- Stay awake and active during the day. Long naps can keep you from feeling sleepy at night.
- Take a walk or get some exercise in the late afternoon.
- Drink warm milk or caffeine-free herbal tea before bed.
- Take a bath close to bedtime.

Ask About Medicines

- Medicine may slow memory loss for a while in some people. It does not cure the disease. For help deciding if this type of medicine is right for you,

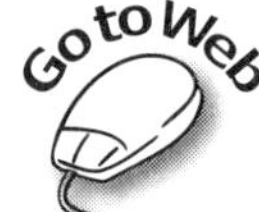

go to the Web site on the back cover and enter **D141** in the search box.

- Do you have trouble sleeping? Are you anxious or depressed? There are medicines that may be able to help with these and other problems. Tell your doctor what problems you're having.

Plan for the Future

You may find comfort in planning now for your future needs. Make sure your legal and financial affairs are in order. Write a living will and name a durable power of attorney for health care if you haven't already done so. Talk with your family and your doctor about what to expect and what care you will need as the disease gets worse.

There's no reason you can't take part in decisions about your future if your judgment is still clear. See Planning for the Future on page 382 for help with these issues.

When a Loved One Has Alzheimer's

Most people who have Alzheimer's disease are cared for at home by family members and friends. Taking care of someone with Alzheimer's disease can be very hard, but there are ways to make it easier. Caregiving can be a positive experience for you and the person you are caring for.

Take Care of Yourself

It's hard to be a good caregiver if you are not well yourself. Don't be afraid to ask for help. See A Caregiver's Guide on page 378.

Help Keep the Person Safe and Healthy

One of your most important tasks as a caregiver is to keep the person safe.

- Make your home safe.
  - Fall-proof your home. See page 364.
  - Use locks on doors and cupboards. Lock up knives, scissors, medicines, cleaning supplies, and other dangerous things.
  - Provide good lighting, especially at night. Put night-lights in bedrooms, halls, and bathrooms.
  - Use hidden switches or controls for the stove, thermostat, water heater, and other appliances, and use child-proofing devices.
- Get a medical ID bracelet for the person so that you can be contacted if he or she gets lost.
- Lock outside doors, and use alarms and other devices to alert you when the person wanders outdoors or into unsafe areas. Provide a safe place, such as an enclosed yard or garden.
- Help the person eat a balanced diet. Serve plenty of whole grains, fruits, and vegetables every day. If the person is not hungry at meals, give snacks at midmorning and in the afternoon. Offer drinks such as Boost, Ensure, or Sustacal if the person is losing weight.
- Encourage exercise. Take walks together.
- Help the person stay active mentally. Read, play games, or do crossword or jigsaw puzzles together.
- Be on the lookout for other health problems. It's easy to get focused on Alzheimer's and miss other issues that come up. Hearing and vision loss, depression, arthritis, thyroid problems, and kidney problems are common in older adults and may make symptoms of Alzheimer's worse. Treating these problems can improve life for you and the person you care for.

More

Should the Person Be in a Nursing Home?

Not everyone can take care of a person with Alzheimer's disease at home. Even if the person starts out at home, it often gets harder with time as the person develops new behaviors or health problems that are hard to manage. You may have health problems of your own, or the stress of caring for the person at home may be too much.

Find out what care options you have, and think about what you and the person with Alzheimer's need and can afford. Do you need part-time help with household tasks? Do you need others to help with caregiving a few times a week or a few hours a day? There are options for all of these needs, from adult day centers to respite services to part-time nursing care at home. Many people need the full support of a nursing home at some point.

Deciding to put a loved one in a nursing home can be very hard. You may feel like you're giving up on the person. But sometimes a nursing home is the best choice. Every family has different needs and feelings to consider.

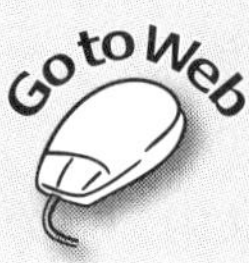

For help with this decision, go to the Web site on the back cover and enter **E866** in the search box.

Help the Person Feel Calm and at Ease

People with Alzheimer's are often easily upset. And they may do or say things that upset you. Here are some ways to reduce and cope with those moments:

- Follow simple routines for bathing, dressing, eating, and other daily tasks.
- Tell the person in advance about changes in his or her regular schedule, such as trips, doctor visits, or visits from friends or family. Remind the person often of upcoming events.
- Keep noise levels low and voices quiet.
- When the person is upset, ask what's wrong. The person might be able to tell you what the problem is, and you might be able to do something about it. (But also realize that the person might not know why he or she gets upset.)
- Remove or avoid things that seem to upset the person, such as certain pictures, objects, music, or TV shows.
- Include some exercise in the person's day. A regular walk, for instance, may help make the person less restless.
- Explain your actions. Break tasks and instructions into clear, simple steps, offered one step at a time.
- Pay attention to your tone of voice. Be calm and supportive. The person is still aware of emotions and may get upset if he or she senses anger or irritation in your voice.

- Don't argue or try to reason with the person. People with Alzheimer's are not able to think the way they used to, and arguing will get you nowhere. Just let it go. Changing the subject is often a good tactic.

Help the Person Enjoy Today

- For as long as he or she is able, let the person make choices about activities, food, clothing, and other things.
- Tailor tasks to the person's abilities. For example, if cooking is no longer safe, ask for help in setting the table, making simple dishes such as salad, or shopping. When the person needs help, offer it gently.
- Be patient. Let the person be independent, even if tasks take more time or are not done perfectly.
- Maintain eye contact and use touch to reassure and show that you are listening. Touch may be better understood than words. Holding the person's hand or putting an arm around his or her shoulder may get through when nothing else can.
- Pay attention to the person's tone of voice and gestures for clues about what the person is feeling. Sometimes the emotion is more important than what is said.
- Treat the person with dignity and respect.

Your relationship with the person will probably change a lot. But you can still have one. Try to focus on the moment. Just sharing a meal or taking a walk can help you connect, even if it's not the way you connected in the past.

When to Call a Doctor

If you or a loved one is having problems with confusion or memory but has not been diagnosed with Alzheimer's or another type of dementia, see Confusion and Memory Loss on page 122.

Call a doctor if:

- A person with Alzheimer's has a sudden, big change in his or her behavior.
- A person with Alzheimer's becomes very hostile or upset, and you can't calm the person down.
- You need help caring for a person with Alzheimer's.

Living Better With Arthritis

Arthritis is a breakdown of the cartilage that cushions your joints. A joint is any place where two or more bones connect, like the knee, hip, wrist, or shoulder. When the cartilage wears down, the bones rub against each other. This causes pain and stiffness.

Osteoarthritis is the most common form of arthritis. Almost everyone older than 65 has it in their hands. A third have it in their knees. It can also affect the joints of the spine, hips, or feet.

When you have arthritis, even simple, everyday movements can hurt. Walking a few steps, opening a door, and even combing your hair can be hard. You may feel especially stiff in the morning until you start moving around.

But there are many things you can do to help with the pain and make it easier for you to move. You can also do things to keep the damage from getting worse. Most people can deal with their symptoms at home with just a little help from their doctor.

What You Can Do

- Take steps to reduce pain and stiffness. This can involve medicines, hot and cold treatments, and other things you can do at home.
- Get regular exercise. This can help make you and your joints stronger, more flexible, and better able to move. Choose activities that are easy on your joints, and avoid or change any activity that causes lasting pain. See page 268.
- Use devices and tools that make it easier for you to do your daily activities. See page 269.
- Reach and stay at a healthy weight. This puts less stress on your joints. If you need help reaching a healthy weight, see page 326.

Reduce Pain and Stiffness

There are several things you can do to help with the pain and stiffness of arthritis.

- Take medicines.
  - If your pain is mild, you may only need pain medicines you can buy without a prescription. These include acetaminophen (Tylenol), aspirin, ibuprofen (Advil, Motrin), and naproxen (Aleve). Talk to your doctor about whether these medicines are safe for you and how much to take.
  - If your pain is severe, you may need stronger prescription medicines. Because you will take these medicines for a long time, you will need to have regular checkups from your doctor.

- Use ice or heat. You may need to try a few approaches until you find what helps you most.
  - Use heat 2 or 3 times a day for 20 to 30 minutes, using a heating pad, hot shower, or hot pack. Heat seems to work well for pain and stiffness caused by not using a joint.
  - Put ice or a cold pack on a painful joint for 10 to 15 minutes. Be sure to put a thin cloth between the ice and your skin. See Ice and Cold Packs on page 51. Ice also is a great pain reliever after you exercise.
  - Try switching between heat and cold.
  - Ask your doctor about heat treatment with paraffin wax. Paraffin wax is a form of moist heat that may help if you have pain and stiffness in your hands or feet. Talk with your doctor before trying this at home.
- If you are stiff when you wake up in the morning, try a warm shower or bath. Keep moving around after you are done so your joints don't stiffen up.

What About Joint Replacement?

If you have severe pain and loss of function because of arthritis, and if other treatments do not help enough, you may want to think about having surgery to replace the joint. This is most often done on hips, knees, or shoulders.

Replacing the joint can mean less pain and better ability to use the joint. But it does not mean that the joint will be the same as it was before you developed arthritis.

Here are a few other things to think about:

- Having a joint replaced is almost never urgent. You have plenty of time to learn more about it and decide whether it's right for you.
- After surgery, it will take several months of rehab and physical therapy to get the best use of your new joint.
- You are likely to get better results if you are in good shape when you have the surgery. It's important to be active and stay at a healthy weight both before and after the surgery.
- Replacement joints do not last forever. You may need to replace the joint again in 10 to 20 years.

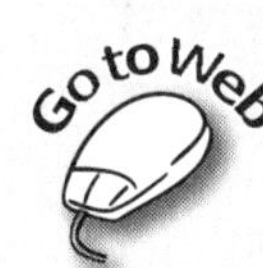

For help deciding whether to have joint replacement surgery, go to the Web site on the back cover and enter **X802** in the search box.

More

Dietary Supplements for Arthritis

Some people with arthritis use the dietary supplements glucosamine or chondroitin for joint pain. Glucosamine and chondroitin come from natural cartilage, which is the tissue that cushions the bones in a joint. You can take these supplements as tablets or capsules or in powder or liquid form.

Studies have shown that glucosamine and chondroitin can help with arthritis pain and improve function. And they seem to have few side effects.

Talk to your doctor before you start taking either of these supplements. It's important to make sure that they are safe for you and that they will not react with any other medicines you might be taking. If you have diabetes, be aware that glucosamine may affect your blood sugar. Check with your doctor before you take it.

Do not take glucosamine if you are allergic to shellfish like shrimp or lobster. Glucosamine is made from shellfish.

Exercising With Arthritis

Regular exercise that is easy on your joints is the best thing you can do for your arthritis. It can help prevent stiffness and improve your ability to do daily activities. It can make you stronger and reduce the stress on your joints. For example, having stronger leg muscles takes some of the stress off the knees and hips. It can also help you feel better and stay at a healthy weight (which is easier on your joints).

Having pain after activity is quite common. It may make you afraid to exercise. But there are things you can do to make it easier to exercise and stay active.

- Balance your exercise with rest. If your joints hurt or you notice redness or swelling, rest your joints, and then try a little exercise.
- Use ice or cold packs on painful joints after you exercise. This can ease pain and swelling.
- Use pain medicines as suggested by your doctor.
- Ask your doctor about using splints or braces for short periods of time to protect your joints.
- Talk to your doctor if you have new or more intense pain. Sharp or unusual pain may be a sign of injury.

In general, swimming, water aerobics, biking, and walking are great ways to be active. They do not irritate your joints as much as other exercises.

Try to do some stretching every day. Put each of your joints through its full range of motion once or twice each day.

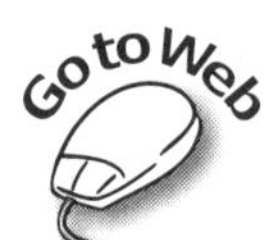

If you're not sure how to get started, go to the Web site on the back cover and enter **K156** in the search box for examples of safe exercises and other tips.

Your doctor or a physical therapist can also help you learn what types of exercise are best. It's always a good idea to check with your doctor before you start an exercise program.

Helpful Hints and Tools

- Use a cane or walker if you need help to get around. These can help rest your joints.
- Put a raised seat on your toilet and risers under low chairs to make it easier to get up.
- Put grab bars in your bathroom to help you get in and out of the shower or tub.
- Place door knob covers on your door knobs to make opening doors easier.
- Buy an electric toothbrush. Or alter your basic toothbrush by putting several layers of duct tape around the handle so that it's bigger and easier to hold.

More

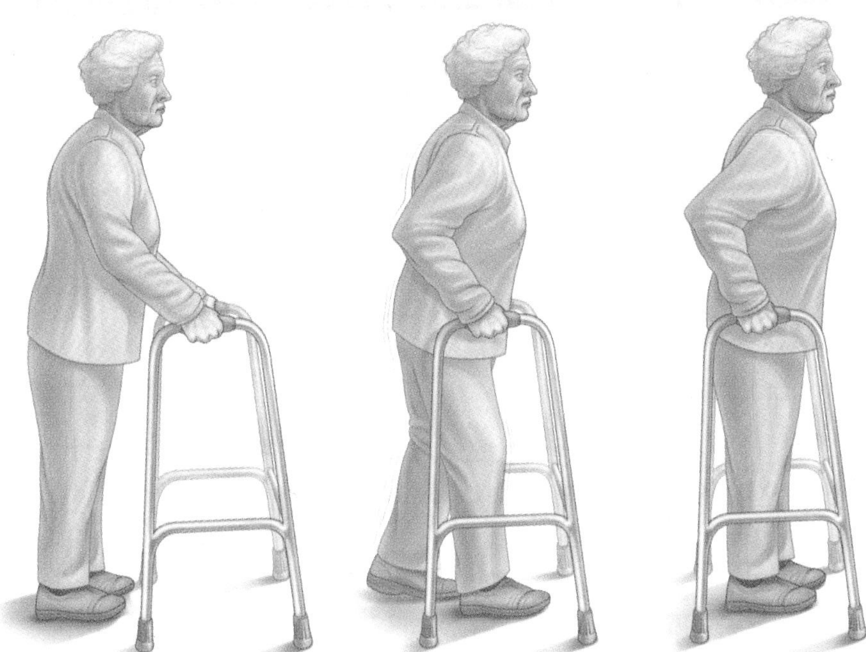

How to use a walker

- Set the walker at arm's length in front of you, with all four legs on the floor. If your walker has wheels on the front legs, just take your weight off your hands and push the walker forward.
- Use the handles of the walker for balance as you move one leg forward to the middle area of the walker. Don't step all the way to the front. If one leg is weaker than the other, step with the weaker leg first.
- Push straight down on the handles of the walker as you bring the other leg forward. Your legs should be even with each other.
- Repeat.

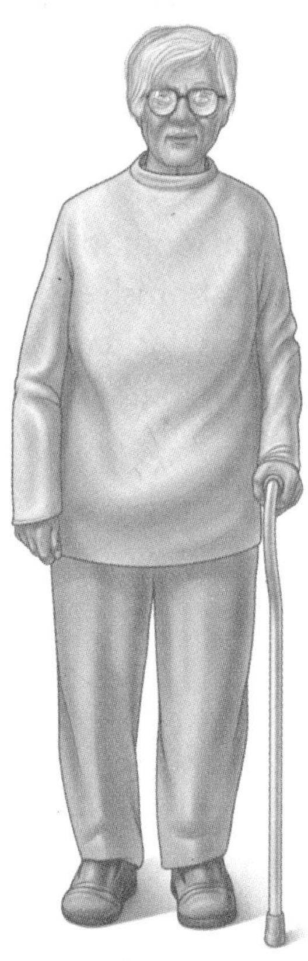

How to use a cane

- If you have a "weaker" side, hold the cane in the opposite hand. (So, if your right leg is weak, hold the cane in your left hand.)
- Set the cane about 4 inches to the side of your stronger leg.
- Put most of your weight on your stronger leg. Move the cane several inches forward while you move your weak leg forward.
- Put weight on your cane to limit the weight on your weak leg, and move your stronger leg forward. Stand up straight as you do this. Do not let your body lean.
- Move your cane about 4 inches in front of you, and start your next step.
- Take small steps.

- If you take several medicines, organize them in a pill box that holds a week's worth of pills.
- Use a reacher to pick up things off the floor or from the back of a cabinet.
- Try some of the kitchen, garden, and writing tools that are designed to help people with arthritis. There are lots of these for sale. See page 380.
- For tasks that you would normally do standing up—such as working in the kitchen—try using a tall stool with wheels instead so you can sit down.

When to Call a Doctor

- You have fever or a skin rash along with severe joint pain.
- You have sudden, unexplained swelling, redness, warmth, or pain in one or more joints.
- A joint hurts so much that you cannot use it.
- Joint pain lasts for more than 6 weeks, and home treatment is not helping.
- You have side effects (stomach pain, nausea, heartburn, or stools that are black or look like tar) from aspirin or other arthritis medicines.

Living Better With Asthma

Whether you have had asthma for years or are new to it, it may help to know just what it is and what it does to your body. Asthma causes inflammation and swelling in the airways (bronchial tubes) that lead to the lungs. This makes the airways narrower, which makes it harder for you to breathe.

How often you have trouble breathing depends on how bad your asthma is and what triggers it. Some people breathe normally most of the time, while others feel as if they are always short of breath. Other people may have trouble breathing only at night or when they exercise.

When you have a lot of trouble breathing, you are having an asthma attack. Your airways are very swollen, and it's hard to get air through them.

Along with the symptoms that asthma can cause from day to day, it also can damage your airways and lungs. Even mild asthma can cause long-term lung problems. And asthma can make illnesses like bronchitis and pneumonia worse.

But asthma does not have to control your life. There are things you can do today and every day to prevent these kinds of problems and to live better with asthma.

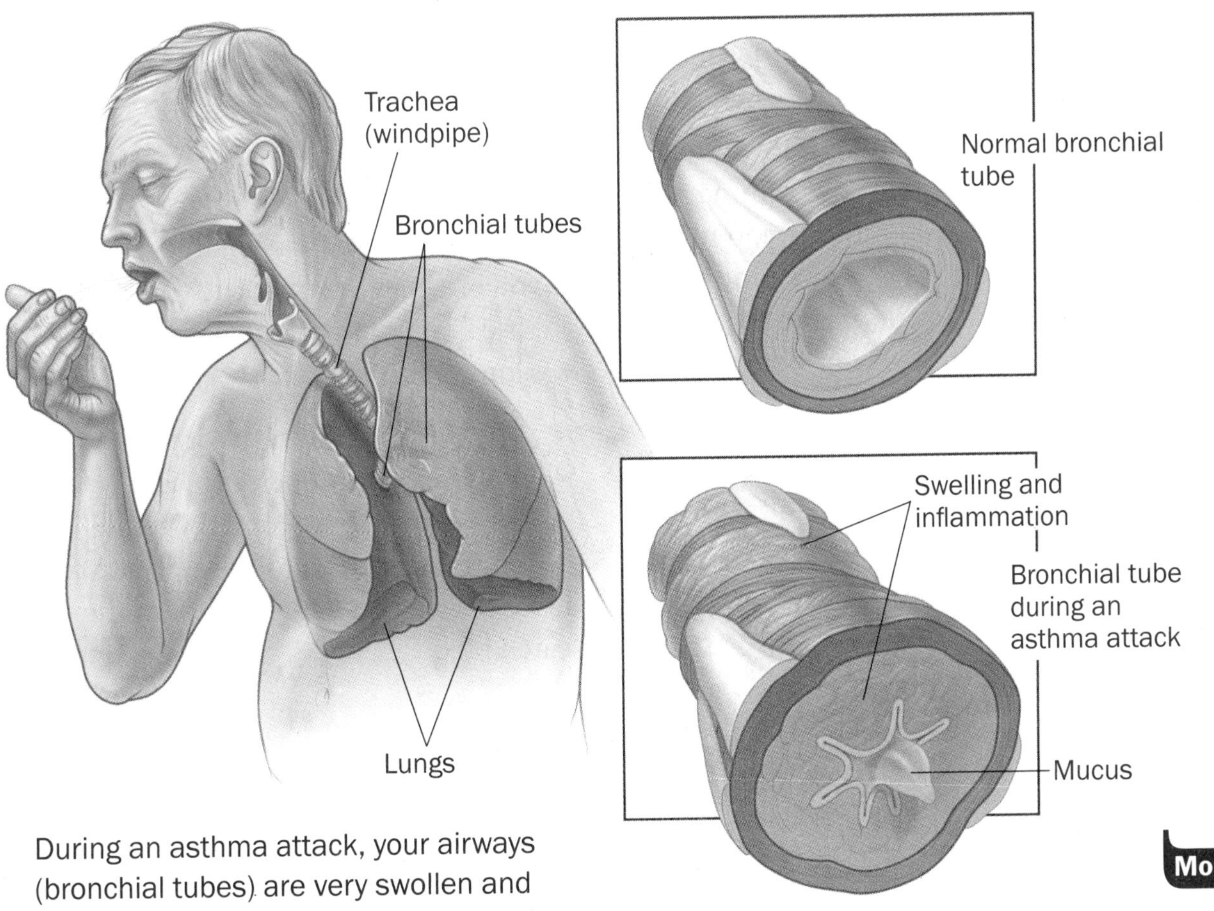

During an asthma attack, your airways (bronchial tubes) are very swollen and inflamed. This is why it's hard to breathe.

More

What You Can Do

- Have and follow an asthma action plan. An asthma action plan can give you much of what you need to manage your asthma. See Your Asthma Action Plan on this page.
- Take your asthma medicines exactly the way your doctor tells you to. If you are not sure how or when to take them, talk to your doctor. See page 273.
- Take part in your care. Use a peak flow meter to check how well your lungs are working (see page 273). Keep track of your symptoms. Do not ignore your asthma just because you feel good.
- Learn what things make your asthma worse or lead to asthma attacks. Avoid these triggers when you can. See page 274.
- See your doctor regularly. How often depends on how bad your asthma is. If you have mild asthma, you may need a checkup every 6 to 12 months. If your asthma is out of control, you may need to see your doctor more often.
- If you smoke, quit. Smoking makes your asthma worse, and it raises your risk for lung cancer and other problems. If you need help quitting, see page 351.

Your Asthma Action Plan

An action plan tells you how to treat an asthma attack. It will help you make good, quick decisions about what to do when your asthma gets worse. It may even save your life.

To use an asthma action plan, you need to know a few things:

- Your peak flow. Peak flow is how fast and well you can breathe out when you try your hardest. It tells you how well your airways and lungs are working. Checking your peak flow is easy. See page 273 to learn how.
- Your personal best peak flow. This number is a baseline for knowing whether you are doing well or getting worse. You find your personal best by taking peak flow readings over 2 to 3 weeks when your asthma is under control.
- Your asthma zones. There are three zones: green, yellow, and red. Your action plan tells you what to do when you are in each zone. The zones are based on your peak flow and your symptoms.

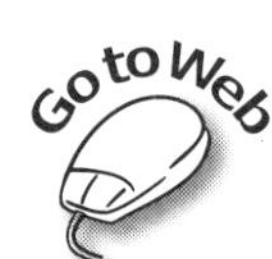

If you don't have a plan now, ask your doctor to help you make one. For help getting started, go to the Web site on the back cover and enter **N298** in the search box.

Quick-Relief Medicine: For Attacks, Not Daily Use

Since quick-relief medicine helps your breathing problems so fast, you may be tempted to use it often to control your asthma instead of taking your controller medicine.

This is not a good idea. Quick-relief medicine is for times when you cannot prevent symptoms and need to treat them. It is not intended as the daily medicine you take to control your asthma—just like controller medicine is not used to treat an attack (it acts too slowly).

Why does it matter?

- The goal is to prevent symptoms before they start. This is the job of controller medicine. Quick-relief medicine does not help as well with this.
- Using quick-relief medicine too often can cause your heart to beat too fast or in an odd rhythm.

Talk to your doctor if you are using quick-relief medicine more than 2 times a week or you go through more than one canister in 3 months.

Note: Some people with asthma need to take quick-relief medicine before they exercise. If your doctor has advised this, it is okay to take it as often as you exercise.

Take Your Medicines

Asthma medicine helps prevent your symptoms and makes you more able to do the things you want to do. It helps you control your asthma instead of your asthma controlling you.

Most people need two types of asthma medicine:

- **Controller medicine.** Take your controller medicine every day, even when you don't have symptoms. It prevents asthma attacks and helps stop problems before they occur.
- **Quick-relief medicine.** Use this when you have symptoms of an asthma attack. It acts fast to treat an attack before it gets bad. Always have some of this medicine with you.

Check Your Peak Flow

Peak flow (peak expiratory flow, or PEF) is how fast and well you can breathe out when you try your hardest. Checking your peak flow regularly can help you:

- Know when an asthma attack is coming, and treat it before it gets bad. This helps you stay healthy and stay out of the hospital.
- Know how well your lungs are working, even if you don't have symptoms.
- Find out what things make your asthma worse. For example, if your peak flow is always worse when you are under stress or when you let your dog sleep in your bedroom, it's a good clue that these things are not good for your asthma.

More

Checking your peak flow is quick and easy. You can do it at home with a simple, low-cost device called a peak flow meter. Here's how:

- Take a breath and blow into the tube on the meter as hard and as fast as you can.
- Write down the number on the meter. Use a notebook or calendar where you can keep track of your peak flow and asthma symptoms over time.
- Do what your asthma action plan (see page 272) says to do based on your peak flow.

Work with your doctor to find out what your peak flow should be and how often to check it. Bring your records of your peak flow readings and symptoms whenever you have a checkup. These can help your doctor know whether you need to change your treatment.

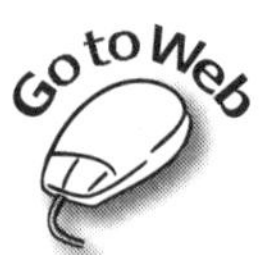

Checking your peak flow is an easy, low-cost step to help you control your asthma and avoid severe attacks. For a complete, step-by-step guide to checking your peak flow, go to the Web site on the back cover and enter **Z611** in the search box.

Using Your Inhaler

Asthma medicine usually comes in an inhaler, a device that lets you breathe the medicine in through your mouth so it goes right to your airways and lungs.

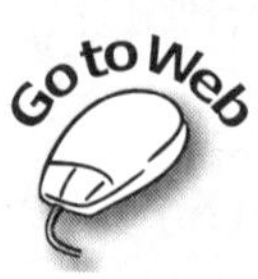

There are two types of inhalers: metered-dose inhalers and dry powder inhalers. Be sure to ask your doctor or pharmacist how to properly use the type that you have. For a step-by-step guide (with pictures), go to the Web site on the back cover and enter **K565** in the search box.

Your doctor may suggest that you use a spacer. A spacer is a piece you attach to the inhaler. It makes using an inhaler easier for many people.

If you still have trouble, tell your doctor. There may be another way you can take your medicine.

Avoid Asthma Triggers

A trigger is anything that makes your asthma worse and can cause an attack. Smoke, pollution, pollen, pet dander, colds, stress, and cold air are triggers for many people.

You can learn what triggers an asthma attack for you by keeping track of your peak flow and your symptoms. When you get worse or better, think about what may have caused it. Is the pollen count high? Did you spend the evening in a smoky bar? Did you go for a walk in the cold air?

After you know what your triggers are, try to prevent or avoid them. These tips may help with the most common triggers:

- If you smoke, quit. See page 351 if you need help quitting. Stay out of smoky places. Do not use a wood-burning stove or fireplace in your home.
- Reduce dust, dust mites, pollen, and mold in your home—especially your bedroom. See page 73 for lots of ideas that can help.
- Do not exercise outside when the air is cold and dry. Try an indoor workout at the gym. Walk at the mall. Get an exercise video you can do at home. (Check with your doctor if you are not sure whether it's safe for you to exercise.)
- Keep pets out of your bedroom. Have your pet stay in areas that have hard floors. They are easier to clean than carpeted ones.

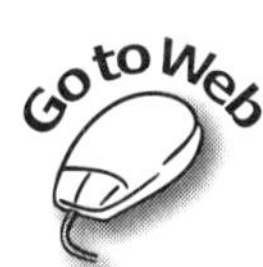

Avoiding your triggers can help prevent asthma attacks and keep you healthy and out of the hospital. For more help finding out what your triggers are and how to deal with them, go to the Web site on the back cover and enter **D990** in the search box.

When to Call a Doctor

Call 911 if:

- You have severe trouble breathing and do not have your asthma medicine with you.
- You have taken your quick-relief medicine and, after 20 to 30 minutes, you do not feel better or your peak flow is still less than 50 percent of your personal best.

Call your doctor if:

- Your symptoms do not get better after you have followed your asthma action plan.
- You cough up yellow, dark brown, or bloody mucus.
- You do not have an asthma action plan and want one.
- You need to use quick-relief medicine more than 2 times a week (for reasons other than exercise).
- You have any problems with your asthma medicine.

Living Better With Cancer

"Cancer" is probably the scariest word in the dictionary. Finding out that you have cancer may make you feel angry, sad, numb, or powerless. Or you may have none of these feelings. Not everyone deals with cancer the same way.

Today, most people with cancer are living longer and better than ever before. Many types of cancer can be cured. For some people, cancer becomes a chronic disease that they live with, like diabetes. As with any chronic disease, living with cancer has its ups and downs.

Getting a diagnosis of cancer changes your life forever. Give yourself time to adjust. You may not be able to do everything you did before. But having a positive outlook, support from loved ones, and a strong, fighting spirit can help you cope with the changes.

What You Can Do

- Learn about the treatments. See this page.
- Manage the side effects. See page 278.
- Stay strong with healthy habits. See page 279.
- Get the support you need. See page 280.
- Get proper follow-up care. See page 280.
- Plan for the future. See page 382.
- Know when to call your doctor. See page 281.

Learn About the Treatments

The treatment may be clear-cut for some cancers. But for others, you may have to decide which treatment or treatments you prefer. The more you know about your options, the better you will be able to decide what is right for you.

Surgery is often done to remove cancer. If the cancer is in a small area, you might have surgery to remove only the cancerous growth (tumor). If the cancer has spread, you may need to have part or all of the affected organs removed. Sometimes doctors also take out some nearby lymph nodes to see if the cancer has spread.

Chemotherapy is the use of medicine to kill cancer cells. The medicines enter the bloodstream and travel throughout the body, so they are a good way to treat cancer that may have spread. Chemotherapy may be given as pills or as shots.

Chemotherapy often works well, but it can cause side effects such as tiredness, nausea, and anemia. And you may get sick more easily. Most of these side effects go away when the treatment is done.

Radiation therapy uses very high doses of X-rays to destroy cancer cells and shrink tumors. This usually works best for cancer that has not spread. Doctors may use it after surgery to destroy any remaining cancer cells. Radiation can also help relieve pain caused by cancer that has spread.

When You Don't Feel Like Eating

Food is one of the most important medicines in fighting cancer. But sometimes it can be hard to eat well. You may not feel hungry, or food may not taste right. Some cancer treatments can cause mouth sores or make you feel sick to your stomach.

Try these tips:

- Eat 5 or 6 small meals or snacks during the day, instead of 3 large meals. Try to always eat breakfast.
- Eat high-protein foods, such as eggs, cottage cheese, meats, fish, and chicken.
- Try meal replacement drinks, such as Ensure or Boost, if you have trouble eating solid food. Soups, smoothies, and milkshakes are also good.
- Eat high-calorie foods. Add honey or brown sugar to foods to make them taste better. Add oil or butter when you cook. Eat peanut butter for snacks.
- Keep snacks on hand that are easy to eat, such as soft granola bars, pudding, and ice cream.
- Drink plenty of water and other fluids. Good choices include ones that have calories but no caffeine or alcohol, such as milk and fruit juices.
- Take a walk before you eat, if possible. It may make you hungrier.

If you keep having trouble, talk to your doctor. There are medicines that can improve your appetite.

Radiation doesn't hurt, but it can cause fatigue, nausea, vomiting, and diarrhea. The side effects usually go away after treatment ends. But you may feel very tired for 4 to 6 weeks after your last treatment.

Watchful waiting is a treatment choice with some types of cancer. It means that you and your doctor will watch your cancer to see if it causes any symptoms or appears to be growing.

It may seem odd to have cancer and not treat it. But sometimes waiting is the best choice. Some cancers grow very slowly, and their treatments are worse than the cancer itself. Treatment may work just as well if you wait until the cancer has grown.

Less common treatments include:

- **Hormone therapy.** This uses hormones to slow the growth of some kinds of cancer. For example, hormone therapy may be used to treat some kinds of breast cancer or prostate cancer.
- **Biological therapy** (also called immunotherapy). This uses substances made by the body or in a lab to boost, direct, or restore your body's natural defenses against disease.

More

Manage Side Effects

Cancer treatments can cause a number of side effects, but you can learn ways to cope with and reduce them.

Nausea and vomiting are common side effects of cancer itself and treatments for it. Your doctor may prescribe medicine that can help control nausea before it starts.

If you feel sick to your stomach, try to eat several small meals a day. When you are feeling better, eat clear soups and mild foods until all symptoms are gone for 12 to 48 hours. Jell-O, dry toast, and crackers are good choices. See page 254.

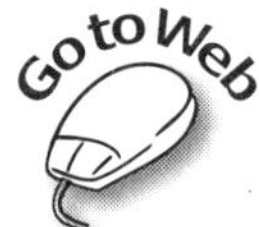

For more tips, go to the Web site on the back cover and enter **P011** in the search box.

Diarrhea may be just a minor problem or a sign of more serious problems. Always tell your doctor if you have diarrhea, especially if you see blood in it.

If you have diarrhea, rest your stomach. Do not eat for several hours or until you are feeling better. Take small sips of water or a rehydration drink and small bites of salty crackers often. See page 30.

Fatigue is often caused by anemia, a problem with your blood (see page 147). Radiation therapy and chemotherapy can cause anemia. If you feel very weak and tired, be sure to tell your doctor. You may need to take medicine for anemia. These tips may help too:

- Slowly increase your exercise. Try walking as your energy allows.
- Limit medicines that might make you more tired, such as tranquilizers and cold and allergy medicines.
- Eat healthy foods. Try not to skip meals, especially breakfast.
- Drink plenty of fluids. Limit alcohol, which can cause dehydration and make you feel more tired.
- Get more rest.

Pain can be caused by cancer and some of its treatments. But that doesn't mean that you have to live with pain. Medicines and other treatments can reduce or stop your pain completely.

If your doctor gives you medicine for pain:

- Take your pain medicines exactly as prescribed. This is very important to keep your pain under control.
- If you take pain medicine "as needed," take it at the first sign of pain. Pain medicine works best if you use it before pain gets bad.
- Don't worry about getting addicted. This is rare if you take your medicine the way your doctor tells you to.
- Tell your doctor if the medicine isn't helping. You are the only person who can say how much pain you have or if a medicine works for you.

There are also other things you can try to control pain. Ask your doctor about:

- Acupuncture. This ancient Chinese technique uses very thin needles to affect energy pathways in the body.
- Progressive muscle relaxation. See page 358.

Dealing With Hair Loss

Hair loss is a common and upsetting side effect of chemotherapy. Some people have mild thinning, while others lose all their hair. Keep in mind that hair almost always grows back after treatment ends.

During treatment:

- Take good care of your scalp and the hair you have. Use a mild shampoo and a soft hairbrush.
- Air-dry your hair. If you have to use a hair dryer, use the low-heat setting.
- Use sunscreen or a hat, scarf, or wig to protect your scalp from the sun.
- Sleep on a satin pillowcase. This will reduce friction on your scalp.
- Think about cutting your hair short. A short style will make your hair look thicker and fuller.
- Do not shave your head. If you cut yourself, you could be at higher risk of bleeding or infection.
- Do not dye your hair or get a permanent.

- Biofeedback. Biofeedback uses the mind to control a body function that the body normally controls on its own, such as muscle tension or heart rate.
- Guided imagery. You can use thoughts and suggestions that direct your mind to a relaxed state.

For more tips on how to reduce or avoid

Go to Web

cancer pain, go to the Web site on the back cover and enter **J643** in the search box.

Stay Strong

It is very important to take good care of yourself when you have cancer. Making healthy lifestyle choices can help you keep up your strength, prevent weight loss, fight infection, and feel better.

- Eat a healthy, balanced diet with plenty of fruits, vegetables, and whole grains. Drink plenty of fluids to prevent dehydration and constipation.
- Get some exercise. Walking is a great way to get moving. Try to do a little more each day, but don't tire yourself out.
- Do not smoke or let others smoke around you. If you need help quitting, see page 351.
- Find ways to lower your stress. See page 356.
- Get enough sleep. If you have trouble sleeping, keep your room dark and quiet, and wear earplugs.
- Spend time with people you care about, and take time to do things that make you happy.

More

Get the Support You Need

When you have cancer, you may feel confused, alone, and scared. But you are not alone. Other people can understand how you feel and can offer support.

- Share your feelings with someone you can trust. Find a good listener who will let you express all your feelings.
- Find a cancer support group in your area or online. These groups can give emotional support as well as practical advice about coping with cancer.
- Talk to your doctors and nurses. They may be able to refer you to support groups or other resources that can help.

You may not have the energy to do all the things you did before. Ask for help when you need it. People who care about you may want to help but not know what they can do. Things they may be able to do include:

- Shopping, cooking, or cleaning.
- Writing bills or doing paperwork.
- Driving you to appointments.

Cancer affects your loved ones too. Encourage them to get counseling or find a support group if they need help.

Get Follow-Up Care

After cancer treatment, you will need follow-up visits and tests for several years or more. How often you need to see your doctor depends on a number of things, including the type of cancer you had. Most people have follow-up appointments every 3 or 4 months for the first 2 or 3 years and then once or twice a year after that.

Be sure you understand:

- How often to see your doctor.
- What follow-up tests you need and how often you need them.
- What symptoms to watch for.
- How to stay healthy and what you can do (if anything) to prevent another cancer.

Will the Cancer Come Back?

If you have had cancer, it is common to feel anxious or scared that it might come back. The best thing you can do is to keep all your appointments, take good care of yourself, and be alert for changes in your health.

- If you have any new symptoms or any new side effects from your treatment, tell your doctor right away.
- If fear or worry keep you from enjoying life, share your feelings with family or friends, or join a support group. Or you may need to talk to your doctor about treatment to help you cope with your feelings.

Deciding to Stop Treatment

All people with cancer hope that treatment will cure the cancer and let them return to a normal life. But sometimes the cancer keeps growing or spreads in spite of treatment. Or the side effects of treatment become too hard to live with. If this happens, you may think about whether you want to keep trying to cure the cancer.

If you decide to stop treatment, you will still see your doctor and get excellent care. But the focus will change from curing the cancer to helping you feel better. This is called **palliative care**. It focuses on controlling pain and other symptoms and improving your quality of life—not just in your body, but also in your mind and spirit. See page 260.

To make the decision about stopping treatment:

- Weigh the benefits of treatment against the side effects. If treatment is not helping and is making you miserable, you may want to stop.
- Find out if there are other types of treatment that you could try. Ask your doctor how likely they are to help.
- Ask your doctor if there are any clinical trials to test new treatments for your type of cancer.

If you are thinking about stopping cancer treatment:

- Talk to your doctor and loved ones about how you feel. A decision to end treatment is hard. But the decision is yours.
- Ask your doctor what to expect if you stop treatment.
- Make plans so you can be sure you get the kind of care you want. To learn more, see Planning for the Future on page 382.
- Remember that you can change your mind. If your health changes or new treatments come out, you can start treatment again.

When to Call a Doctor

- You feel depressed or hopeless.
- You are worried that your cancer is coming back.
- You have any symptom that worries you.
- You have questions about your cancer treatment or its side effects.

Living Better With COPD

COPD (chronic obstructive pulmonary disease) is a long-term illness that makes it hard to breathe. When you have COPD, air does not flow easily out of your lungs. You may be short of breath, cough a lot, and have a lot of mucus in your airways.

If you have emphysema or chronic bronchitis, you have a form of COPD.

With time, breathing problems get worse, and it gets harder to do everyday activities. COPD can lead to heart problems and to death.

But you can make a difference in your health. Good self-care can help you stay healthier for a longer time. For example, regular exercise, special breathing techniques, and rest breaks during the day may help you feel better from day to day. Taking the medicines your doctor prescribes may help with your breathing.

The best thing you can do is stop smoking. This is the only sure way to slow the disease. But it may also be the hardest step to take when you have COPD.

Talk to your doctor about stop-smoking programs and medicines that can help. Also see Quitting Smoking on page 351.

Take Your Medicines

COPD medicines reduce shortness of breath, control coughing and wheezing, and can prevent or reduce a flare-up. Most people with COPD find that using their medicine makes breathing easier.

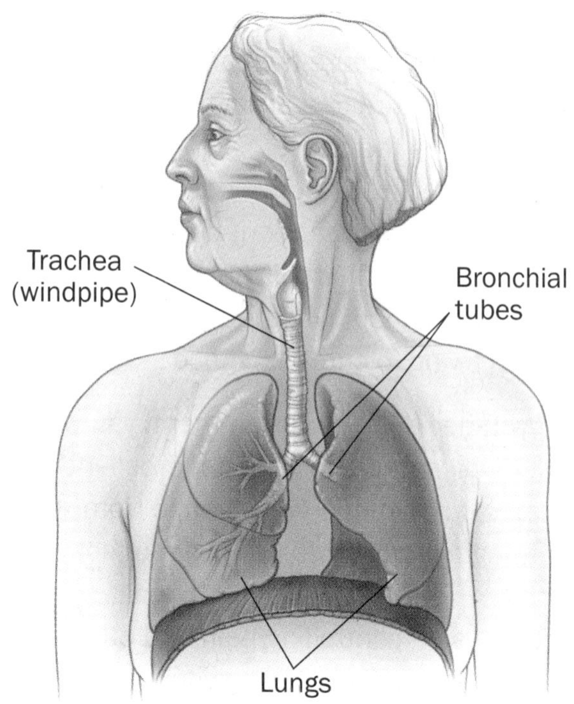

When you have COPD, the airways (trachea and bronchial tubes) leading to the lungs may be blocked by swelling, damage, and mucus. This makes it hard to breathe.

COPD medicines usually come as an inhaler—a device that lets you breathe the medicine in through your mouth so it goes right to your airways and lungs.

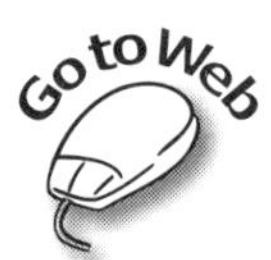

Be sure you are using your inhaler correctly. For a step-by-step guide (with pictures), go to the Web site on the back cover and enter **P588** in the search box. You can also ask your doctor or pharmacist for help.

If you still have trouble using an inhaler, talk to your doctor. There may be another way you can take your medicine.

COPD Flare-Ups

Sometimes your usual shortness of breath will suddenly get worse. You may start coughing more and have more mucus. This is called a COPD flare-up or exacerbation.

Air pollution or a lung infection can cause a flare-up. Sometimes a flare-up may happen after a quick change in temperature or when you are around chemicals.

A COPD flare-up can be life-threatening. If you have one:

- Use your inhaler medicine first.
- If your symptoms do not get better after you use your medicine, have someone take you to the emergency room. Call 911 if you have to.

You may need to be treated in a hospital until you can breathe better on your own. With the right treatment, most people recover from a flare-up, and their breathing is no worse than it was before.

Do everything you can do to avoid flare-ups and stay out of the hospital:

- Take your medicines.
- Avoid "triggers" like smoke, poor air quality, and chemicals.
- Stay as healthy as you can.

Breathe Clean Air at Home

Many things can make your symptoms worse or cause flare-ups—smoke, poor air quality, dust, pollen, even the weather. Some of these COPD "triggers" are out of your control. But you can make your home a place where you can breathe easier.

- Do not let anyone smoke in your home. That means you too.
- Use air-conditioning so you don't have to open the windows. Fresh air may seem like a good idea, but pollen, mold, and air pollution can make your COPD worse.
- Use an air conditioner or air purifier with a HEPA filter.
- Make sure gas appliances are vented well and have tight-fitting doors. Check flues and chimneys for cracks. Don't use an open fireplace or wood-burning stove. Wood smoke is bad for your breathing.
- Do not use strong chemicals or aerosol sprays in your home, and do not mix cleaning products. Try natural cleaners like vinegar, lemon juice, boric acid, or baking soda.
- Do not keep items for recycling indoors. Newspapers, rags, cans, and bottles can give off fumes.
- Reduce the dust in your house as much as you can. See page 73.
- Make sure outdoor fresh-air intake vents for heating and air-conditioning systems are above ground. Keep cars, trucks, and other sources of pollution away from the vents.

More

Breathing Lessons

People with COPD tend to take quick, short breaths. Breathing this way makes it harder to get air into your lungs. But you can learn some other ways to breathe that make it easier. Use these methods when you are more short of breath than normal. Practice them every day so you can do them well.

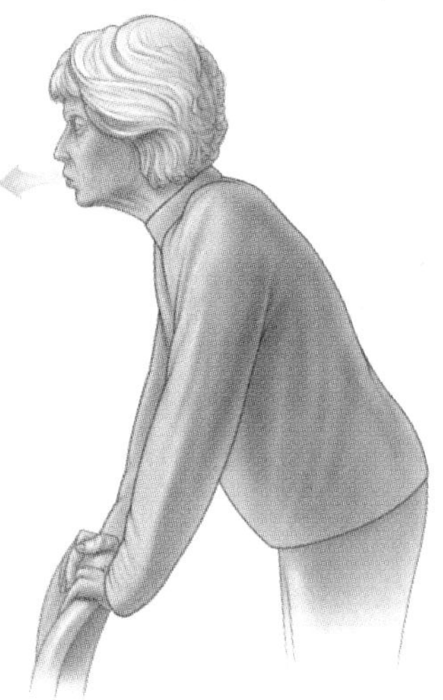

Pursed-lip breathing while bending forward

Pursed-lip breathing

Breathe in through your nose and out through your mouth while almost closing your lips. Breathe in for about 4 seconds, and breathe out for 6 to 8 seconds.

Pursed-lip breathing helps you breathe more air out so that your next breath can be deeper. It makes you less short of breath and lets you exercise more.

Breathing while bending

Bending forward at the waist may make it easier for you to breathe. It can reduce shortness of breath while you are exercising or resting.

Breathing with your diaphragm

Breathing with your diaphragm helps your lungs expand so that they take in more air.

- Lie on your back or prop yourself up on several pillows.
- With one hand on your belly and the other on your chest, breathe in. Push your belly out as far as you can. You should feel the hand on your belly move out, while the hand on your chest should not move. When you breathe out, the hand on your belly should move in.
- After you learn to do this lying down, you can learn to do it while sitting or standing.

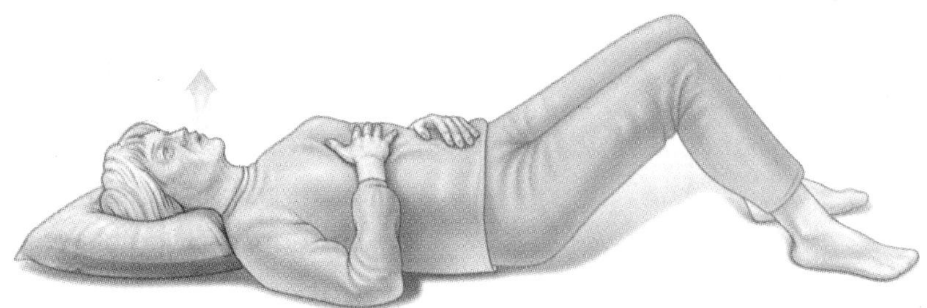

Breathing with your diaphragm

Stay Healthy, Feel Better

There are things you can do that will help you be able to do more and give you more energy.

- Stop smoking. This is the most important step you can take to feel better and live longer. See page 351 to get started.
- Avoid colds, the flu, and pneumonia.
  - Get a flu shot each fall. Ask those you live or work with to do the same, so they don't get the flu and pass it to you.
  - Wash your hands often, especially during cold and flu season.
  - Get a pneumococcal vaccine shot every 5 to 10 years or as advised by your doctor. This can help prevent serious illness from pneumonia.
- Avoid smoke; cold, dry air; hot, humid air; and high altitudes. Stay inside with the windows closed when air pollution is bad.
- Exercise most days of the week. Walking is a great way to be more active. To learn what other kinds of exercise are good for people with COPD, go to the Web site on the back cover and enter **T179** in the search box.

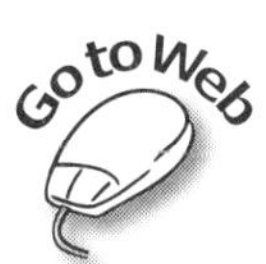

- Ask your doctor whether a pulmonary rehab program would be good for you. In rehab, you work with a team to learn how to breathe easier, exercise, and eat well. Many people with COPD find these programs helpful. To learn more, go to the Web site on the back cover and enter **C825** in the search box.

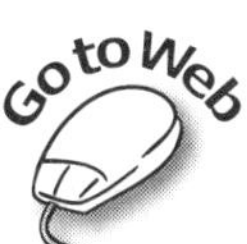

- Take short rest breaks when you are doing chores and other activities. This will help your breathing and help you avoid getting too tired.
- Eat regular, healthy meals. People with COPD often find it hard to eat because of their breathing problems, but there are some simple ways to make it easier. To learn how, go to the Web site on the back cover and enter **G407** in the search box.

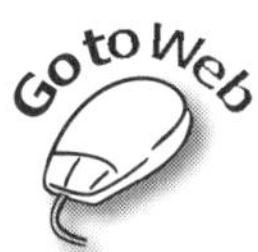

Planning for the Future

Over time, your breathing and your overall health are probably going to get worse no matter what you do. It's normal to feel frightened, angry, hopeless, or even guilty. Talk to your family, friends, or a therapist about how you feel, or join a support group. Talking about your feelings can help you cope.

You may also feel a little more at peace with the future if you plan for it. Talk to your doctor and your family about what you want to happen when your health gets worse. Write out advance directives, such as a living will, so that you get to decide what kind of treatment you have at the end of your life.

For help with end-of-life planning, see page 382.

More

What About Oxygen Therapy?

At some point you may need oxygen therapy. By boosting the oxygen in your blood, this treatment helps you breathe easier and gives you more energy. It may also help you live longer and stay out of the hospital.

You can use oxygen therapy while you move around and do daily tasks. You may breathe the oxygen through a flexible plastic tube in your nostrils (nasal cannula), a face mask, or a tube put into your windpipe.

The oxygen can be supplied in several ways: an oxygen gas tank, liquid oxygen in small containers, or a machine called an oxygen concentrator. Each has its pros and cons in terms of weight, cost, how much oxygen it holds, and how dangerous it is. (There is a risk of fire if you use oxygen around a lit cigarette or an open flame.)

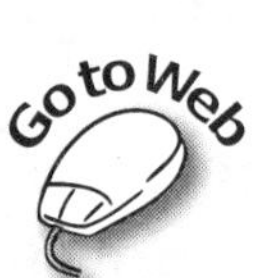

You may need oxygen only when you exercise or when you are asleep. Or you may need it all the time. If you and your doctor decide that you need oxygen to prolong your life and make you more comfortable, work together to decide what is best for you. To learn how to use oxygen at home, go to the Web site on the back cover and enter **S093** in the search box.

When to Call a Doctor

Call 911 if you have severe trouble breathing.

Call your doctor if:

- You have shortness of breath or wheezing that is quickly getting worse.
- You are coughing more deeply or more often than usual.
- You cough up blood.
- Swelling in your legs or belly gets worse.
- You have a fever.
- Your medicine does not seem to be working as well as it had been.

Living Better With Coronary Artery Disease

Coronary artery disease (CAD) means that the blood vessels that bring blood to the heart (coronary arteries) have become narrow or blocked. They usually get blocked by **plaque**, which is a buildup of fat and other substances.

When you have CAD, your arteries cannot bring as much blood and oxygen to your heart. Poor blood flow can cause **angina** (chest pain) when you force your heart to work harder. If the blood flow gets completely blocked, you may have a heart attack.

With poor blood flow over time, your heart may get weaker and not pump as well as it should. This can lead to dangerous heartbeat problems and heart failure.

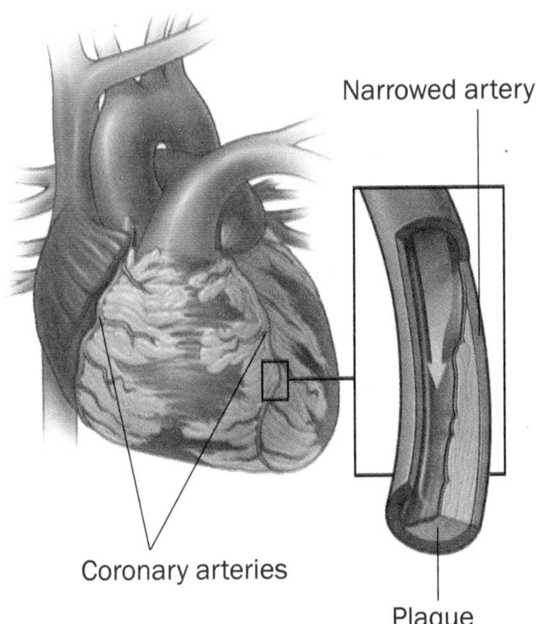

Plaque is a buildup of fat and other substances that can block your arteries.

You may not feel sick at all until your heart disease gets a lot worse. Some people have CAD for years without having chest pain or any other symptoms. This may make it hard to feel like you need to pay attention to the problem.

But try not to ignore the fact that you have heart disease, even if you feel fine right now. The goal is to keep feeling good for a long time. You have a better chance of doing that if you start living healthier today. What you do can make a big difference.

How to Avoid a Heart Attack

For many people with CAD, their biggest fear is a heart attack. To avoid a heart attack and live longer and better, you will need to take steps to improve your health. The good news is that you are in control.

Here are things you can do now to get healthy and stay that way:

- If you smoke, quit. See page 290.
- Eat healthy food. Eat more fiber, and cut down on cholesterol, saturated fat, and salt. See page 289.
- Get some exercise most days of the week. Start with short walks or any other activity you enjoy. See page 290.
- Take any medicines your doctor prescribes.

More

What Is Angioplasty?

Angioplasty is a way to widen a narrow or blocked coronary artery and improve blood flow to your heart without surgery. It is often used during or soon after a heart attack. It can also help prevent a heart attack for some people with coronary artery disease.

During angioplasty, your doctor threads a thin tube called a catheter into the blocked or narrow artery. At the end of the catheter is a tiny balloon. The doctor inflates the balloon inside the artery to open the blocked area.

The doctor may also put a stent in the artery. A stent is a small, wire-mesh tube that expands and pushes out against the walls of the artery to keep it open. Some stents also release a drug that helps keep the artery open.

Whether you need angioplasty depends on how many blocked arteries you have, how badly they are blocked, other problems you may have, and other issues.

Dealing With Angina

Many people with CAD have no symptoms. But others may feel chest pain or pressure when they do things that make their heart work harder. This type of chest pain is called angina.

Angina is a signal that your heart is not getting enough oxygen. The pain usually is mild at first and gets worse over several minutes. It may spread to your belly, upper back, shoulders, neck, jaws, or arms.

If you have had angina for a while, you may be able to predict almost exactly how much activity will cause pain. You know what things cause your angina, and you know what to expect and what to do when it happens. This is called stable angina.

Watch for changes in your angina. If your angina is worse or lasts longer than usual, or you start getting it more often, it could mean that your heart disease is getting worse. Call your doctor right away. You may need a checkup or tests, or your doctor may need to change your treatment.

What to do when you have chest pain

- Stop what you are doing. Sit down and rest.
- If your doctor has prescribed a medicine like nitroglycerin, take one dose.
- If you are not feeling better within 5 minutes, **call 911**. Stay on the phone. The emergency operator will tell you what to do next.

If you take nitroglycerin

Nitroglycerin is a medicine that opens blood vessels to improve blood flow. This relieves chest pain and reduces how hard the heart has to work.

Your doctor will tell you when to use your nitroglycerin. You may need to take it:

- To relieve sudden angina.
- Before stressful activities that can cause angina, such as exercise or sex.

Do not take erection-producing medicines such as Viagra, Levitra, or Cialis if you are taking nitroglycerin. Taking any of them with nitroglycerin can be very dangerous. If you get chest pain and have taken one of these erection-producing medicines, tell your doctor so that you are not given nitroglycerin or a similar medicine.

Eat a Heart-Healthy Diet

Most experts agree that the best diet for your heart is high in fiber, low in cholesterol and saturated fat, and low in salt.

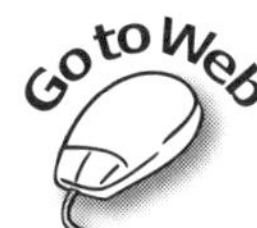

The tips in the chart on this page can help you get started. To learn even more about heart-healthy foods, go to the Web site on the back cover and enter **P493** in the search box.

Your doctor may suggest that you follow the DASH (Dietary Approaches to Stop Hypertension) diet or something similar. To learn what this diet is and

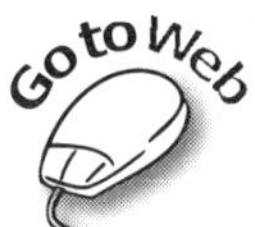

how it can help you, go to the Web site on the back cover and enter **X209** in the search box.

More

Eating a Heart-Healthy Diet

Instead of:	Try this:
Frying your food	Bake, broil, steam, poach, or grill your food.
Eating convenience foods (canned soups, TV dinners, frozen pizza)	Eat fresh fish, skinless chicken, fruits, and vegetables.
Using butter or oil high in saturated fat	Use products low in saturated fat, such as olive oil, vegetable oil, canola oil, or chicken broth.
Using salt, soy sauce, or barbecue sauce	Use salt-free spices.
Eating all of the meat product	Trim fat from meat and skin from chicken.
Eating egg yolks	Eat egg whites or egg substitutes.

An Aspirin a Day?

Taking 1 aspirin a day may help you avoid a heart attack or stroke. If you have not discussed this with your doctor, ask about it at your next visit to make sure it's safe for you.

Stop Smoking

Quitting smoking is one of the best things you can do if you don't want to die of heart disease. Your risk of dying from heart attack or stroke will start to go down very soon after you quit. Within several years, your risk will be about the same as that of someone who has never smoked.

If you have had angioplasty or bypass surgery to fix blocked arteries, those arteries will be less likely to get blocked again if you quit smoking.

You will also feel better after you quit smoking. Your angina may get better. You will have more energy and breathe easier. And you may feel more hopeful about your future and have less fear of getting cancer or dying suddenly from heart disease.

Smoking is bad for everyone, but it is even worse for people with coronary artery disease.

- It makes your blood cells more likely to form clots. This can cause a heart attack or stroke.
- It can cause a sudden narrowing in your coronary arteries, which can reduce the blood flow to your heart.
- It can make your heart beat in an odd rhythm.
- It lowers "good" (HDL) cholesterol and lets "bad" (LDL) cholesterol build up in your arteries more easily.
- It reduces how much oxygen your blood can carry. This means your heart (and the rest of your body) may not get enough oxygen.

Quitting smoking is not easy. Many people have to try several times before they quit for good. But the point is that they do finally succeed. And with the right help, so can you.

See Quitting Smoking on page 351 to learn how to get started.

Exercise Your Heart

If you are not active right now, starting to exercise may seem hard. But it is worth it. You don't have to do a lot to make a difference.

Being more active can:

- Help you control your weight, blood pressure, and cholesterol.
- Make your heart stronger and reduce symptoms like chest pain.
- Help you avoid a heart attack or stroke and live longer.
- Reduce stress and give you more energy.

Walking is a great, easy way to get exercise. If your doctor says it's safe, start out with some short walks. Make the walks a little bit longer until you are walking 20 to 30 minutes at a time.

If you don't enjoy walking, you might try swimming, biking, or water aerobics. Your doctor can help you make a plan.

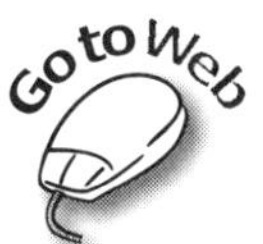

The important thing is to try to get some exercise several days a week. Even a little bit of exercise can help if you have not been active at all. For some ideas that might work for you, go to the Web site on the back cover and enter **P836** in the search box.

You might also ask your doctor about joining a **cardiac rehab** program. In cardiac rehab, you work with a team of doctors, nurses, and therapists to learn how to stay healthier and feel better.

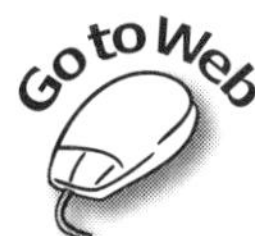

Many people with heart disease find this type of program helpful. To learn more about whether cardiac rehab might be right for you, go to the Web site on the back cover and enter **W065** in the search box.

Be safe when you exercise

See your doctor before you start exercising. He or she may want to do a test to see how much activity your heart can handle.

If your doctor has prescribed nitroglycerin for you, be sure to have it with you whenever you exercise. Stop what you are doing right away if you have any chest pain or start to feel bad.

When to Call a Doctor

Call 911 if:

- You have chest pain or pressure with other signs of a heart attack. These may include:
  - Sweating.
  - Shortness of breath.
  - Nausea or vomiting.
  - Pain in your upper back, upper belly, neck, jaw, or arms.
  - Feeling dizzy or lightheaded.
  - A fast or uneven heartbeat.

  After calling 911, chew 1 adult aspirin (unless you are allergic to aspirin). If you cannot get an ambulance, have someone drive you to the hospital. Do not drive yourself.
- You have been diagnosed with angina, and you have chest pain or pressure that does not go away with rest or within 5 minutes after you take nitroglycerin.
- You faint.

Call your doctor if:

- You have chest pain (angina) more often than usual, or the pain is worse or different than usual.
- You have had any chest pain, even if it has gone away.
- You have any problems with your medicines.

Living Better With Depression

Depression takes the joy out of life and can leave you feeling sad and hopeless. Many things can bring on depression:

- Having a stroke or a chronic disease such as cancer or diabetes
- Losing someone you love
- Going through a major life change like divorce, retirement, or moving
- The stress of caring for someone who is sick
- Taking certain medicines
- Abusing alcohol or drugs

Sometimes people get depression without an obvious cause or change in their life.

Depression is very common in older adults. Yet many people do not get the help they need. Doctors may not recognize the signs of depression in older adults. And many people don't ask for help, because they're embarrassed or think they'll get better on their own. If you think you may be depressed but you have not been diagnosed, see Are You Depressed? on page 146.

Depression is a medical problem, not a character flaw or weakness. If you are depressed, there is no reason for you to suffer. Treatment works very well for most people. With counseling, medicines, good self-care, and a little time, you can feel a lot better. Treatment can also help you avoid future problems with depression.

Counseling Can Help

The words "counseling" or "therapy" may make you think of lying on a leather couch and talking about your childhood. But the most common kind of counseling does not look for hidden feelings or memories. It deals with how you think about things and how you act each day. It helps you replace thoughts or actions that make you feel bad with ones that make you feel better. Over time, these changes turn into habits.

If you decide to see a counselor to help with your depression, know that sometimes it takes a number of meetings before you start to feel better. And you may need to see a counselor regularly for several months or longer to get the best results.

Choosing a counselor

Your counselor may be a psychiatrist (a medical doctor), a psychologist, or a licensed counselor. When you choose a counselor:

- Be sure the person has experience and training in treating depression. Also make sure that he or she has a license to practice in your state. Some states have strict rules about who can work as a counselor.
- Choose someone you like and trust. For counseling to work, you have to talk honestly about your feelings. Having a counselor you feel comfortable with makes this easier. If you meet with someone and don't feel good about it, try someone else.

What About St. John's Wort?

St. John's wort is an herbal supplement sold in health food stores and drugstores. Europeans have used it for centuries to treat depression. But in the United States, it is still being tested.

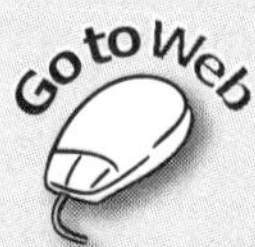

High-quality St. John's wort may help with mild or moderate depression. After talking to your doctor about it, you may want to see if it works for you. Go to the Web site on the back cover and enter **Y764** in the search box to learn more.

Do not take St. John's wort with antidepressants or any other medicines unless your doctor has told you it's safe. St. John's wort can cause dangerous reactions if you use it with other medicines.

Keep in mind that herbal supplements are not tested and controlled the way medicines are. Each pill may not have the same amount of active ingredient. Always tell your doctor if you're using an herbal product. You could have serious side effects. See Vitamins, Herbs, and Other Supplements on page 370.

Medicines for Depression

Antidepressant medicines help many people with depression get better. They can help keep the chemicals in your brain in balance. They do not change your personality. To see if medicine

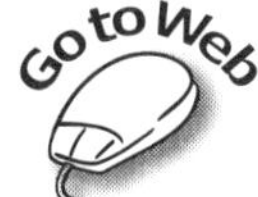

might be right for you, go to the Web site on the back cover and enter **Q515** in the search box.

There are many medicines for depression, and there is no proof that one works better than another. But they have different side effects and treat different symptoms of depression.

Your doctor will consider many things when deciding which drug to give you:

- How did you respond to medicines used in the past?
- Are you taking medicine for other health problems? Your doctor will not give you a drug that will react badly with any other drugs you're taking.
- Will the drug make any other illness you have worse or harder to treat?
- How old are you? How is your overall health? Older adults may need lower doses.
- How much are the side effects likely to bother you?

You may need to take antidepressants for at least a few months to feel completely well. But you may start to feel better much sooner. Here are some things to keep in mind:

More

- You may start to feel better within 1 to 3 weeks of starting an antidepressant. But it can take 6 to 8 weeks before you see more improvement.
- Often the first drug the doctor prescribes will work well. If not, there are other choices. You may need to try several before you find the one that works best for you.
- The medicine may have side effects. Many of these will go away as you get used to the medicine. If they continue, or if they bother you too much, talk to your doctor. You may need a different drug.
- Make sure to tell your doctor if you take any other medicines or herbal products. Tell your doctor about any other health problems you have.
- After you start to feel better, you may need to take your medicine for at least several more months. This can help keep depression from coming back.
- When you think you're ready to quit taking antidepressants, you will need to work with your doctor to slowly lower the dose. Stopping suddenly can cause serious problems or a return of depression. See Feeling Better? on page 295.

Do not stop taking antidepressants on your own unless you have chest pain, hives, trouble breathing or swallowing, or swelling of your lips. Call your doctor right away or go to the emergency room if you have any of these serious side effects.

Seasonal Affective Disorder

Some people feel more depressed during the winter months when there is less sunlight. This is sometimes called seasonal affective disorder (SAD).

It may help to:

- Go out in the sun as often as you can. (Remember to protect your skin.)
- Get regular exercise, either outdoors or indoors near a sunny window.
- Ask your doctor about light therapy. This involves sitting or working in front of special lights for up to several hours a day.

As with other forms of depression, medicine and counseling can also help.

While You Recover

Your mood will improve, but it takes time. In the meantime:

- Take your medicines as prescribed, and go to your counseling sessions. It may take several weeks before you notice a change.
- Take good care of yourself. Eat healthy meals. Get enough sleep. If you have problems sleeping, see the tips starting on page 233. Do not take sleeping pills.
- Stay active. Get outside and take walks. Go to a movie, concert, or ball game.

- Spend time with friends and family. Take part in social events or church.
- Do not drink alcohol or use illegal drugs. And don't take medicines that have not been prescribed for you.
- Break large tasks into smaller steps that you can handle. Do what you can.
- If possible, put off major decisions like marriage, divorce, or a job change until you feel better. Talk over big changes with friends and loved ones who can offer other points of view.
- If you have another illness, like diabetes or heart disease, keep treating it.

Ask for help if you need it. And if you ever have thoughts of hurting yourself, get help right away.

Feeling Better?

If you are feeling better, you may think it's okay to stop going to counseling or to quit taking your medicine.

Wait! Talk to your doctor before you do this. To keep depression from coming back, you may need to continue with treatment even after you feel better. Some people need to take medicines for years.

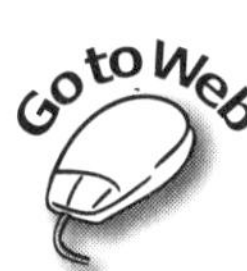

For help deciding whether medicines are still right for you, go to the Web site on the back cover and enter **U844** in the search box.

How to Prevent a Relapse

- Do not stop taking your medicine too soon. It may help to keep taking it after you feel better. Some people need to take medicine for the rest of their lives to stay healthy.
- Do not stop taking your medicine suddenly. If you want to stop taking it, ask your doctor whether this is safe for you and how best to do it.
- Keep seeing your counselor after you stop the medicine. This helps some people avoid a relapse.
- Eat a healthy diet, and get regular exercise. Stick to a regular sleep schedule.
- Avoid alcohol and illegal drugs.
- See your doctor right away if you have new symptoms or feel worse.

When to Call a Doctor

- You feel hopeless and cannot stop thinking about hurting yourself or someone else. **Call 911 or the national suicide hotline at 1-800-784-2433.**
- You hear voices.
- You think you are depressed, and you have not talked to your doctor about it.
- Your depression gets worse even with treatment.
- You have been taking an antidepressant for 3 weeks and have not started to feel better.
- You have any problems with your medicine.

Living Better With Diabetes

Whether you've been dealing with diabetes for years or have just found out that you have it, it's important to understand what happens and how to take care of yourself. Having diabetes means that your body may not make enough of a hormone called **insulin** or may not use insulin properly. Insulin helps your body use sugar from your food as energy or store it for later use. When this doesn't happen, too much sugar stays in your blood.

Over time, high blood sugar can lead to serious problems.

- It can harm your eyes (retinopathy), nerves (neuropathy), and kidneys (nephropathy).
- It can damage your blood vessels, leading to heart disease and stroke.
- It can reduce blood flow to parts of your body, especially your feet. This can cause pain and slow healing.

How can you prevent these problems? What can you do to keep them from getting worse if you already have one or more of them? Here are the most important things to do:

- Take your diabetes medicines.
- Check your blood sugar as often as your doctor recommends. See page 298.
- Eat healthy, balanced meals and snacks. See page 300.
- Exercise on most days of the week. See page 301.
- See your doctor for checkups and tests on a regular schedule. See page 299.
- If you have high blood pressure or high cholesterol, take the medicines your doctor prescribed to control the problem.
- If you smoke, quit. This will reduce the risk of damage to your blood vessels. If you need help quitting, see page 351.

Living with diabetes day after day can be a struggle. Watching what you eat, checking your blood sugar, taking your medicine on time—there will be times when you just can't do it all. Don't be too hard on yourself. Just try to get back on track.

And if you're already doing what you need to, keep it up!

Medicines for Diabetes

Some people with type 2 diabetes need medicine to help their bodies make more insulin or use insulin properly. Pills for type 2 diabetes can also slow down how the body absorbs sugar. This can help keep your blood sugar at a safe level.

You may need to take one or more pills more than once a day. Some people need medicine for only a short time. Some have to take it for the rest of their lives. What you need will depend on how well your blood sugar stays in a safe range. Weight loss, exercise, and healthy eating can sometimes reduce your need for medicine by bringing your blood sugar down.

People with type 1 diabetes have to take insulin throughout their lives to control their blood sugar. If you have type 2 diabetes, you may be able to avoid or delay the need for insulin with careful eating, regular exercise, and proper use of other diabetes medicines. Many people with type 2 diabetes do end up needing to take insulin at some point.

Cost tips for medicines

Your diabetes medicine helps you to stay healthy and avoid more serious, costly problems. While the costs of the medicine can add up, there may be ways to get your diabetes medicine for less.

You can buy most diabetes medicines either by their brand names or as generic drugs. (For example, many people with diabetes take the drug metformin. You may know it by its brand name, Glucophage.) There can be a big cost difference between these. If you are taking a brand-name drug, ask your doctor whether the generic one would work just as well for you.

Some diabetes medicines are sold as a combination pill, with two different drugs in a single dose. While this may be convenient, it may cost more than getting each drug on its own, especially if you can buy one or both of the medicines as generics.

See page 3 for other suggestions on how to save money on your medicines—like buying in bulk and using online drugstores.

Five Things to Do Today

1. **Take an aspirin** (if you have talked to your doctor about it). An aspirin a day may help you avoid a heart attack or stroke. If you have not discussed this with your doctor, ask about it at your next visit to make sure it's safe for you.
2. **Get a medical alert bracelet** online or at your local drugstore. If you have a health emergency and cannot speak, this ID will let medical staff know that you have diabetes. This is even more important if you take insulin or often have problems with low blood sugar.
3. **Check your feet** for small cuts, sores, or toenail problems. Small problems can become big ones if you don't deal with them. See Foot Care on page 209. For more tips, Go to Web go to the Web site on the back cover and enter **A691** in the search box.
4. **Take a walk.** Regular exercise can help you control your blood sugar and reduce your need for medicine. Make sure you wear sturdy shoes.
5. **Get support.** Call your local hospital and ask if it has a support group or classes for people with diabetes. Or visit the Web site of the American Diabetes Association, www.diabetes.org. It has recipes, exercise tips, and all kinds of information that can help you.

More

Check Your Blood Sugar

You may not like having to check your blood sugar every day and keep track of the results over time. But it can really help you keep your diabetes under control.

- Checking how your blood sugar rises or falls in response to certain foods, exercise, and other things can help you reduce symptoms and prevent blood sugar emergencies.
- Having a record of your blood sugar over time can help you and your doctor know how well your treatment is working and whether you need to make any changes.

Simply put, you have a better chance of keeping your blood sugar in a safe range if you know what it is from day to day. Controlling your blood sugar will help you feel better and will slow down the long-term damage to your eyes, kidneys, and heart that can result when your blood sugar is not controlled.

Many people are able to do a good job of tracking their blood sugar after they get in the habit. It helps to:

- Know how and when to check your blood sugar.
- Have the right supplies and know how to use them.
- Have an easy way to keep track of your results.

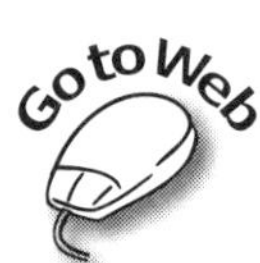

For help setting up a routine that works for you, go to the Web site on the back cover and enter **Z203** in the search box.

If You Have Prediabetes

If you have prediabetes (impaired glucose tolerance), your blood sugar level is higher than normal, but it is not as high as it would be if you had diabetes. Prediabetes is a warning sign for type 2 diabetes. Think of it as a wake-up call. Most people who get type 2 diabetes have prediabetes first.

If you have prediabetes, you may be able to avoid or delay type 2 diabetes (and the problems it can cause) by making some changes in your lifestyle.

- Eat a balanced, healthy diet. Try to eat an even amount of carbohydrate all through the day. This can help you avoid sudden peaks in blood sugar.
- Get at least 30 minutes of exercise on most days of the week. Exercise helps control your blood sugar. It also helps you control your weight. Walking is a good choice for many people. You also may want to try swimming, cycling, or other activities. See page 340.
- Try to stay at a healthy weight. If you need to lose weight, keep in mind that even a small loss of 5 to 10 pounds can help. See page 326.
- If you smoke, quit. Smoking can make prediabetes worse. If you need help quitting, see page 351.

Tests That Can Help You

Seeing your doctor and having certain tests on a regular schedule can help you watch for and avoid many of the problems caused by diabetes. Diabetes can damage many different parts of your body, but you may not have symptoms of the damage until it's too late to do much about it. Tests give you and your doctor a chance to find problems early, when they are easier to treat.

The table below lists some of the tests a typical person with diabetes may need. Talk with your doctor about what test schedule is right for you.

Schedule for Tests and Exams

Test	Why you need it	How often to get it
Hemoglobin A1c blood test	Checks average blood sugar over past 3 months; best way to see how well treatment and self-care are working	Every 3 to 6 months
Blood pressure test	Need to monitor blood pressure; high blood pressure increases risk of blood vessel and nerve damage	Every 3 to 6 months
Sensory foot exam	Reduced feeling in feet can be sign of nerve damage (neuropathy)	At least every year
Eye exam by an ophthalmologist	Diabetes can damage vision (retinopathy); does not cause symptoms until severe	Every year (your main doctor may also check your eyes at each visit)
Fasting cholesterol test	Diabetes puts you at risk for high cholesterol and heart disease	Every year (more often if you take medicine for high cholesterol)
Urine test for protein	Protein in urine may be the only sign of early kidney damage (nephropathy)	Every year
Dental exam and cleaning	Diabetes increases risk of gum problems and infection	Every 6 months

More

What About Carbohydrate and Sugar?

When you have diabetes, you have to be careful about how much carbohydrate you eat at one time. If you eat too much at once, your blood sugar will quickly rise (and then later may drop sharply).

Carbohydrate is an important nutrient you get from food. It is a great source of energy for your body and helps your brain and nervous system work at their best.

It comes in two forms:

- Starch (complex carbohydrate). Starch is in foods such as breads, cereals, grains, pasta, rice, flour, beans, and vegetables.
- Sugar (simple carbohydrate). Sugar is in foods such as fruits, juices, milk, honey, desserts, and candy.

All forms of carbohydrate raise your blood sugar, depending on how much carbohydrate is in the food.

The goal is to keep your blood sugar steady and avoid high blood sugar after meals. You can help by spreading your carbohydrate throughout the day, rather than eating a lot at once. This will also keep you from getting too hungry. See Meal Planning: What Does Your Plate Look Like? on this page to learn more about this.

Unlike what you may have heard, you can eat foods that have sugar when you have diabetes. But if foods that are high in sugar make up a large part of your diet, you are probably not eating enough of other, healthier foods. And your blood sugar levels may be too unsteady.

Meal Planning: What Does Your Plate Look Like?

Eating right helps keep your blood sugar in a safe range. For some people, healthy eating and regular exercise are enough to keep their diabetes under control without medicines. If you take medicine, eating right can help the medicine work better.

Meal planning for diabetes includes eating certain amounts and kinds of foods at regular meals and snacks. You may have heard about the need to count your carbohydrate grams and use diabetic exchange lists and food guides. It may seem overwhelming.

But there's an easy way to get started: the **plate format**. The plate format is a great way to learn about meal planning and get used to measuring how much you eat.

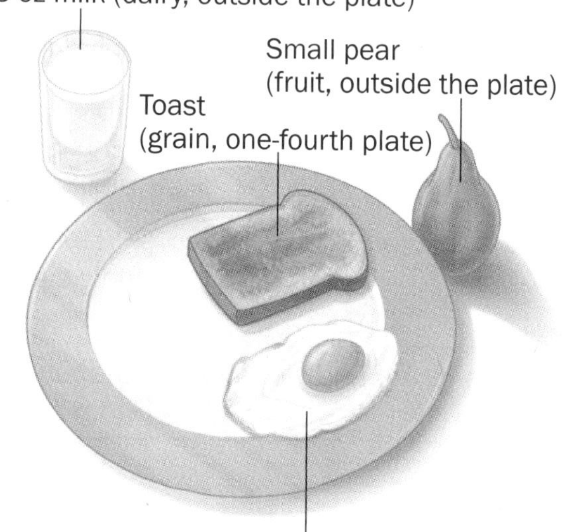

Sample plate for breakfast

8 oz milk (dairy, outside the plate)

½ c. peaches
(fruit, outside the plate)

Brown rice
(grain, one-fourth plate)

Carrots, asparagus, mushrooms (veggies, half plate)

Salmon
(protein, one-fourth plate)

Sample plate for dinner

Using a plate format lets you picture what a meal should look like and how much space each food should take up on your plate. This can help you eat balanced meals. It also can stop you from eating too much carbohydrate at once.

For example, a typical healthy plate for lunch or dinner will have:

- Bread, starchy foods, or grain on one-fourth of the plate.
- Meat or another form of protein (like beans or an egg) on one-fourth of the plate.
- Vegetables on half the plate.
- 1 small piece of fruit outside the plate.
- 1 cup of milk or yogurt or ½ cup of pudding or ice cream outside the plate.

Post a sample plate format on your refrigerator until you get used to what a healthy plate looks like. When you can picture your plate, you can use the method anywhere, even when you eat out.

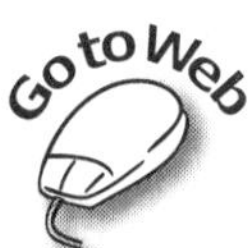

To learn how to use the plate format for all your meals and snacks, go to the Web site on the back cover and enter **B106** in the search box. And when you are ready to learn more about meal planning, talk with a registered dietitian or diabetes educator about other methods.

Safe Exercise

Exercise helps control your blood sugar. It also helps you stay at a healthy weight, raises "good" (HDL) cholesterol, and lowers high blood pressure. These benefits help prevent heart disease, the main cause of death in people who have diabetes.

Try to get at least 30 minutes of exercise on most days. You may need to slowly work up to this if you are not used to being active. Even small amounts of exercise can help.

Walking, running, bike riding, and swimming are great for most people with diabetes. But some activities may not be safe. For instance, if you have diabetic eye disease (retinopathy), it may not be safe to lift weights. If you have nerve disease (neuropathy), running may cause foot problems.

More

Before you start a new exercise program, check with your doctor to find out what activities are best for you.

Here are some other safety tips:

- Check your blood sugar before you exercise, and be careful about what you eat. This is especially true if you take insulin or other medicines for diabetes. Do not exercise when your blood sugar is too low (less than 60 mg/dL).
- Try to exercise at about the same time each day to keep your blood sugar steady. If you want to exercise more, slowly increase how hard or long you exercise.
- Have someone with you when you exercise, or exercise at a gym. You may need help if your blood sugar drops too low.
- Keep some type of quick-sugar food with you. You may get symptoms of low blood sugar during exercise or up to 24 hours later.
- Use proper footwear and the right equipment.
- Pay attention to your body. If you are used to exercise and notice that you cannot do as much as usual, talk to your doctor.

When to Call a Doctor

Call 911 if:

- Your blood sugar stays below 60 mg/dL after you treat low blood sugar, or you are getting more sleepy or confused.
- Your blood sugar is very high, you are becoming less alert, and your breathing is fast and deep.
- You have chest pain or pressure, especially if it occurs with other signs of a heart attack. See page 38.

Call your doctor if:

- You often have problems with your blood sugar being too high or too low. Your doctor may need to change your medicine.
- You have burning pain, tingling, numbness, or swelling in your feet or hands.
- You have vision changes or pain in your eyes.
- A wound looks infected or will not heal.
- You often have a lot of bloating, belching, constipation, nausea and vomiting, or belly pain after you eat.
- You have a hard time knowing when your blood sugar is low.

Living Better With Heart Failure

When you have heart failure, your heart does not pump as much blood as your body needs. Failure does not mean your heart has stopped pumping. It means your heart is not pumping as well as it should.

Your body has an amazing ability to make up for heart failure. It may do such a good job at first that you may not feel like you have a disease.

But at some point, your body will not be able to keep up. Then fluid will slowly build up in your body and cause symptoms like weakness and shortness of breath. This fluid buildup is called congestion.

What You Can Do

Heart failure usually gets worse over time. But there are many steps you can take to feel better and stay healthy longer. These are the most important:

- Take your medicines as prescribed. This gives them the best chance of helping you. See Take Your Medicines on this page.
- Limit salt (sodium). This helps keep fluid from building up and makes it easier for your heart to pump. See page 304.
- Watch for signs that you're getting worse so that your doctor can help you. Weighing yourself every day is one of the best ways to do this. Weight gain may be a sign that your body is holding on to too much fluid. See page 305.
- Try to exercise most days of the week. Exercise makes your heart stronger and can help you avoid symptoms. See page 305.
- Find out what your triggers are, and learn to avoid them. Triggers are things that make your heart failure worse, often suddenly. A trigger may be eating too much salt, missing a dose of your medicine, or exercising too hard.

There are other things you can do to help too, like eating right, not smoking, not drinking much alcohol, controlling your blood pressure, and staying at a healthy weight. These things make it easier for your heart to keep pumping. They will also reduce your risk of heart attack and stroke.

Take Your Medicines

You will probably take several medicines for heart failure. You may also need medicine to treat the problem that caused your heart failure, such as high blood pressure, heart disease, or a heart attack.

- Take your medicines exactly as your doctor tells you to. If you can't do this, or if you think you need to stop or change your medicine, talk to your doctor about it.

More

- If you have any problems with the medicines, tell your doctor. Ask your doctor what side effects you may have and what problems to watch for.
- See your doctor regularly so that he or she can check whether your medicine is working or needs to be changed.
- Always ask your doctor before you take any new medicines, including those you can buy without a prescription. Some medicines can make heart failure worse.

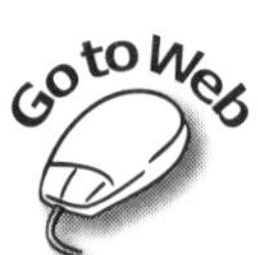

To get the best results from your medicines, be sure to take them properly. This can be tricky when you have to take more than one. For tips that can help, go to the Web site on the back cover and enter **G687** in the search box.

Cost tips for medicines

You will need medicine for the rest of your life to control your heart failure. This can get very expensive. But there may be ways you can reduce the cost—using generic instead of brand-name drugs and shopping for the best prices, for example. For help controlling costs, see page 3.

Cut the Salt

Eating less salt (sodium) can help you feel better and stay out of the hospital. Salt makes your body retain water, makes your legs swell, and makes it harder for your heart to pump.

Five Ways to Reduce Salt

1. Read food labels. Salt may be "hidden" in foods under many different names, such as sodium bicarbonate, disodium phosphate, and monosodium glutamate (MSG). Buy foods labeled "no salt added," "sodium-free" (less than 5 mg per serving), or "low-sodium" (less than 140 mg per serving).
2. Eat lots of fresh or frozen fruits and vegetables. They have very little salt, and they're good for you.
3. If you use canned vegetables or beans, rinse them before you use them. They are very high in salt unless you buy low-sodium or sodium-free kinds.
4. Flavor your food with garlic, lemon juice, onion, vinegar, healthy oils (olive, walnut), herbs, and spices instead of salt. Do not use soy sauce, steak sauce, onion salt, garlic salt, mustard, or ketchup on your food. They all have a lot of salt.
5. Eat fewer processed foods. These include anything that's not fresh, such as canned foods, packaged lunch meats and hot dogs, bottled sauces, boxed frozen meals, chips and pretzels, and pizza. Eat less often at restaurants, especially fast-food ones.

Your doctor may want you to eat less than 2,000 mg (2 g) of salt each day. That's less than 1 teaspoon. You can stay under this number by limiting the salt you eat at home and by watching for "hidden" sodium when you eat out or shop for food.

Write down what you eat and how much salt it has. That way you will know when you are close to (or over) your limit.

Eating less salt can be hard, but it has a big reward: feeling better and staying out of the hospital. The tips on page 304 can help you get started. If you are ready for even more ideas—or want an easy way to keep track of what you eat—go to the Web site on the back cover and enter **A181** in the search box.

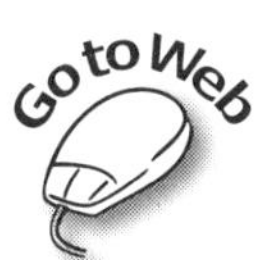

Check Your Weight Every Day

Get in the habit of weighing yourself every day and writing down your weight. Sudden weight gain may mean that fluid is building up in your body and your heart failure is getting worse.

- Weigh yourself at the same time each day, using the same scale on a hard, flat surface. The best time is in the morning after you go to the bathroom and before you eat or drink anything.
- Wear the same thing each time you weigh yourself, or always wear nothing. Do not wear shoes.
- Keep a calendar by the scale. Write your weight on it each day, and take it with you when you see your doctor.
- Keep notes on how you feel each day. Is your shortness of breath worse? Are your feet and ankles swollen? Do your legs seem puffy? Do you have to prop yourself up more at night to breathe, or do you wake up suddenly in the middle of the night feeling out of breath?

Call your doctor if you gain more than 2 pounds over 2 days. If you are gaining weight slowly, tell your doctor at your next visit.

Exercise Your Heart

If you are not active right now, starting to exercise may seem hard. But it's worth it. Regular exercise:

- Makes your heart stronger.
- Makes it easier to breathe.
- Helps you feel better and have more energy.
- Helps control your weight, blood pressure, and cholesterol.

See your doctor before you start exercising. He or she may want to do a test to see how much activity your heart can handle so you don't push too hard.

Walking is a great way to get exercise. If your doctor says it's safe, start out by walking a few minutes at a time. Slowly extend your walks until you are walking 20 to 30 minutes at a time. Swimming, cycling, or water aerobics might be other good choices. Your doctor can help you make a plan.

More

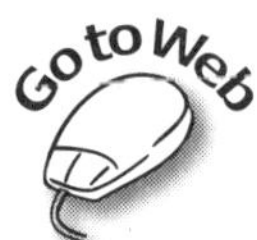

The important thing is to exercise regularly (3 to 5 times a week) and not to overdo it. There are many ways you can exercise safely with heart failure. For some ideas that might work for you, go to the Web site on the back cover and enter **U755** in the search box.

If You Have to Limit Fluids

Your doctor may give you "water pills" called diuretics to help get fluid out of your body. For many people, taking this medicine and reducing salt is enough.

If you have advanced heart failure, you may also need to limit how much fluid you drink. This can reduce symptoms and help you stay out of the hospital.

Your doctor will tell you how much fluid you can have each day. Usually, it will range from 4 to 8 cups (32 to 64 fl oz), which is about 1 to 2 liters. You will need to keep track of your fluids so you do not take in more than your body can handle.

- You might simply write down how much you drink every time you do. Measure how much fluid your regular drinking glasses hold. When you know this, you will not have to measure every time.
- Some people keep a container (like a pitcher or large plastic bottle) filled with the amount of fluid they can have for the day. If they drink from a source other than the container, then they pour out that amount. When the container is empty, they stop drinking.
- Count any food that will melt or that has a lot of liquid as part of your fluid for the day. That means you need to measure and count ice cream, gelatin, ice, juicy fruits, and soup.
- If you feel thirsty, try chewing gum or sucking on hard candy, breath mints, or frozen grapes or berries. If your lips feel dry, use lip balm.

What About Cardiac Rehab?

You might ask your doctor about joining a cardiac rehab program. In cardiac rehab, you work with a team of doctors, nurses, and therapists to learn how to stay healthier and feel better.

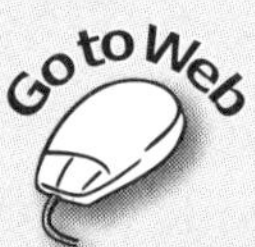

Many people with heart failure find cardiac rehab helpful. For help deciding whether this might be a good idea for you, go to the Web site on the back cover and enter **W065** in the search box.

When to Call a Doctor

Call 911 if:

- You have chest pain or pressure that has not gone away with rest or within 5 minutes after you take nitroglycerin, especially if the pain occurs with shortness of breath, sweating, and nausea.
- You have symptoms of a stroke (see page 54). These may include:
  - Sudden weakness, numbness, or loss of movement on one side of your body.
  - Sudden loss or change in vision.
  - Sudden trouble speaking or understanding simple statements.
  - A sudden, severe headache.
  - Sudden, severe dizziness, loss of balance, or loss of coordination.
- You have severe trouble breathing.
- You cough up foamy, pink mucus.
- You faint.
- Your heart suddenly starts to beat very fast or unevenly, and you feel dizzy, nauseated, or like you are going to faint.

Call your doctor if you have signs that your heart failure is getting worse. For example:

- You gain more than 2 pounds over 2 days.
- You have new or worse swelling in your feet, ankles, or legs.
- Your breathing gets worse. Activities that did not make you short of breath before are hard for you now.
- Your breathing when you lie down is worse than usual, or you wake up at night needing to catch your breath.

Living Better With Chronic Kidney Disease

Having chronic kidney disease means that for some time your kidneys have not been working the way they should. Your kidneys have the important job of filtering your blood. They remove waste products and extra fluid and flush them from your body as urine. When your kidneys don't work right, wastes build up in your blood and make you sick.

Chronic kidney disease may seem to have come on suddenly. But it has probably been happening bit by bit for many years as a result of damage to your kidneys. Diabetes and high blood pressure are by far the most common causes.

Kidney disease is a complex problem that can get worse over time. To stay as healthy as you can, work closely with your doctor. There are also many things you can do to slow or stop the damage to your kidneys and help you feel better.

What You Can Do

- Keep your blood pressure below 130/80. See pages 183 and 310.
- If you have diabetes, keep your blood sugar as close to normal as you can. See pages 296 and 310.
- Take your medicines as prescribed. See page 309. And talk to your doctor before you take any new medicine. Some medicines can damage your kidneys. See Be Careful With Medicines on page 309.
- Follow an eating plan that is good for your kidneys. Most people need to limit salt, and some may need to limit protein. See page 311. Some people may also need to limit how much fluid they drink every day. See page 310.
- Be careful not to get dehydrated. It could put you in the hospital and cause lasting kidney damage. Get treatment right away for diarrhea, vomiting, or fever. Be careful when you exercise or during hot weather. See Dehydration on page 29.
- Do not smoke or chew tobacco. Smoking can reduce blood flow to the kidneys. If you need help quitting, see page 351.

There are other steps you can take too, like staying at a healthy weight and getting some exercise every day. These things can protect your kidneys by helping you control or prevent high blood pressure and diabetes. They also lower your risk for other diseases.

Take Your Medicines

You may have to take several medicines. Some of them may treat problems caused by kidney disease, such as anemia. Others may help treat the problem that caused your kidney disease, such as high blood pressure or diabetes. Medicines can help you feel better and slow the disease.

- Take your medicines exactly as your doctor tells you to. Be sure you understand how much of each medicine to take and when to take each one.
- If you have any problems with your medicines, tell your doctor. Ask your doctor what side effects you may have and what problems to watch for. If you think you need to change or stop a medicine, talk to your doctor first.
- See your doctor regularly so he or she can check whether your medicines are working or need to be changed.

If you take several medicines at different times of day, it can be hard to remember to take them all. So try to make it as simple as you can. Plan to take your medicines when you are doing other things, like eating a meal or getting ready for bed. See page 367 for other tips.

Cost tips for medicines

You will need medicine for the rest of your life to control your kidney disease. This can get very expensive. But there may be ways you can reduce the cost—using generic instead of brand-name drugs and shopping for the best prices, for example. For help controlling costs, see page 3.

More

Be Careful With Medicines

Some medicines can hurt your kidneys. Common ones include:

- Nonprescription pain relievers that also reduce swelling (anti-inflammatories). Examples include aspirin, ibuprofen (Motrin, Advil), and naproxen (Aleve).
- Antibiotics such as penicillins and sulfa drugs.
- Medicines used to treat cancer (chemotherapy).

To be safe:

- Talk to your doctor before you take any new medicine. This includes both nonprescription and prescription drugs, vitamins, or herbs.
- Make sure that all your doctors know that you have kidney disease.
- Keep a list of the medicines and supplements you take, and review it with your doctor at each visit.

Limiting Fluids

When you have kidney disease, your kidneys have trouble getting rid of extra fluid. Extra fluid can raise your blood pressure and force your heart to work harder.

If you need to limit fluids, your doctor will tell you how much you can drink each day. You will need to keep track of your fluids so you do not take in more than your body can handle. These tips may help:

- You might simply write down how much you drink every time you do. Measure how much fluid your regular drinking glasses hold. When you know this, you will not have to measure every time.
- Some people keep a container (like a pitcher or large plastic bottle) filled with the amount of fluid they can have for the day. If they drink from a source other than the container, then they pour out that amount. When the container is empty, they stop drinking.
- Count any food that will melt or that has a lot of liquid as part of your fluid for the day. That means you need to measure and count ice cream, gelatin, ice, juicy fruits, and soup.
- If you feel thirsty, try chewing gum or sucking on hard candy, breath mints, or frozen grapes or berries. If your lips feel dry, use lip balm.

Control Blood Pressure and Diabetes

One of the most important parts of treating kidney disease is to control the disease that caused it. If you have diabetes or high blood pressure, getting your blood sugar or blood pressure under control can help protect your kidneys from more damage. It can also improve your overall health.

- Keep your blood pressure below 130/80. To be sure you are doing this, check your blood pressure at home. To learn how, go to the Web site on the back cover and enter **L311** in the search box.

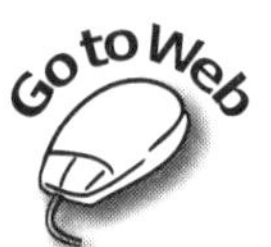

- Keep your blood sugar as close to normal as you can. You have the best chance of keeping your blood sugar in a safe range if you check it yourself every day. For help learning how to do this, go to the Web site on the back cover and enter **Z203** in the search box.
- Take medicines for diabetes or high blood pressure as prescribed.
- Stay at a healthy weight. To learn how, see Reaching a Healthy Weight on page 326.
- Try to get at least 30 minutes of exercise on most days of the week.
- Don't drink alcohol. Alcohol can keep your medicines from working well and can affect your blood sugar.

For more tips on managing diabetes, see page 296. To learn about home treatment for high blood pressure, see page 184.

Manage How You Eat

A dietitian can help you plan a diet based on how well your kidneys are working. You may need to limit salt (sodium), fluids, and protein. Some people also have to limit minerals such as potassium and phosphorus.

It may be hard to change your diet. You may have to give up many foods you like. But it is very important to make these changes so you can stay healthy as long as possible.

There is no one diet that is right for everyone with chronic kidney disease. And your diet may change over time as the disease changes. But here are some basic ideas that may help you follow your kidney diet.

Note: These diet tips are not for you if you are on dialysis or have had a kidney transplant. Follow the special diet your doctor gave you.

Get the right amount of protein

Eating too much protein can stress the kidneys. But if you don't get enough, you can become weak, tired, and more likely to get infections. To get the right amount of protein:

- Learn which foods contain protein. High-protein foods include meat, poultry, seafood, and eggs. Other foods with protein are milk and milk products, beans, nuts, breads, pastas, cereals, and vegetables.
- Know how much protein you can have each day. Limit high-protein foods to 5 to 7 ounces a day, or less, if your doctor or dietitian tells you to. A 3-ounce serving of protein is about the size of a deck of cards.

More

What Is Glomerular Filtration Rate (GFR)?

Glomerular filtration rate (GFR) is a number that tells your doctor how well your kidneys are working. Your doctor figures your GFR based on your age, your sex, your race, your size, and the amount of creatinine in your blood. Creatinine is a chemical that builds up in your blood when your kidneys are not working well.

A GFR below 60 is a sign of kidney disease. The lower the GFR number, the worse the kidneys are working. A person with a GFR below 15 has severe kidney failure and may need to start dialysis or have a kidney transplant.

Your doctor will schedule regular visits to check how well your kidneys are working. Be sure to keep all your appointments.

Limit salt (sodium)

Salt helps you keep the right balance of fluids in your body. But your kidneys have trouble clearing extra salt from your body. Eating too much sodium can cause fluids to build up.

To limit salt:

- Read food labels. Salt may be "hidden" in foods under different names, such as monosodium glutamate (MSG), sodium citrate, and sodium bicarbonate. Buy foods that are labeled "no salt added," "sodium-free" (less than 5 mg per serving), or "low sodium" (less than 140 mg per serving).
- Use lemon juice, garlic, vinegar, healthy oils (olive, walnut), herbs, and spices to flavor your food. Do not use soy sauce, onion salt, garlic salt, mustard, or ketchup. They all have a lot of salt.
- Choose fresh or frozen fruits and vegetables. If you use canned vegetables or beans, rinse them well before you use them. They can be high in salt.
- Eat fewer processed foods. These include anything that's not fresh, such as canned foods, lunch meats and hot dogs, bottled sauces, frozen meals, chips, and pretzels. Eat less often at restaurants, especially at fast-food places.

Get the right balance of minerals

Healthy kidneys keep the right balance of minerals such as phosphorus and potassium in the blood. You may need to keep track of these minerals in your diet so you don't get either too much or too little.

If you need to limit potassium:

- Choose low-potassium fruits such as apples, grapes, berries, and tangerines. You can also eat canned fruits, such as fruit cocktail, peaches, pears, and pineapple.
- Choose low-potassium vegetables such as asparagus, bean sprouts, cabbage, cucumber, green beans, and lettuce.

If you need to limit phosphorus:

- Know how much milk and dairy products you can have. Milk and dairy products such as cheese, yogurt, and ice cream have a lot of phosphorus.
- Limit high-phosphorus foods such as nuts, peanut butter, seeds, lentils, beans, sardines, and cured meats like sausages, bologna, and hot dogs.
- Avoid colas and soft drinks that have phosphate or phosphoric acid.
- Avoid bran in breads, muffins, and cereals.

Other tips

- Don't skip meals or go for many hours without eating. If you don't feel very hungry, try to eat 4 or 5 small meals instead of 2 or 3 bigger meals.
- If you have trouble keeping your weight up, talk to your doctor or dietitian about ways to add calories to your diet. Healthy fats such as olive or canola oil may be good choices.

Unless you have diabetes, you can use honey and sugar to add calories and increase energy.

- Ask your doctor if you should take vitamin and mineral supplements. Do not take any supplements or medicines without talking to your doctor first.

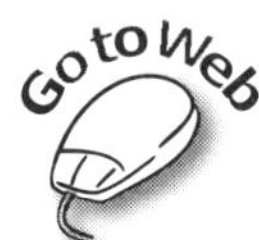

To learn how to eat well when you have kidney disease, go to the Web Site on the back cover and enter **K815** in the search box.

More

Looking Ahead: Dialysis and Transplant

If chronic kidney disease gets worse, you could develop kidney failure. Kidney failure affects your whole body. It can cause serious heart, bone, and brain problems and make you feel very sick.

There are two treatments for kidney failure: dialysis and kidney transplant.

- **Dialysis** is a process that does the work for your kidneys. It is not a cure for kidney failure, but it can help you feel better and live longer.
- **Kidney transplant** may be the best choice if you are otherwise healthy. But the wait to get a kidney may be long. Most people start dialysis while they wait.

There are two types of dialysis: hemodialysis and peritoneal dialysis. Both types have pros and cons. For example:

- Hemodialysis is usually done in a hospital or dialysis center. Peritoneal dialysis can be done at home.
- Hemodialysis is usually done 3 times a week. Peritoneal dialysis has to be done every day.

It may be hard to decide which type of dialysis is best for you. For help with

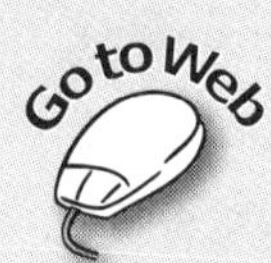

this decision, go to the Web site on the back cover and enter **Q707** in the search box.

Many people have successful kidney transplants or live for years using dialysis. But at this point, it is a good idea to talk with your family and your doctor about what you want to happen if your health gets worse. You can write a living will and choose a health care agent to make decisions if you are not able. It can be comforting to know that you will get the care you want.

To learn more about planning for the future, see page 382.

When to Call a Doctor

Call 911 if:

- You faint.
- Your heart is beating very slow or very fast.
- You have chest pain or are very short of breath.
- Your muscles feel very weak.
- You have signs of severe dehydration. These include little or no urine for 12 hours; sunken eyes, no tears, and a dry mouth and tongue; skin that sags when you pinch it; feeling very dizzy or lightheaded; fast breathing and heartbeat; and not feeling or acting alert.

Call your doctor if:

- You have trouble urinating or can urinate only very small amounts.
- You have nausea and vomiting.
- You have new or worse swelling in your arms or feet.
- You are confused or have trouble thinking clearly.
- You are losing weight and don't feel like eating.
- You feel weaker or more tired than usual.

Living Better After a Stroke

A stroke occurs when a blood vessel in the brain is blocked or bursts. Without blood and the oxygen it carries, part of the brain starts to die. The part of the body controlled by the damaged area of the brain can't work properly. Quick treatment can often help limit the damage.

A stroke can cause problems such as trouble walking or moving, pain or numbness on one side of the body, and trouble speaking, writing, or understanding language. Some people also have bladder or bowel problems or trouble eating or swallowing.

Some people have permanent problems after a stroke. But many people are able to get back most of the skills and abilities they lost. You will make the most progress in the first few months after your stroke. But you can keep getting better for years. It just may happen more slowly.

The key to getting better after a stroke is to start stroke rehabilitation ("rehab") right away. In stroke rehab, a team of doctors, nurses, and therapists works with you to regain skills you lost as the result of a stroke. There are also many things you can do on your own to get better.

What You Can Do

For most people, recovering from a stroke is a lifelong process. To do your best:

- Learn ways to adapt to the problems the stroke caused. See this page.
- Take your medicines as prescribed. This gives them the best chance of helping you. See page 316.
- Adopt healthy lifestyle habits to help prevent a future stroke. See page 316.
- Make your home safer to prevent falls. See Preventing Falls on page 364.
- Deal with your emotions so they don't slow down your recovery. See page 318.

Adapt to the Changes

The problems you have after a stroke depend upon what part of your brain was affected and how much damage the stroke caused. Soon after a stroke, a stroke rehab team works to help you learn ways to adapt to your problems. You can keep working on these skills after you go home.

A stroke can cause a range of problems, but here are ideas for dealing with some common ones.

Getting dressed

- Choose clothing that has Velcro closures or snaps and elastic waistbands.
- Use devices such as stocking or sock spreaders, rings or strings attached to zipper pulls, and buttonhooks.
- Sit down while you get dressed.
- Put your weaker arm or leg into the piece of clothing first, before the stronger arm or leg. When you undress, remove the stronger arm or leg first.

Trouble with eating or swallowing

- Eat foods that smell good. This can increase saliva and help you swallow.
- Eat soft foods or finely chopped solid foods.
- Thicken liquids with nonfat dry milk powder. This makes them easier to feel in your mouth and throat.
- Eat small bites of food. Place food in the unaffected side of your mouth.
- Avoid foods that are sticky or hard to swallow, like bananas and peanut butter, and dry foods, like crackers and toast.

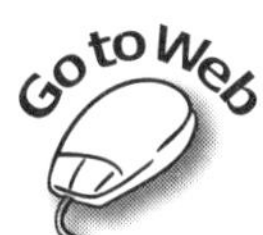

For more ideas on dealing with eating problems, go to the Web site on the back cover and enter **A253** in the search box.

If you can't move an arm or leg

If you have an arm or leg that you can't move well, you need to protect it.

- Change its position often.
- Check your skin every day, especially over bony areas where pressure sores can form. See page 213.
- Exercise all your joints at least 2 times a day.
- Do not lie on your affected arm or leg.

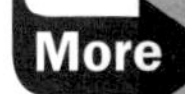

- Bathe and do dishes in lukewarm water. Test water with your unaffected hand.
- To prevent swelling, prop up the affected arm or leg anytime you sit or lie down.

Take Your Medicines

You will probably need to take several medicines. Some can help prevent a future stroke. Others may decrease pain, treat sleep problems, or help speed your recovery. To get the best results:

- Take your medicines exactly as your doctor tells you to. If you can't do this, or if you think you need to stop or change a medicine, talk to your doctor about it first.
- If you have any problems with your medicines, tell your doctor. Ask what side effects you may have and what problems to watch for.
- See your doctor regularly so that he or she can check whether your medicines are working or need to be changed.
- Always ask your doctor before you take any new medicines. This includes both nonprescription and prescription drugs, vitamins, and herbs.

If you take several medicines at different times of day, it can be hard to remember to take them all. Try to make it as simple as you can. See page 367 for tips.

Prevent a Future Stroke

After you have had a stroke, you are more likely to have another one. But there are changes you can make that can reduce your risk. They can also help you control other diseases, such as high blood pressure and heart disease, and help you live a longer, healthier life.

- Do not smoke, and avoid secondhand smoke. Smoking can more than double your risk of stroke. If you need help quitting, see page 351.

Can You Drive After a Stroke?

After a stroke, do not drive until your doctor says that you can. This may be hard to accept. But a stroke can affect your vision or your ability to move quickly, and this can make it unsafe to drive. You need your doctor's okay for the safety of yourself and others.

After your doctor says that you can drive, check with the motor vehicle department. You may need to take classes, be tested again, or have changes made to your car. Some stroke rehab centers give driver training classes.

If you can't drive because of problems from your stroke, check with your stroke rehab center for other options. Some programs offer special vans that can take you to and from places. Senior groups and volunteer agencies may also have ride services.

- Eat heart-healthy foods. Get plenty of high-fiber fruits, vegetables, beans, and grains. Cut back on cholesterol, saturated fat, and salt. See pages 289 and 333.
- Get some exercise most days of the week. Your doctor can suggest a safe level of exercise for you. See page 340.
- Stay at a healthy weight. See page 326.
- Limit alcohol. Having more than 2 drinks a day increases the risk of stroke.
- Learn the signs of stroke, and get help right away if you have any of them. See page 54.
- Check your blood pressure regularly. See your doctor if your blood pressure is higher than 140/90. See page 183.
- Take all the medicines your doctor prescribes. See page 316.

More

If You Are a Caregiver

Taking care of someone who has had a stroke can be hard in many ways. The rehab team is there to help. They can teach you how to help the person get dressed, go to the bathroom, eat, and do other activities. They can also help you find a caregiver support group and learn about ways to pay for rehab.

Here are some things you can do to help the person you take care of get better:

- Help the person take part in rehab. Go to the rehab sessions as often as you can.
- Help the person learn and practice new skills.
- Find out what the person can do on his or her own. Don't do those tasks that he or she can do without your help.
- Visit and talk with the person often. Play cards or watch TV together. Ask family and friends to visit.

Caring for another person can be exhausting. Often, caregivers take on too much and end up depressed or ill themselves. If you want to give good care, you have to take care of yourself first. See A Caregiver's Guide on page 378.

Whether you can care for a loved one at home depends on many things, including your own health and how much support you have from family or outside help. Some people simply cannot give the care needed at home.

Go to Web

Still, it can be hard to decide to put a loved one in a nursing home. For help deciding if this is the best choice for you, go to the Web site on the back cover and enter **D619** in the search box.

Deal With Your Emotions

You may find it hard to control your emotions after a stroke. Some people cry more easily or have sudden mood swings. These changes may be the result of injury to the brain, and they often get better in time.

Other feelings are a natural response to a life-changing event like a stroke. You may feel:

- Sad or angry about the loss of the lifestyle you had before.
- Isolated by speech and language problems.
- Frustrated by the slow pace of your recovery.
- Worried about the future.

These feelings are normal and expected. But if you feel sad or hopeless, you may be depressed. Depression can be treated. If you think you might be depressed, see Are You Depressed? on page 146. Then talk to your doctor.

To deal with your emotions:

- Be easy on yourself. Let go of mistakes.
- Give yourself credit for the progress you have made.
- Make time for things that you enjoy.
- Talk to people who can understand how you feel. This may be family, friends, or a counselor.
- Join a stroke support group. Your rehab team or local hospital can help you find one.

Recovering from a stroke is hard work, and you are the only one who can do it. Your mood and energy will be highest if you:

- Take good care of yourself. Get some exercise every day, eat well, and get plenty of rest.
- Feel good about yourself. Get dressed every day, and keep yourself clean.

When to Call a Doctor

Call 911 if you think you might be having another stroke. See page 54.

Call your doctor if:

- You take a blood thinner such as warfarin (Coumadin), and you have signs of bleeding problems, such as:
  - Blood in your stools, or stools that are black or look like tar.
  - Bleeding from your nose or gums.
  - Blood in your urine.
  - Any vaginal bleeding after menopause.
  - New bruises or blood spots under your skin.
- You have new symptoms that may be related to your stroke, such as falling or trouble swallowing.
- You think you may be depressed.

Staying Healthy

Get Immunized 320

Wellness Exams and Screening Tests 321

Reaching a Healthy Weight 326

Healthy Eating 333

Exercise for Health 340

Quitting Smoking 351

Take Care of Your Teeth 354

Managing Stress 356

Keep Your Brain Healthy 359

Sex and Aging 361

Safe Sex 363

Preventing Falls 364

Driving: Are You Safe?. 365

Master Your Medicines 367

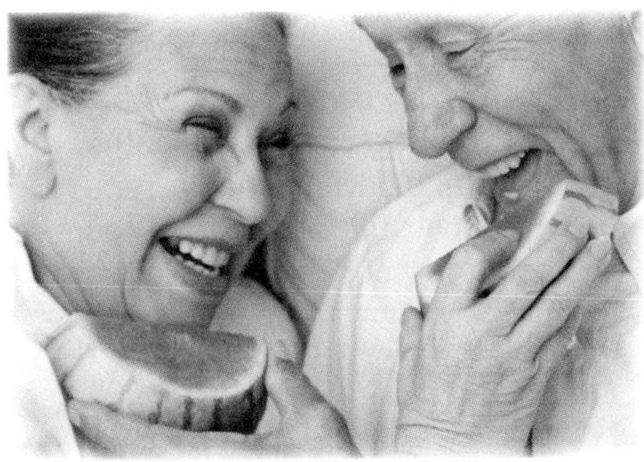

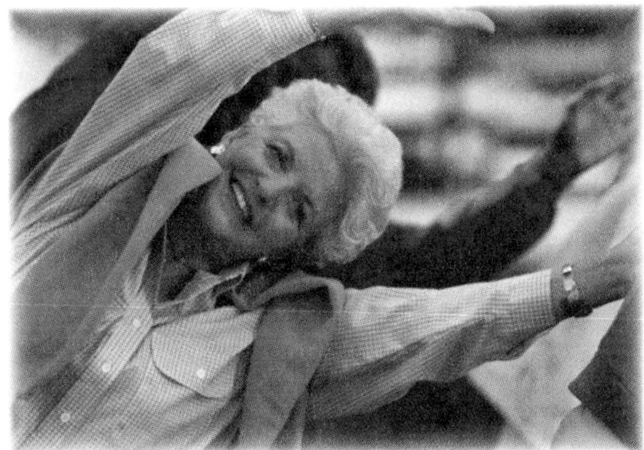

Get Immunized

Immunizations (vaccinations) help protect the body from diseases. When you get a vaccine, your body learns to find and attack the bacteria or virus that causes the disease before it can cause problems.

Immunizations save lives. They help prevent many serious illnesses. They cost less than treating the diseases they protect against. And the risk of serious side effects from the vaccines is much lower than the risk of serious illness if you do not get the vaccines.

Be sure to get the immunizations you need. Each year thousands of adults are hospitalized, and many die, because of flu and other diseases that vaccines can prevent. Use the chart on this page as a guide for which shots you need, and then talk to your doctor. The recommendations change from time to time.

Immunizations		
Immunization	**Who should have it?**	**How often?**
Flu shot	All adults 50 and older	Every year in the fall
Pneumococcal vaccine (PPV)	All adults 65 and older, and anyone under 65 who has a chronic disease (such as heart or lung disease) or has a damaged or missing spleen	1 time only for most; some people need a booster shot after 5 years
Shingles vaccine	All adults 60 and older	1 time only
Tetanus and diphtheria (Td) vaccine	All adults, and anyone who gets a deep, dirty wound and hasn't had a booster in the past 5 years	Every 10 years for life
Tetanus, diphtheria, and pertussis (Tdap) vaccine	All adults 64 and younger	1 time in place of 1 Td booster; if you plan to have close contact with a baby younger than 12 months and have not had a Td booster in the past 2 years, get your Tdap booster now

To be sure you have the most recent

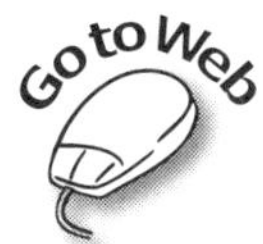

information about vaccines, go to the Web site on the back cover and enter **T275** in the search box.

Special Concerns

Call your local health department if you are in close contact with people who have contagious diseases or you are planning to travel to places where malaria, typhoid, cholera, yellow fever, or other illnesses are common. You may need to get other shots.

Reactions to Immunizations

Brief, mild reactions are common.

- If you get a slight fever, take acetaminophen (Tylenol) or ibuprofen (Advil, Motrin). Also see Fever on page 150.
- The area around the shot may swell and hurt a little. Put ice or a cold pack on it for 10 to 15 minutes. Put a thin cloth between the ice and your skin.

Call your doctor right away if you have more than just a mild reaction.

Wellness Exams and Screening Tests

One way to protect your health is to watch for changes in your body and find problems early, when they may be easier to treat.

Preventive health care can help you do this. This type of care includes:

- **Wellness exams.** These are checkups you have when you are healthy. They are focused on your overall health.
- **Screening tests.** Screening tests look for signs of disease before you have symptoms. Pap tests, mammograms, and PSA (prostate-specific antigen) tests are examples of screening tests for cancer. See page 322.

The recommendations for wellness exams and screening tests here are for mostly healthy people at average risk for health problems. Some of the things that affect your level of risk include your overall health, your family history (whether your close relatives have had certain diseases), and lifestyle factors, such as smoking, exercise habits, and sexual history.

If you have a chronic illness or other health problems, you may need checkups and tests more often. Work with your doctor to decide on the best schedule for you.

The schedule on pages 322 and 323 lists some of the most common screening tests. Most adults need some or all of these tests. Talk with your doctor about which tests you may need.

More

Sample Health Screening Schedule

Screening	Who should have it?	How often?
Blood pressure	All adults	Every 1 to 2 years. More often if you are at risk for high blood pressure. See page 185.
Cholesterol	All adults	Talk to your doctor. See page 186.
Type 2 diabetes (fasting blood sugar test)	All adults who have high cholesterol or high blood pressure	Every 3 years. More often if you are at high risk. Talk to your doctor.
Vision problems, especially glaucoma (see page 162)	All adults	Talk to your doctor. Need for exams increases with age.
Hearing problems	All adults	Talk to your doctor. Need for exams increases with age.
Colorectal cancer (colonoscopy, flexible sigmoidoscopy, fecal occult blood test, or barium enema)	All adults starting at age 50	Depends on which tests you have. See page 121.
Breast cancer (mammogram and clinical breast exam)	All women	Mammogram: Every 1 to 2 years. See page 324. Clinical breast exam: Every year. See page 325.
Pap test for cervical cancer	All women	Every 1 to 3 years for women at average risk. See page 323.
Osteoporosis	All women over 65; women age 60 or older who are at high risk	Talk to your doctor. See page 207.

Sample Health Screening Schedule		
Screening	**Who should have it?**	**How often?**
Prostate cancer (PSA test or digital rectal exam)	Some men. See Should You Be Tested? on page 214.	Talk to your doctor.
Ultrasound test for abdominal aortic aneurysm	Men ages 65 to 75 who have ever smoked	Talk to your doctor.
Other things you and your doctor may want to keep an eye on include weight (see page 330), thyroid level (see page 239), and skin changes that could be cancer (see page 230).		

For Women: Pelvic Exams and Pap Tests

A **pelvic exam** looks for early signs of problems in the reproductive organs. The exam usually includes:

- An external genital exam. The doctor looks at the genital area for skin changes, sores, or other problems.
- A Pap test.
- A manual exam. The doctor inserts two gloved fingers into your vagina and presses on your lower belly with the other hand to check the shape and size of your ovaries and uterus.

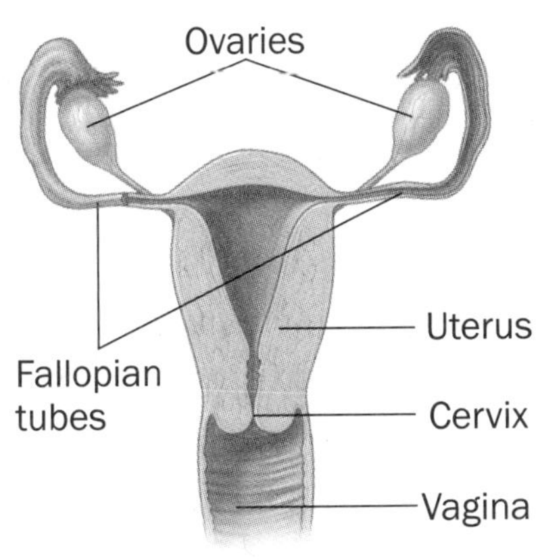

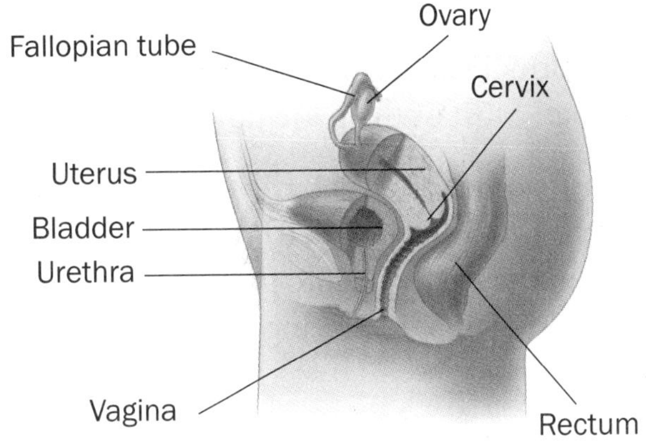

The female pelvic organs (front and side views)

The **Pap test** is a screening test for cancer of the cervix (the lower part of the uterus that opens into the vagina). The test looks for changes in the cells that could lead to cancer. When done regularly, Pap tests can find most cervical cancers early enough that they can be cured.

More

To do the test, the doctor inserts an instrument called a speculum into your vagina to spread apart the vaginal walls. He or she then collects cell samples from your cervix with a wooden or plastic device that gently scrapes some cells off the surface. The cells are sent to a lab.

Your doctor should let you know the results of your Pap test when they come back from the lab. If your results are abnormal, you may need to return for more tests. You may need another Pap test, or you may need a test called a colposcopy. This gives a more complete view of the cervix.

Abnormal Pap results can mean many things. Most of them are not cancer.

Most women should have a Pap test every 1 to 3 years. Talk to your doctor about the best schedule for you. Also see When to Stop Having Pap Tests on on this page.

You may not need a Pap test every year if:

- You have had normal Pap results at least 3 years in a row.
- You have not had cervical cancer.
- You do not have a sexually transmitted disease such as genital warts or HIV infection.
- You were not exposed to the drug diethylstilbestrol (DES).

Do not douche, have sex, or use feminine hygiene products for at least 24 hours before a Pap test, because it may affect the test results.

When to Stop Having Pap Tests

It may be okay to stop having Pap tests if:

- You are over 65 and have had three normal Pap tests in the past 10 years.
- Your cervix was removed during a hysterectomy for a reason other than cancer.

You and your doctor can decide on the right age to stop being tested, based on your health history.

For Women: Mammograms and Clinical Breast Exams

Breast cancer can often be cured if it is found early. The most common ways to look for early breast cancer are mammograms and clinical breast exams.

A **mammogram** is a breast X-ray that can find cancer while it is still too small to be felt in a breast exam.

- Have a mammogram every 1 to 2 years if you are not at high risk for breast cancer.
- Have a mammogram every year if you have already had breast cancer or are at high risk for breast cancer. You are at high risk if your mother, a sister, or another close female relative had breast cancer before menopause.

Some women don't get mammograms because they are afraid it will hurt. But it's worth a few minutes of discomfort to catch breast cancer early, when it can be cured. Mammograms save lives.

To prepare for a mammogram:

- Do not wear deodorant, perfume, powder, or lotion. They can affect the quality of the X-ray.
- Wear clothing that lets you easily undress from the waist up.
- If your last mammogram was at a different facility, have the original X-ray sent before your test, or pick it up and take it with you.

During a **clinical breast exam**, a doctor or nurse looks at your breasts and gently feels them for lumps or other changes. Have a clinical breast exam every year or anytime you have a problem with your breasts.

Talk to your doctor if you find a lump or have a problem with your breasts. See Breast Problems on page 99. You may need a breast exam or a mammogram to help find the cause.

What about breast self-exams?

Breast self-exams are a good way for you to learn what your breasts normally look and feel like. When you know what's normal for you, you'll be better able to notice changes and know when to get help early instead of waiting for your next checkup. But a self-exam does not take the place of a mammogram or a clinical breast exam.

A breast self-exam is easy to do. If you do not know how to do a breast self-exam, ask your doctor or nurse to show you. Your doctor's office may have the instructions printed on a sheet or card that you can take with you.

Reaching a Healthy Weight

A healthy weight is a weight at which you feel good about yourself and have energy for work and play. It's also one that does not put you at risk for weight-related problems like heart disease, diabetes, stroke, arthritis, and cancer.

Many people are not at a healthy weight but want to get there. Does this sound like you? If it does, there are things you can do today to move toward your goal.

Here are the big ideas to keep in mind as you get started:

- Focus on health first.
- Choose healthier foods.
- Be careful about how much you eat.
- Be more active.
- If you are overweight, decide not to gain any more weight. When you're ready, try to lose some weight.

Too Thin?

Most of the information that follows is focused on people who are overweight. But being too far below a healthy weight is not healthy either. Healthy foods and exercise are just as important for your health if you are underweight. If you are underweight, see page 330.

Focus on Health First

Eating healthier and being more active will probably help you lose weight. Even if you don't lose much weight, these changes can help you feel better, have more energy, and prevent disease.

Focus on these healthy changes rather than weight loss. Losing weight is very hard for most people, and it takes time. But you can take steps to be healthier right now.

Eat Healthier Foods

The kinds of foods you eat have a big impact on both your weight and your health. Reaching and staying at a healthy weight is not about going on a diet. It's about choosing healthier foods every day and changing your diet for good.

Pages 333 to 340 have information that can help you make healthier food choices at home and when you eat out. In general, fruits and vegetables, whole grains, lean protein (lean meats, fish, beans), and low-fat dairy foods should be most of what you eat.

But there's also room for a few sugary and high-fat foods in most people's diets. Most foods can be part of a healthy diet as long as you don't eat too much of them.

Watch How Much You Eat

Many people eat more than their bodies need. Part of controlling your weight means learning how much food you really need from day to day and not eating more than that. Even healthy foods can lead to weight gain if you eat too much.

- Pay attention to how much food is on your plate.
- Read food labels to learn what a serving size is.
- Slow down. Think about what you are eating, and enjoy every bite.
- Don't go back for seconds.
- If you eat out a lot, know that most restaurants serve much bigger portions than most people need.

With time, you can get used to eating less.

Be More Active

When people think of losing weight, they most often think of food or diets. But a big part of weight control is exercise. When you change what you eat *and* you exercise, you increase your chances for success.

Start With Small Changes in Your Diet

Changing your diet is a big step. But you can break it into lots of small ones like these.

- Eat a healthy breakfast every day. Try whole-grain cereal with low-fat or skim milk and fruit, or whole wheat toast with an egg and a small glass of juice.
- Use a smaller dinner plate.
- Avoid buffets. If you go to a buffet, make one trip only. Forget about "getting your money's worth."
- Make a healthy lunch instead of eating out.
- Save money and calories when you eat out. Split an entrée with someone, or ask for half of it in a to-go box. Order a lunch portion instead of a dinner one.
- Bring a healthy snack to work: fruit, carrot or celery sticks with low-fat dip, or whole-grain crackers with string cheese. A good snack may keep you from overeating later.
- Drink water or nonfat milk with meals. If you drink soft drinks, choose diet soda.

With time, these small changes may become routine. Look at every step you take as a success.

More

Exercise helps in three ways:

1. It reduces your risk for health problems like heart disease, high blood pressure, stroke, and diabetes.
2. It burns calories. This makes it easier to lose weight and keep it off. To see how many calories you can burn when you exercise, go to the Web site on the back cover and enter **M278** in the search box.

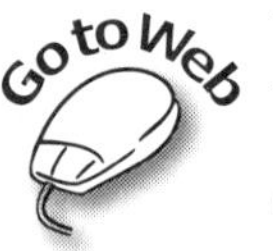

3. It gives you more energy, makes you stronger, and lets you do more with less effort. For most people, the more active they are, the better they feel.

Pages 340 to 351 are all about how to be more active. For those who can't picture themselves "working out," there are tips on how to be more active that don't involve traditional exercise. You'll also find ideas for how to work around some of the things that may keep you from being active: having a busy schedule, feeling too out of shape, having a disability or limited movement, or not knowing how to get started.

Just being a little more active can make a difference. You can do it. Lots of people have.

Avoid Weight Gain

You may not be ready to try to lose weight. But if you are like many people, you can take a big step toward better health by making sure your weight stays right where it is.

Losing weight can be hard. But most people can gain weight without thinking about it.

- They often gain weight so slowly that they don't even notice.
- Most people tend to put on weight as they get older unless they are very careful. And as their weight creeps up, so does their risk for health problems.

How can you avoid this? Start by weighing yourself today. Use that as your weight limit, and then make sure you stay within a few pounds of that number. If you start to put on weight, cut back on calories a bit or get a little more exercise so you can get back under your weight limit.

Do not weigh yourself every day. Weight can go up and down a little from day to day without meaning that you are gaining or losing weight.

Try to Lose Weight

Weight loss seems like it should be simple. Burn more calories than you eat, and you will lose weight. But for most people, it's not simple at all.

The good news is:

- You don't have to reach an "ideal" weight to be healthier.
- Losing as little as 5 to 10 percent of your weight can make a difference. For someone who weighs 200 pounds, that's only 10 to 20 pounds.

Which Diet Is Best?

By themselves, formal "diets" are not usually enough to lose weight and keep it off over the long run. The key is to make healthy food choices, not eat more than your body needs, and get regular exercise. If you stick with this approach most of the time, you will have the best chance of reaching a healthy weight and staying there.

Formal diets may help some people get started. If you think this might work for you, be sure to choose a sensible, healthy one. The best diets:

- Rely on normal, everyday foods. If you have to eat special foods while you're on the diet, it may be hard to keep weight off once you go back to "regular" food.
- Do not cut out entire food groups. Most foods can be—and should be—part of a healthy eating plan, even when you are trying to lose weight.
- Work on changing your eating habits for good.
- Focus on slow, steady weight loss. Fast, extreme weight loss is not good for your body. It can even be dangerous. And most people can't keep the weight off when they lose it that way.

Go to Web

To make sure you are on a safe path to weight loss, go to the Web site on the back cover and enter **Z310** in the search box.

You may want and need to lose more than that. But for most people, setting small goals and building on small successes is easier than trying to reach one big goal. Feel good about all your efforts, big and small, to take better care of yourself.

Plan to Succeed

1. Think about what stops you, and look for solutions. Do you feel too busy to exercise or cook healthier meals? Are you afraid you are too out of shape and will look silly or hurt yourself? Do you not have the support you need? There are ways to get around all of these barriers.

2. Start small. For most people, it's easier to tackle a series of small changes than one or two big changes. Small successes add up. And if you don't succeed with a small change, it will be only a minor setback—one that's easy to get past so you can try again.

3. Be specific. Simply planning to work out more and eat better is too general and too hard to follow. Instead, set specific goals you can measure (and reach). At the end of the day or the week or the month, you should be able to say "Yes, I met my goal" or "No, I did not meet my goal." For example:

- Make a plan to walk 2 days a week for 20 minutes each time.
- Replace your lunchtime soda with water or a low-calorie drink every day.

More

- Twice a week, bring a healthy lunch to work instead of eating out.
- Eat a piece of fruit in place of your regular dessert 3 nights each week.

Set goals like these that are right for you. When you have met them, set new ones.

4. Track your progress. It may help to write down what you eat and when and how long you exercise, at least in the beginning. This helps you do two things: feel good when you reach a goal, and know where you went wrong when you don't. Be sure to reward yourself when you succeed—perhaps with new clothes or new exercise gear.

5. Make new habits part of your daily life. Schedule exercise time on your calendar. Have your family eat the same healthy foods you do. It will be easier to stick to exercise and healthy eating when you think of them as part of a normal day rather than as extras.

Controlling your weight takes daily effort. Some days you just won't feel like exercising. Some days you'll want a cheeseburger, not lean turkey on whole wheat. That's okay. Just don't let those days add up.

Are You at a Healthy Weight?

There are two measurements that can tell you whether your weight is healthy. Neither is perfect, but they can help you know if your weight is putting you at risk for disease.

They are:

- Your BMI (body mass index).
- Your waist size (circumference).

When You Don't Weigh Enough

Being underweight can cause problems. As you lose weight, you lose muscle and can get weaker. Keeping your weight in a normal range may help you be stronger, have more energy, and stay healthier.

If you have lost weight and muscle, you may need to eat a high-calorie, high-protein diet. This may be easier to do if you eat 3 meals plus 2 or 3 snacks a day. But talk to your doctor or dietitian before you make any changes to your diet to be sure they are safe for you.

It's also important to exercise. It can help you rebuild your muscles and keep your heart healthy. See page 340.

Some people lose weight because they have diseases such as a high thyroid level, a serious infection, Crohn's disease, COPD, or cancer. Some medicines can also cause weight loss. Call your doctor if you are losing weight and you don't know why.

BMI

BMI is a measure of your weight compared to your height. Your risk of weight-related disease may be higher if you are above or below a healthy BMI range. For adults, the healthy range is from 18.5 to 24.9.

Use the chart on this page to find your height and weight and find your BMI.

BMI is not always an accurate sign of your health risk. For example, an athlete with a lot of muscle may have a high BMI but still be at a very healthy weight. A frail person with little muscle may have a low BMI but still have too much body fat.

But for the average person, BMI is a good guide, especially when you look at it with waist size.

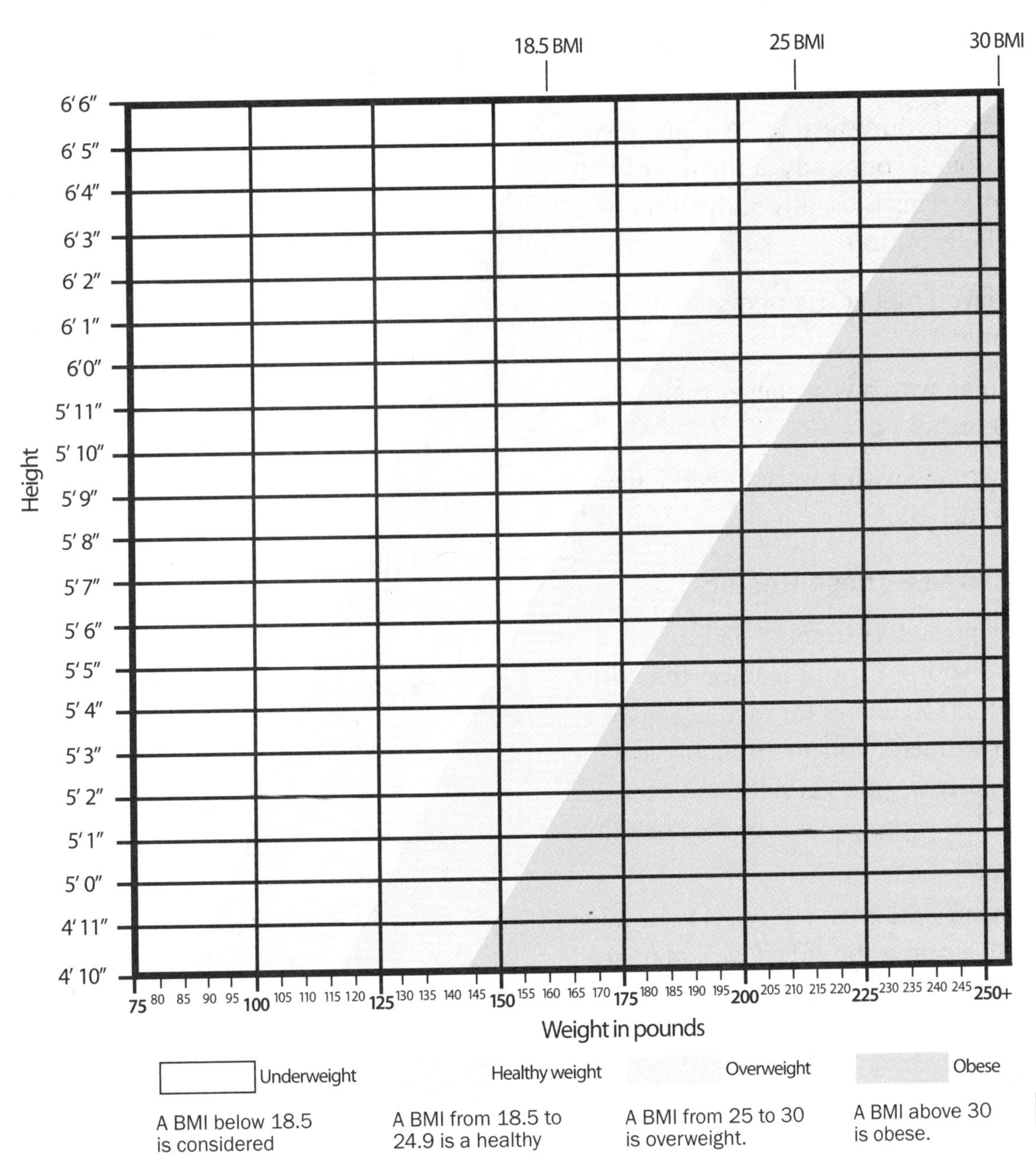

More

Waist Size: Apple or Pear?

Where you store fat in your body makes a difference to your health.

- Some people store most of their fat around their hips. These folks are sometimes called "pear-shaped."
- Others store their fat around their belly, so they are "apple-shaped."

Of these two shapes, "apples" are more likely to have weight-related diseases.

One way to find out whether your body fat is putting you at risk is to measure the size of your waist. Place a tape measure around your body at the top of your hipbone. This is usually at the level of your belly button.

You have a higher risk of disease if you are:

- A man with a waist larger than 40 inches.
- A woman with a waist larger than 35 inches.

How to Use These Results

- If your BMI is from 18.5 to 24.9 and your waist size is lower than the cutoff (40 inches for men, 35 inches for women), you are probably at a healthy weight. Eat right and exercise so that your weight stays in a healthy range.
- If your BMI is over 25, or if your waist size is above the cutoff, you may need to lose some weight. Even a small weight loss can help.

Also talk to your doctor about any other risk factors for disease, such as smoking, high blood pressure, and high cholesterol. If you have these in addition to being overweight, you are at higher risk.

Weight Is Not the Only Thing That Matters

Weight is only one measure of your health.

- You can be a little overweight and still be healthy if you eat right and are active.
- If you do not eat right or exercise, you may not be healthy no matter what you weigh.

Healthy bodies come in many shapes and sizes. Everyone can get healthier by eating better and being more active. Most of us will never look like fashion models or world-class athletes. But if you treat your body well—feed it healthy food and move it in the ways it's built to move—you can feel good about it.

Healthy Eating

Healthy eating means eating a variety of foods from the basic food groups in reasonable amounts. It's not about "going on a diet." Food is one of life's great pleasures. Almost any food can be part of a healthy eating plan if it's eaten in sensible amounts.

Here are some basic ways to start eating healthier:

- Eat more fruits and vegetables. See this page.
- Learn which fats are good for you and which ones to avoid. See page 334.
- Add more whole grains and fiber to your diet. See page 335.
- Choose lean sources of protein. See page 337.
- Cut back on salt. See page 338.
- Don't eat too much sugar. See page 338.
- Get plenty of water. See page 339.

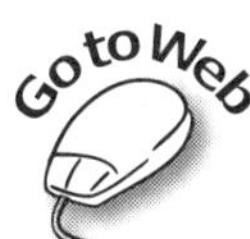

When you're ready to learn more about healthy food choices, go to the Web site on the back cover and enter **M494** in the search box.

Eat More Fruits and Vegetables

A healthy diet includes plenty of fruits and vegetables. Nearly everyone could benefit from eating more of them. They're full of vitamins, minerals, and fiber, and most are very low in fat and calories. They also have substances that help prevent heart disease, high blood pressure, and some types of cancer.

Easy Ways to Add Fruits and Veggies to Your Diet

- Add fresh or frozen berries or a sliced banana to breakfast cereal or yogurt. Put apple slices in oatmeal.
- Have a glass of juice with breakfast. One 6-ounce glass is a serving. (But don't depend on juice for all of your fruit servings. Juice has more calories than plain fruit. And fruit also gives you fiber that juice doesn't.)
- Add lettuce, tomato, cucumber, and bell peppers to sandwiches. Get pizza with veggies—try mushrooms, peppers, spinach, or broccoli.
- Add vegetables to soups, stews, and stir-fries. Purée them in a blender or food processor first if it makes them easier to use.
- Keep carrots, celery, and other veggies handy for snacks. Buy them already sliced and ready to eat if it makes you more likely to eat them.
- Have a salad with dinner every night. Make sure the salad is mostly vegetables, rather than mostly cheese, croutons, and salad dressing.
- Have fruit for dessert. If plain fruit doesn't seem like dessert to you, try baked apples or pears with cinnamon, or have fresh berries or melon with some vanilla yogurt.

More

Healthy Ways to Cook

How you cook affects how you eat. For many people, "cooking" means frying. This often means using lard, shortening, butter, or lots of oil to make food taste good. But there are healthier methods you can use and still have great-tasting food.

Here are some low-fat ways to cook. Try one for your next meal.

- Bake in aluminum foil. This keeps food juicy and full of flavor. Wrap meat or fish in foil with some herbs for seasoning and even a little wine or broth. Add some vegetables too.
- Before you eat chicken or meat, cut off the fat. If you eat red meat, choose the leanest cuts. Lean cuts usually have the word "round" or "loin" in them.
- Stir-fry. To stir-fry, cut meat, chicken, or vegetables into small pieces so they cook fast. Use a nonstick pan or a wok over medium-high heat. Add the food and constantly stir and turn it. If the food sticks, add a little peanut or sesame oil; cooking spray; or water, wine, or broth.
- Try fat-free or low-fat yogurt, sour cream, or cottage cheese in place of full-fat cream and sour cream.
- Poach. Put chicken or fish in one layer in a pan. Cover it with water or broth, and add herbs or a little wine for flavor. Bring the liquid to a boil. Then lower the heat and simmer for 10 to 12 minutes until the food is done.

- Make a fruit smoothie. Blend bananas, berries, or oranges with fat-free or low-fat yogurt or milk.
- Keep frozen and canned fruits and vegetables on hand. They are as good for you as fresh ones and can be an easy way to add more fruits and vegetables to your diet.

Learn About Fats

Except for some fruits and vegetables and skim milk, almost everything you eat has some kind of fat. Your body needs some fat to work properly. But not all fats are the same. Some are better for you than others. For many people, the least healthy types of fats—saturated and trans fats—make up too much of their diet.

A healthy eating plan can and should include healthy fats in reasonable amounts. The kinds of fat in nuts, seeds, and vegetable oils can help lower your cholesterol and may reduce your risk of some diseases. Oily fish like salmon, trout, and herring contain heart-healthy omega-3 fats. Eating 2 servings of these fish each week may help reduce your risk of heart attack.

Understanding Fats

Type of fats	What foods are they in?
Healthy fats: Monounsaturated fats Polyunsaturated fats Omega-3 fats	**Monounsaturated fats:** ◆ Avocados, olives, olive oil, peanut oil **Polyunsaturated fats:** ◆ Canola, corn, safflower, sunflower, and walnut oils **Omega-3 fats:** ◆ Fish (salmon, trout, herring, mackerel) ◆ Some plant foods (flaxseed, canola oil, walnuts) Soybeans and most nuts and seeds contain healthy fats.
Unhealthy fats: Saturated fats Cholesterol Trans fats	**Saturated fats and cholesterol:** ◆ Whole milk, whole-milk cheese, whole-milk yogurt ◆ Butter, margarine, lard (and foods cooked in these) ◆ Red meat (such as beef), chicken skin **Saturated fats and trans fats:** ◆ Packaged cookies, crackers, pies, cakes, and chips ◆ Shortening, stick margarine, hydrogenated vegetable oil ◆ Nondairy whipped topping and creamer ◆ Coconut and palm oils

With unhealthy fats, it's best to avoid them as much as you can. Besides having a lot of calories, they also raise your cholesterol and increase your risk of heart disease.

Use the Understanding Fats chart on this page to learn which fats to avoid and which to enjoy. But remember, all fats are high in calories, so watch your serving sizes.

How much fat should you eat? If you're eating an average diet of about 1,800 calories a day:

- Aim for about 60 grams of fat each day. Most of that should be monounsaturated fats.
- Eat less than 20 grams of saturated fats a day.
- Try to avoid all trans fats. Check food labels, and choose ones with 0% trans fat.

Get More Whole Grains

Whole grains like whole wheat, oats, and brown rice are full of B vitamins, minerals, and fiber and are a great source of energy. They're also very filling. **Refined grains** like white flour, white rice, and pasta have fewer vitamins and minerals. They're not as filling because they don't have much fiber.

More

How do you know if it's whole grain?

- Read the food label. The first ingredient should be whole wheat, whole grain, or whole oats. "Enriched wheat flour" is a refined grain, not a whole grain. Multi-grain breads and crackers are not always whole grains.
- Don't go by color alone. Bread can be brown but not be whole-grain or whole wheat.

You can add whole grains to your diet by choosing whole wheat bread instead of white bread; whole-grain crackers and cereals; oatmeal; brown rice instead of white rice; and whole wheat pasta. Try other whole grains like bulgur, barley, and quinoa.

Add Fiber to Your Diet

Fiber is the part of fruits, vegetables, and grains that your body cannot digest. It is found only in plants. Foods that come from animals (meats, milk and dairy foods, eggs) do not have fiber.

Eating plenty of fiber helps keep your digestive tract healthy. If you are often constipated, adding more fiber to your diet will help. People who eat a lot of fiber have fewer problems with the colon (large intestine).

A high-fiber diet can also help keep your blood sugar steady, lower your cholesterol, and reduce your chance of heart disease.

High-Fiber Foods

Type of food	Examples
Breads and grain products (especially whole-grain foods)	Oatmeal Whole wheat breads, whole wheat or corn tortillas, and whole-grain cereals Brown rice Barley, bulgur, millet, and quinoa
Vegetables	Dried beans and peas Cabbage, brussels sprouts Broccoli, cauliflower Beets, turnips, carrots Baked potato with skin
Fruits	Fruits with skin or seeds that you eat (apples, pears, strawberries, kiwifruit, figs, blueberries) Oranges, grapefruit

How to Get More Fiber

Most adults need about 20 to 30 grams of fiber each day. To reach that amount:

- Choose whole-grain breads and cereals that have at least 2 grams of fiber in each serving. Read the label on the package.
- Buy bread that lists whole wheat, stone-ground whole wheat, or cracked wheat first in the ingredient list.
- Eat brown rice, bulgur, or millet instead of white rice.
- Eat more fresh fruits every day. See the list of high-fiber fruits in the chart on page 336.
- Eat more vegetables every day.
- Eat cooked beans, peas, and lentils more often.

Choose Lean Protein

Protein is vital to your health. It helps keep your muscles, bones, skin, hair, blood, and internal organs healthy. But some forms of protein tend to have too much cholesterol and unhealthy fats. So it's best to choose lean sources of protein, such as:

- Fish, skinless chicken, and the leanest cuts of beef.
- Dried beans, peas, and lentils.
- Fat-free or low-fat dairy products.
- Eggs (yolks in moderation).
- Tofu and other soy products.

Most adults in North America get all the protein they need in their diets. If you eat animal products, your diet probably has plenty of protein. If you are a vegetarian, make sure you get protein from plant sources like dried beans, grains, and soy.

More

Should You Take Supplements?

For most people, the best way to get all the nutrients they need is to eat a healthy diet that includes a variety of foods.

Supplements can't make up for a poor diet. But they can help fill in the nutrition gap for people who have special needs. For example, older adults tend to have trouble absorbing enough vitamin D and calcium from their diets, so they may need a supplement. Some older people have trouble absorbing vitamin B_{12} and need to take B_{12} shots.

Talk to your doctor or a dietitian about whether you need vitamin or mineral supplements. If you decide to take a supplement:

- Unless your doctor recommends a specific vitamin or mineral, choose a balanced multivitamin-mineral supplement that has close to 100 percent of the Daily Values (DVs).
- Do not take a specific mineral unless your doctor recommends it. Taking some minerals as supplements can upset the way your body absorbs other minerals.

Cut Back on Salt

You need some salt (sodium) in your diet, but most people get far more than they need. Lowering your salt intake can help you keep your blood pressure under control.

For tips on how to reduce salt in your diet, see Five Ways to Reduce Salt on page 304.

Don't Eat Too Much Sugar

A little sugar is fine. It tastes good, and it's not harmful for most people. But most sweets also have a lot of "empty" calories—they don't fill you up or have much nutritional value. If too many of your calories come from sugar, you may not be getting enough of the healthy foods you need. (You may also gain weight.)

Using the USDA's MyPyramid

The USDA's MyPyramid aims to help you make healthy food choices and be active every day. It is based on the idea that your calorie and nutrient needs depend on your age, sex, and activity level. For example:

- A woman over 60 who gets more than 60 minutes of physical activity on most days may need about 2,000 calories a day.
- A woman over 60 who gets less than 30 minutes of daily exercise may need only about 1,600 calories a day.

Both women need to eat a variety of healthy foods from all the food groups—grains, vegetables, fruits, milk, meat and beans, and healthy fats. But they don't need the same amounts of those foods. Eating more food (and thus more calories) than you need can lead to weight gain.

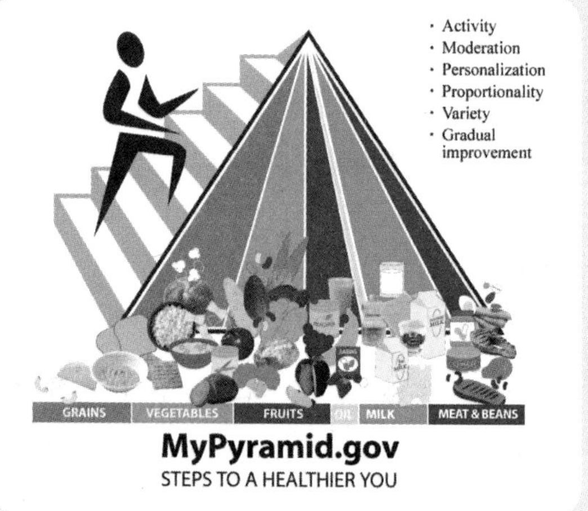

Want to know what's right for you? Go to www.MyPyramid.gov to:

- Figure out what kinds and amounts of food you should eat each day.
- Get help with meal plans and serving sizes.
- Track your progress toward healthier eating.

Many people need to cut down on sugar. Here are a few things that can make a big difference:

- Drink fewer sugar-sweetened drinks, such as soft drinks, lemonade, and fruit juices. Try sparkling water, unsweetened tea, or sugar-free soda instead. Or stick to plain water and milk.
- Make it a habit to eat fruit instead of sugary desserts and snacks most of the time. Have a bowl of strawberries instead of a bowl of ice cream. Grab an apple instead of a candy bar.
- Check the labels on food packages before you buy things. Yogurt, cereal, and canned fruits often have sugar added. Look for cereals that have 6 grams or less of sugar in each serving.

Get Plenty of Water

Unless your doctor has told you to limit fluids, make sure you get enough water every day. Many older adults don't get the fluids they need. As you age, you may lose some of your sense of thirst, so you can get dehydrated without knowing it. Dehydration can be a serious problem, especially in older adults.

Don't wait until you are thirsty to drink. Keep a glass or water bottle nearby, and take sips often. Water is the best choice. Nonfat milk can give you extra calcium and is also a good choice.

If you have bladder control problems, don't stop drinking plenty of water. But do talk to your doctor about ways to manage your problem. See page 92.

Eating Alone?

Many older adults live alone. Often this means they don't eat as well as they should. They are more likely to eat a limited range of foods or skip meals.

If this sounds like you, try these tips:

- Plan your meals for a week, and shop from a list. You are more likely to eat if you have planned your meals and have what you need to make them.
- Make a big pot of soup or stew. Eat it for a few meals and freeze the leftovers.
- Find a friend who will take turns cooking and eating with you. Or start a potluck supper club.
- Call your local senior center. Many of them serve healthy, low-cost meals.
- Find out if your area has a "Meals on Wheels" program that will bring a hot meal to your home once a day.

More

If You Have Trouble Eating

Some people have health problems that make it hard to eat, or they take medicines that reduce their appetite. If you have trouble eating enough to stay at a healthy weight, try these tips:

- Eat 3 regular meals, and try to add 2 or 3 snacks a day.
- Drink high-calorie liquid supplements, such as Ensure Plus or Boost Plus.
- Choose high-calorie items from each food group. For example, drink whole milk instead of low-fat milk.
- At each meal, eat the food that has the most calories first.
- Add calories to your diet. Healthy fats such as olive or canola oil may be good choices. Unless you have diabetes, you can use honey and sugar to add calories and increase energy.
- If you have trouble chewing foods, choose softer foods from all food groups. Don't leave out a food group because it is hard to eat.

Exercise for Health

Being more active is one of the best things you can do to improve your health and your quality of life. And it becomes even more important as you age. It can help you to:

- Feel stronger and have more energy. (And look better too!)
- Lower your risk for heart disease, stroke, certain cancers, diabetes, and high blood pressure. If you already have these diseases, it can help you get them under control.
- Reach and stay at a healthy weight.
- Keep your bones, muscles, and joints strong, and relieve arthritis pain.
- Handle stress, fight depression, and sleep better.
- Do daily tasks more easily—carry groceries, climb stairs, clean house.
- Keep your mind sharp.

If you are already in good health, regular exercise can help you stay that way. But if you are not in good health, or if you have a long-term health problem, just a little more exercise every day can make a big difference.

It's never too late to become more active. And it's never too late to get the benefits that exercise can bring. No matter how old you are, how fit you are, or what health problems you have, there is a form of exercise that will work for you.

Attitude Counts

Starting or changing an exercise routine doesn't have to be hard. Lots of people find ways to be more active that work for them. Success starts with the right attitude.

"I'll never be too old to exercise."

Exercise helps at any age. In fact, being active can help you avoid some of the problems that often come as we get older. Talk to your doctor about what kinds of activity might be best for you.

"I can find time for a little more exercise."

Even the busiest people can find time. If you're worried about not having enough time:

- Focus on being more active. You don't have to do formal "exercise" to improve your fitness. You just need to move more.
- Spread your workout throughout the day. You don't have to do all your exercise at once. For example, walk for 10 minutes 3 times a day.
- Get up early to walk, do a workout video, or go to a class at your local health club. It may seem hard at first, but you'll get used to it. You might even start to like it.
- Look for ways to be more active in your everyday life. Take the stairs instead of the elevator. Park farther away from work or the mall. Move faster through chores like cleaning, yard work, or vacuuming. Do daily tasks at a pace that gets your heart beating faster and gets you breathing harder. This can give you a good workout.
- Be creative. Instead of e-mailing or phoning a coworker or neighbor, walk over. When meeting with someone, suggest that you take a walk instead of staying inside.

"I'll have more energy if I exercise."

At first, exercise may make you feel tired because you're not used to it. Start by doing a little bit at a time, and stick with it. You may be surprised at how much more energetic you'll start to feel.

"Exercise doesn't have to hurt."

Even gentle exercise can improve your health. If you are new to exercise, at first your muscles may ache and your lungs may "burn" a little when you are breathing hard. Start slowly, and your body

More

Have a Long-Term Health Problem?

You may think that because you have a health problem like high blood pressure, arthritis, or diabetes, exercise is not for you. But exercise can help almost everyone. It may even be part of the treatment for your health problem.

You may not be able to do certain kinds of exercise. But there are dozens of ways to be more active. You only need to find a few. Talk to your doctor about what exercises are safe for you and how much exercise you should get.

will adapt. Talk with your doctor if you have chest pain or if your joints hurt.

"Exercise is for large people too."

No matter what your size, exercise can make you healthier and happier. At first you may get tired quickly and not be able to move or bend very well if you are overweight and unfit. You might feel self-conscious. Just remember to take one small step at a time. Those steps will quickly start to add up.

Should You See Your Doctor First?

Moderate exercise is safe for most people, but it's always a good idea to talk to your doctor before you get started. This is especially important if:

- You are older than 60 and are not used to exercise.
- You have heart trouble or high blood pressure, or you often have chest pain or pressure.
- You often feel faint or dizzy.
- You have arthritis or other bone or joint problems.
- You have diabetes (you may need to adjust your medicine).
- You have two or more risk factors for heart disease. These include high cholesterol, high blood pressure, smoking, obesity, an inactive lifestyle, and a family history of heart disease before age 50.

"Exercise doesn't have to cost much."

You do not need to spend a lot to get fit.

- Start walking. It's free.
- Get home workout videos from the library, a thrift store, or a used bookstore.
- Apply for a reduced-cost membership at your local YMCA. Some gyms offer a senior discount.
- Shop for used exercise equipment in the newspaper or at yard sales. Make sure it's in safe condition.
- Check with your local senior center. It may offer free or low-cost exercise classes for older adults.

"Exercise can help me avoid a heart attack."

If you have a heart problem, you may worry that you could have a heart attack or stroke while exercising. You are probably more likely to have one if you do *not* exercise. There may be some limits on what you should do, but regular, safe workouts will strengthen your heart, blood vessels, and lungs. See your doctor before you get started.

"Exercise can be fun!"

- Look for something you enjoy. Try new things until you find something you like. Ride a bike. Take a dance or water exercise class. Go hiking. If you like what you're doing, you are much more likely to stick with it.

- Don't do the same thing every day. Variety can keep you motivated, and it's good for your body. Swim one day, and take a walk the next. Try a yoga class.
- Get a partner, or join a group or class. For many people, the social part makes their workout more fun.

"It never hurts to try."

Don't worry about failing, no matter what your past experience with exercise has been. Just go slowly, and set small goals. When you meet those goals, set new ones. And if you don't meet a goal, think about what might have helped you meet it. Then try again.

Make Your Heart Stronger

When exercise gets your heart beating faster and gets you breathing harder, it makes your heart stronger. Whether you call it aerobic exercise, cardio exercise, or just "exercising your heart," it all means the same thing. And just a little more every day can reduce your risk for heart attack, stroke, and other problems.

What kinds of workouts are good for your heart? Anything that raises your heart rate and keeps it there counts:

- Walking, hiking, and jogging
- Biking (outside or indoors)
- Swimming and water aerobics
- Dancing
- Doing household chores or yard work at a fast pace
- Climbing stairs

A simple way to tell if you are working your heart is the "talk-sing" test. If you are too short of breath to talk while you exercise, you may be pushing too hard. If you can sing while you exercise, you might do more for your heart by working just a bit harder. If your heart rate is increased but you can still talk, your heart is getting a good workout.

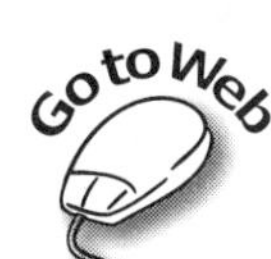

Getting started can be as simple as taking a walk a few times a week. For help making a plan to get more fit, go to the Web site on the back cover and enter **Z704** in the search box.

More

Three Types of Exercise

The ideal exercise program includes the three types of exercise:

- Activities that make your heart stronger (aerobic exercise).
- Strength training to tone and strengthen your muscles.
- Stretching to help you be more flexible and avoid injuries.

It's easy to include them all:

- Stretch for a few minutes to warm up your muscles.
- Get some aerobic exercise. Take a brisk walk, bike ride, or swim.
- Use light weights to tone and strengthen your muscles.
- Then spend a few minutes cooling down. Do some light stretches or balance exercises.

Walking Works!

Want to start making your heart stronger today? Take a walk. Walking is one of the easiest ways to be more active and improve your health.

- Start with small, short-term goals you can reach. For example, if you have not been active in a long time, start with 15-minute walks 3 times a week. The next week, increase your walks to 20 minutes.
- Start each walk with a warm-up. Pick up your pace in the middle of the walk, and then slow down at the end.
- Walk fast enough to raise your heart rate and make you breathe harder, but not so fast that you can't talk.
- Wear comfortable shoes with good arch support.

The tips below have helped lots of people stick to their walking routines. They can help you too.

- Find a friend, family member, or coworker to walk with. You will be less likely to skip your walk if you know someone is expecting you.
- Get a step counter or pedometer, a small device that counts your steps. Set a daily step goal, and wear your pedometer all day. Park your car a little farther away, use the stairs instead of the elevator, or walk to the store instead of driving there. You may be surprised how fast the steps add up.
- Get a dog. Dogs love to walk, and taking your dog for a walk once or twice a day is a great way to fit walking into your life.

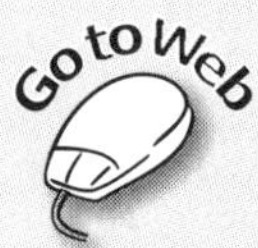

For more tips on how to start a walking program, go to the Web site on the back cover and enter **A687** in the search box.

Make Your Body Stronger

Muscles get weak if they aren't used. Strength exercises help tone your muscles, strengthen your bones, and protect your joints. Your goal may be to be able to get around better. Maybe you want to reduce body fat and stay trim. Or you may want to stay strong so you can live on your own as long as possible.

Doing a few simple exercises twice a week can make a difference. For a guide to

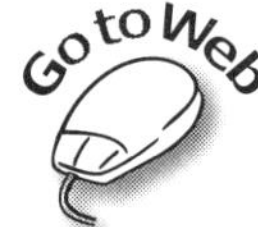

some basic exercises, go to the Web site on the back cover and enter **G736** in the search box.

The exercises and stretches on the next few pages are good ones to start with if you have not been active in a long time. Many of them will work for people who cannot move well.

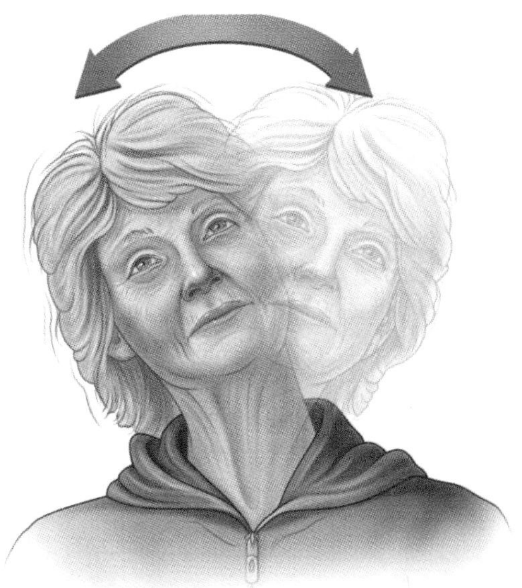

Neck stretches

Gently lower your right ear toward your right shoulder. Hold for 5 counts. Bring your head back to center. Lower your chin to your chest. Hold for 5 counts. Return to center. Lower your left ear toward your left shoulder. Hold for 5 counts. Return to center.

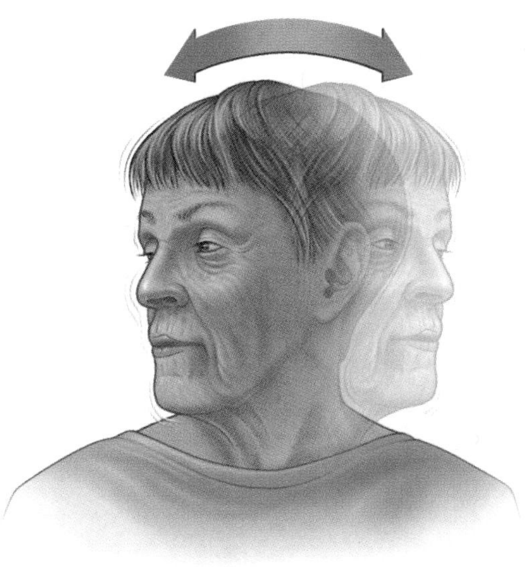

Head half-circles

Keep your chin level. Gently turn your head to the right. (Try to look over your shoulder.) Hold for 2 counts. Now turn your head to the left. Hold for 2 counts.

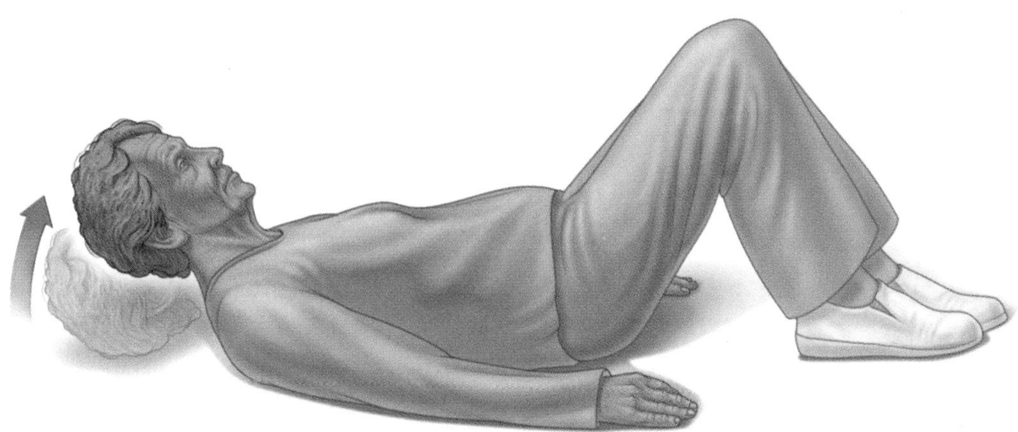

Head and shoulder curl

Lie on your back with your knees slightly bent. Keep your arms at your sides. Curl your head and shoulders off the floor. Hold for 5 counts. Return to the starting position. Do this 10 times. Get up from the floor slowly.

More

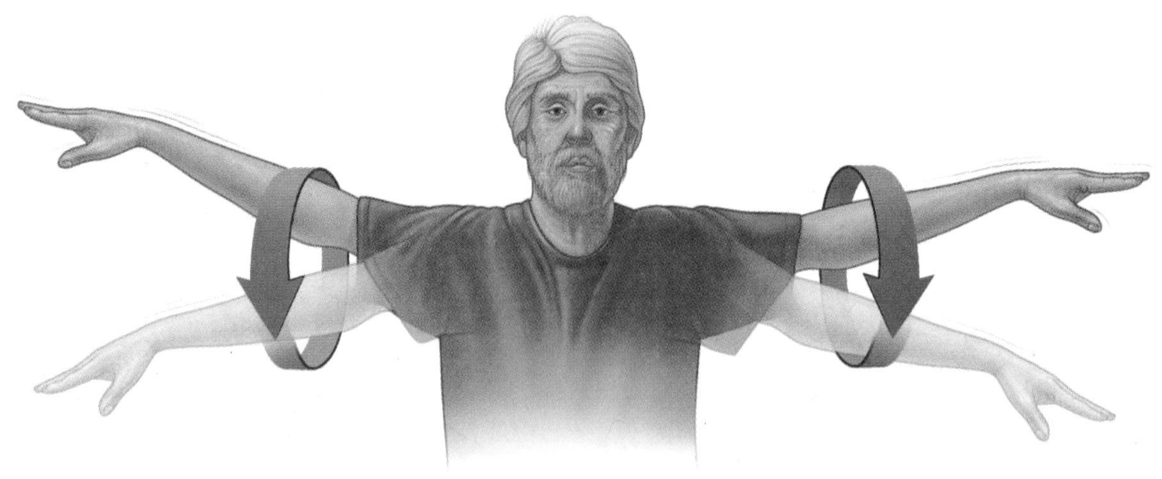

Arm circles

Raise your arms out to the sides at shoulder level. Keeping your arms straight, make 10 small circles forward, then 10 backward.

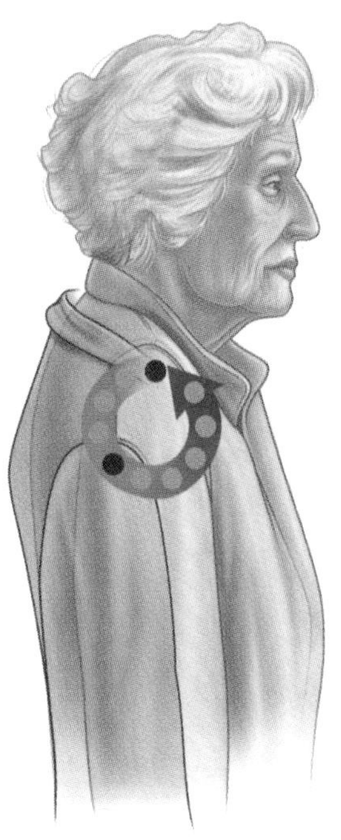

Shoulder rolls

Keep your arms relaxed and at your sides. Roll your shoulders forward, making large circles with them. Roll forward 5 times, then backward 5 times.

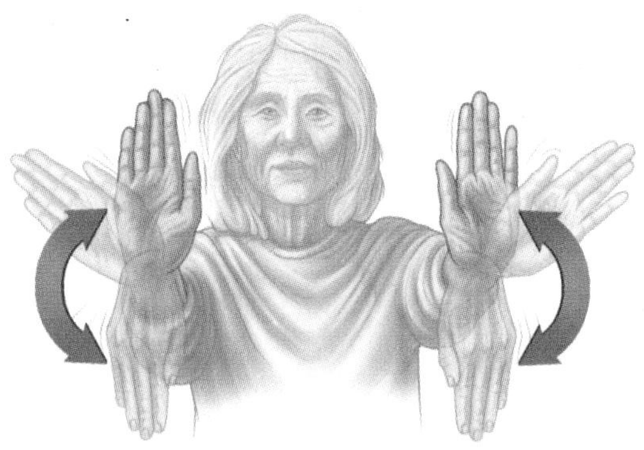

Hand circles

Extend your arms out in front of you at shoulder level. Keeping your arms straight, rotate your wrists in small circles. Do 10 circles to the right, then 10 to the left.

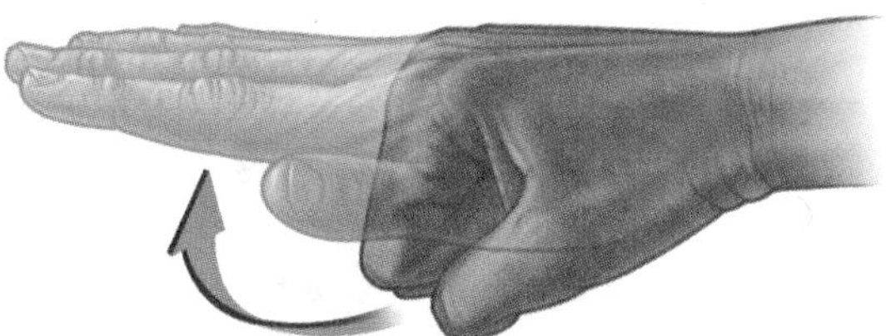

Finger squeezes

Extend your arms out in front of you at shoulder level, palms down. Slowly squeeze your fingers to make a fist, then release. Do this 5 times. Then turn your palms up. Make a fist and release. Do this 5 times.

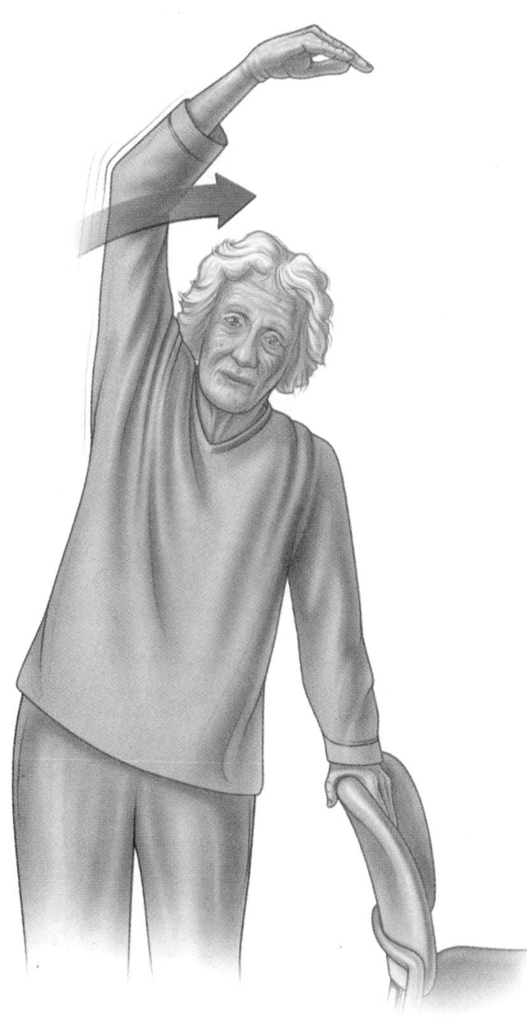

Side stretch

Hold on to the back of a chair with your left hand. Stand with your feet shoulder-width apart. Bring your right arm up and over your head. Slowly bend over to the left. Feel the stretch in your right side. Make sure to keep your weight on both legs. Hold for 10 counts. Repeat on the left side.

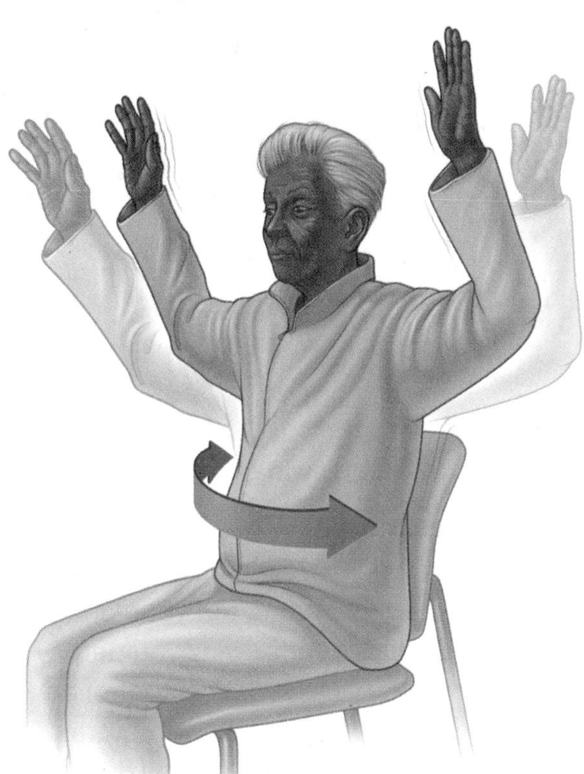

Spine twist

Sit or stand with your back and neck straight. Raise your arms out at your sides at shoulder level, and bend your elbows so your palms are facing forward. Keep your knees and hips facing forward, and slowly twist at your waist to the right. Hold for 5 counts. Return to center, then twist to the left. Hold for 5 counts.

More

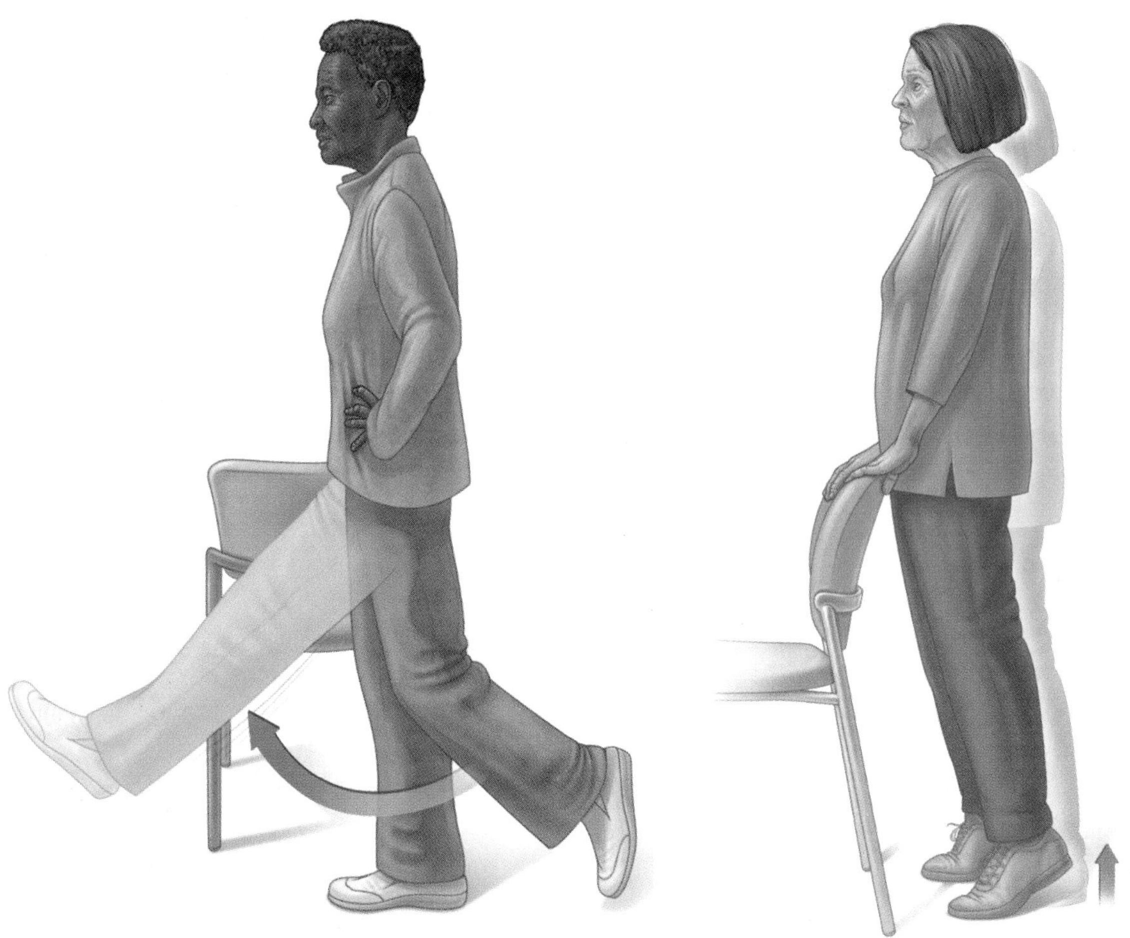

Leg swings

Stand up straight with your right leg next to the back of a chair. Hold on to the chair with your right hand. Put your left hand on your hip. Gently swing your left leg forward and backward. Use controlled movements. Don't let your body move to the back or front when you swing your leg. Do this 10 times with each leg.

Heel raises

Hold on to the back of a chair for support. Rise up on your toes. Hold for a count of 5, then lower your heels to the ground. Do this 10 times.

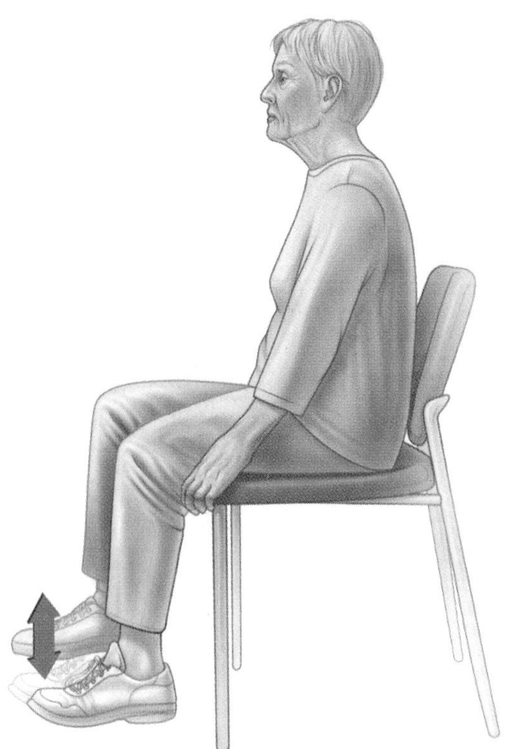

Leg lifts

Sit in a chair with both feet on the floor. Lift your right knee as high as you can. Do not pull up or push down on the chair with your hands. Set your foot back on the floor. Repeat with your left knee. Repeat 5 times for each leg.

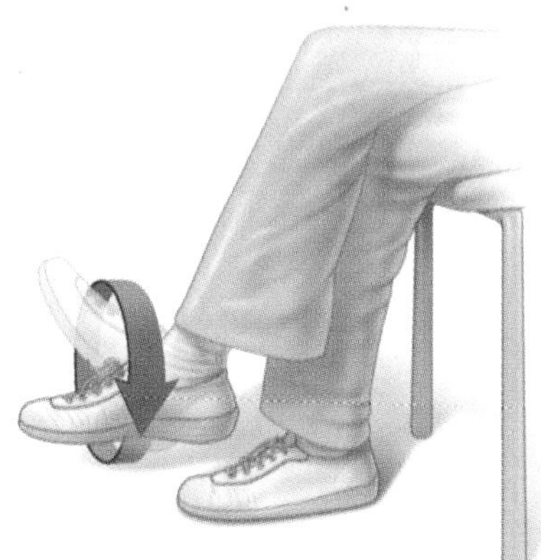

Ankle and foot circles

Sit in a chair and cross your right leg over your left knee. Slowly make large circles with your right foot. Then switch to the other side. For each foot, do 10 circles to the right and 10 to the left.

Stretch

Stretching keeps you flexible and helps with sore or tense muscles. It improves your balance and posture and can also be a great way to relax. And you can do it for free, anywhere, without any equipment.

There are lots of ways to bring stretching into your life:

- Stretch at home when you first get up in the morning or before you go to bed (or both). If you need help, get a video you can follow, or find a good fitness book or magazine that explains some stretches.
- Take a stretching class at a gym or health club or at a senior center.
- Try yoga or tai chi. These are great ways to stay flexible, improve balance, and reduce stress.

Basic stretches are easy to learn. The pictures on the next page show some simple stretches you can do on your own. The shaded area in each shows where you should feel the stretch. Here are a few tips to get you started:

- Ease into each stretch. Stretching is not about going fast or making sudden movements.
- Hold each stretch for at least 20 to 30 seconds. You should feel a gentle pull in the area you are stretching, but you should not feel sharp pain.
- Do not hold your breath during a stretch.

More

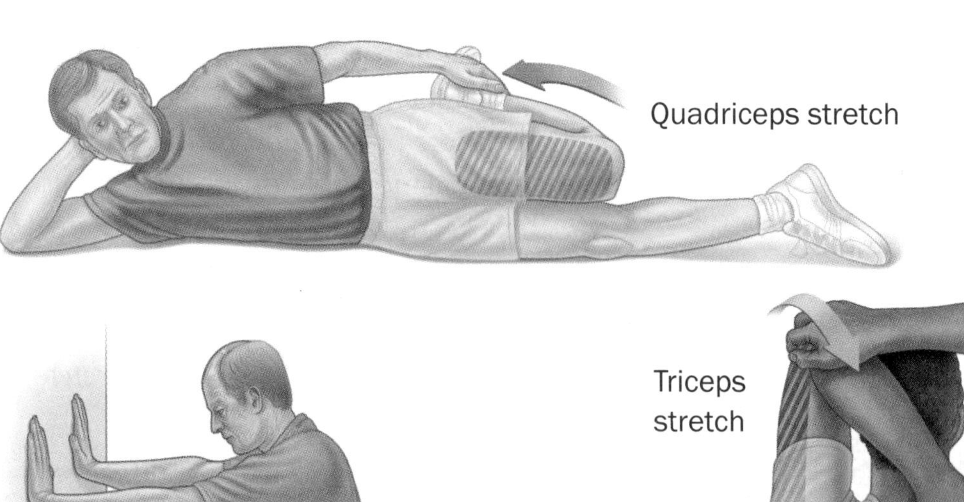

Quadriceps stretch

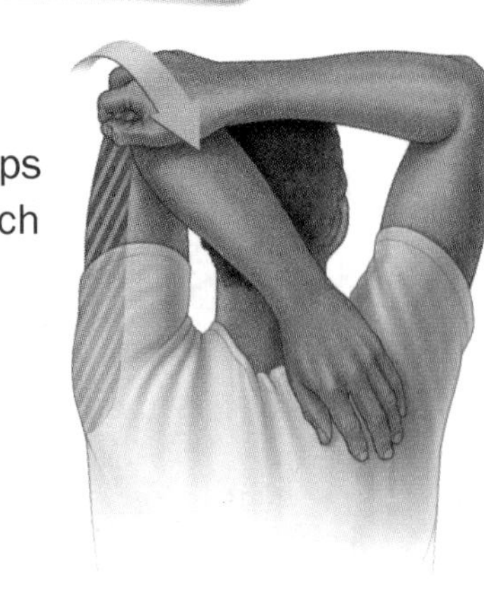

Triceps stretch

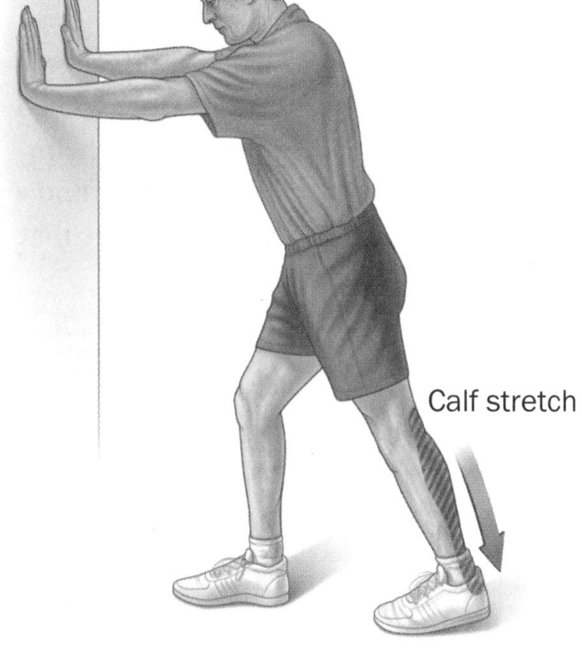

Calf stretch

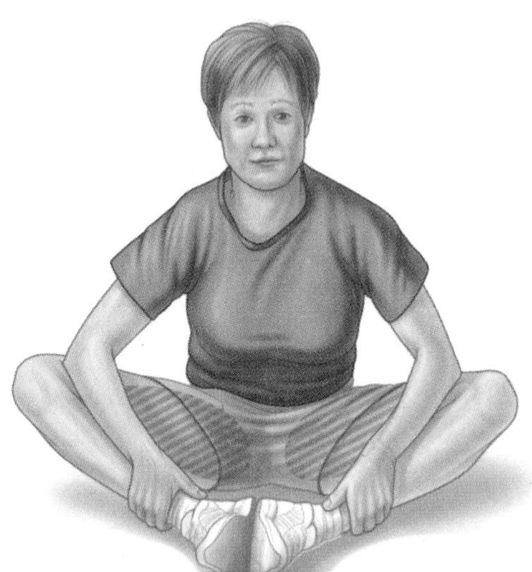

Groin stretch

Hip, buttocks, and hamstring stretch

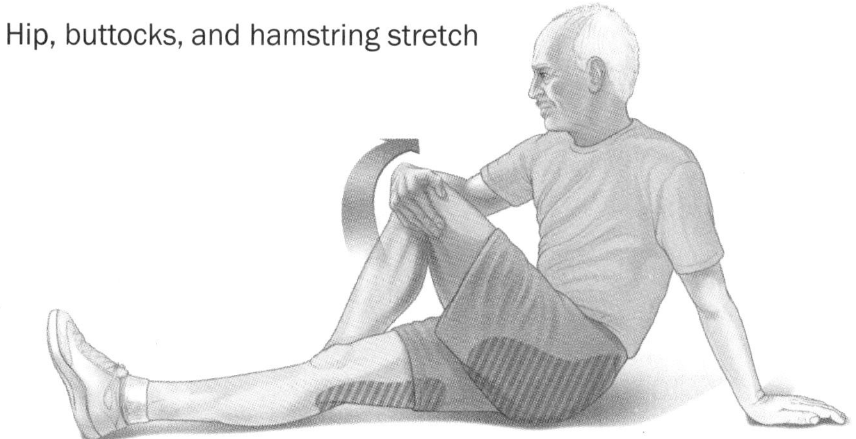

Improve Your Balance

As you age, your balance tends to get worse. This increases your chance of falling. Falls are a leading cause of injury and disability in older adults.

Some simple exercises can help you improve your balance.

- To start, stand up straight and hold onto a counter or sturdy chair with one hand.
- Bend one knee so your foot comes up behind you. Lower your foot to the floor. Repeat using the other leg.
- Rise up on your toes. Hold for a few seconds. Lower your heels to the floor. (See the picture on page 348.)
- Keeping your legs straight, lift one leg a few inches to the side. Hold for a few seconds. Lower your leg. Repeat on the other side.

Repeat each exercise several times. As you feel more steady, try the exercise without holding on.

Quitting Smoking

Millions of people have quit smoking. Some quit on their own. Some quit with the help of stop-smoking programs or support groups. Some used nicotine replacement products.

The point is that people find ways to quit for good. So can you.

But you have to be ready. Giving up tobacco is a big change, and the process of deciding that you will quit may take time. If you aren't sure you're ready, go to the Web site on the back cover and

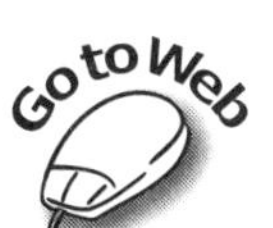

enter **Z175** in the search box. You can take a quiz to help you figure out where you are in the process.

It's Never Too Late

Anyone who smokes has good reason to stop—even if you have smoked for decades. No matter how long you've smoked, your risk of a heart attack and other health problems will start to go down once you quit. You will start to feel better and breathe easier.

It can be hard to break a long-time habit. But you can do it, just like millions of other people who have quit.

More

It's Not Just Cigarettes

Some people think they are safe because they only smoke cigars or use spit tobacco. Think again. Pipes, cigars, chewing tobacco, snuff—all of them are dangerous:

- They contain chemicals that can lead to cancer.
- They contain nicotine, which is addictive.
- They raise your risk of heart disease, high blood pressure, and other serious diseases.

If you use any of these products, you can use the information in this section to help you quit.

Thinking About Quitting?

If you're thinking about quitting, you're already on your way. It may help to know that you don't have to quit smoking through willpower alone.

- Treatments can help with the physical effects of giving up smoking and nicotine.
- Resources can help with the emotional side of quitting smoking.

These approaches have helped many people stop smoking for good. They can help you too.

Nicotine Replacement and Medicines

When you try to stop smoking, you may have trouble sleeping, crave nicotine, or feel grumpy, depressed, or restless. These symptoms of withdrawal are at their worst during the first couple of days after you quit, but they may last up to a few weeks. Cravings may last even longer.

Treatment can reduce withdrawal symptoms and help you beat your body's nicotine addiction.

- Nicotine replacement products, such as gums, patches, inhalers, sprays, and lozenges, help your body slowly get used to less nicotine until you don't need it at all. You can buy these products without a prescription.
- Medicines such as bupropion (Zyban) or varenicline (Chantix) can help you cope with cravings and mood swings. They do not have nicotine. Your doctor can prescribe one of these for you.

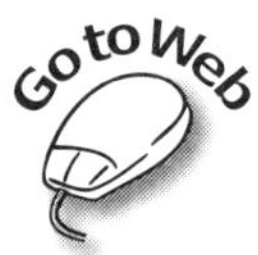

Using these treatments makes it much more likely that you will quit for good. For help in deciding whether to try them, go to the Web site on the back cover and enter **U285** in the search box.

It's Not Just the Nicotine

If you are like many smokers, smoking is part of your daily routine. You enjoy it. It's relaxing. When you quit smoking, you have to give all that up (or at least find something to replace it).

The good news is that you don't have to do it alone. You can get support from:

- Stop-smoking programs. Call your health plan, your local hospital, or the American Lung Association to find out what programs are offered in your area.

- Telephone "quitlines," such as 1-800-QUITNOW (1-800-784-8669). These connect you to trained counselors who can help you make a plan for how to quit.
- Online quit groups. Like quitlines, these are convenient since you can get help from home at nearly any hour.
- Support groups, such as Nicotine Anonymous.
- Counseling from doctors, nurses, or therapists.

This kind of support can help you change your habits. Think about whether any of these options appeal to you, and give one a try. If it's not for you, try something else.

When You've Decided to Quit

No one approach works for everybody. But for many people, it helps to:

- **Set a quit date.** Pick a date within the next month. Give yourself time to get ready (but not too much time).

More

10 Reasons to Quit

1. Live longer and better. On average, people who smoke die nearly 7 years earlier than people who do not smoke. But it is not as simple as just dying a little younger. Smoking can affect the quality of your life as well. Having chronic lung disease is not an easy or pleasant way to live or die.
2. Breathe easier and cough less. You may have more energy and stamina after you stop smoking.
3. Reduce your risk of erection problems. Smoking can damage your blood vessels, including those that bring blood to the penis.
4. Cut your risk of heart attack in half within 1 year. Five years after quitting, your risk will be about the same as that of someone who never smoked.
5. Reduce your risk for lung cancer, mouth and throat cancer, gum disease, and dental problems.
6. Get fewer colds, and be less likely to get the flu or pneumonia. If you have asthma, you will have fewer and less severe asthma attacks.
7. Set a good example for your children and grandchildren.
8. Stop having to find places to smoke at work or in public and exposing others to secondhand smoke.
9. Have a brighter smile, better sense of taste and smell, and fewer wrinkles.
10. Save money by not buying cigarettes. (Also, as a nonsmoker, you may pay less for health insurance.)

- **Plan.** Will you go to a class or use nicotine replacement? Make sure you have low-calorie snacks on hand. Clean your clothes, carpet, furniture, and car to get rid of the smoke smell. If you know you tend to smoke in certain situations, plan for ways to avoid them.
- **Quit!** Stick to your quit date. That day, get rid of cigarettes, ashtrays, and lighters.

For more ideas that can help you get ready to quit and then stop smoking for good, go to the Web site on the back cover and enter **R520** in the search box.

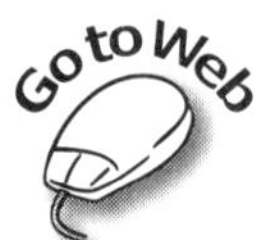

Started Smoking Again?

You're not alone. Many people who have quit smoking had to try several times before they were able to quit for good. The good news is that each time you try to quit—whether it's your second attempt or your tenth—you can get closer to quitting for good.

Think about why you started smoking again. Was it stress? Were you with a certain group of people or in a certain situation? What might have triggered you to smoke? Learn from what worked for you and what didn't.

Knowing what went wrong can help you when you are ready to quit again. The important thing is to keep trying.

Take Care of Your Teeth

Your teeth and gums will last a lifetime if you take good care of them.

- Brush your teeth 2 times a day, and floss once a day.
- Brush your tongue too. This will leave your breath fresher.
- Use a toothbrush with soft bristles that have rounded ends, or use an electric toothbrush. If you use an electric toothbrush, look for one that has the American Dental Association (ADA) seal of approval. Replace your toothbrush or the head of an electric toothbrush every 3 to 4 months.
- Use a fluoride toothpaste. Fluoride makes teeth stronger and helps prevent tooth decay.
- Check for signs of gum disease. These include gums that bleed when you brush your teeth or when you eat firm foods, such as apples. See page 164.

To make sure your teeth and gums stay healthy:

- See your dentist every 6 months to get your teeth cleaned and checked. Tell your dentist if you are taking any new medicines.

- Eat a healthy diet that includes whole grains, vegetables, and fruits and that is low in saturated fat and salt.
- Do not smoke or chew tobacco. This can cause gum disease and oral cancer. Even breathing someone else's smoke can cause problems.

Many older adults feel that they cannot afford dental care. However, many towns and cities have programs in which dentists reduce their fees for some older adults. Contact the public health department or social services to find out about dental care in your area.

Denture Care

You need to clean and care for your dentures every day.

- Clean your dentures with a brush and a denture cleaner, such as Polident or Efferdent. Clean fixed bridges with a floss threader, special floss with a stiff threader section, or a special brush.
- Store dentures in lukewarm water or denture-cleansing liquid at night. Do not let them dry out.
- Dentures can be fragile. Stand over a folded towel or sinkful of water when you take them out. This way if you drop them, they won't break.

To keep your mouth healthy:

- Brush your gums, tongue, and the roof of your mouth every day before you put in your dentures. Use a toothbrush with soft bristles.
- Give your mouth at least 6 hours of rest from your dentures every day. Your mouth heals more slowly as you age and needs time to recover from the rubbing caused by wearing your dentures.
- Check your gums every day before you put in your dentures. If your gums are red or swollen, let them heal before you wear your dentures again. Call your dentist if the redness does not go away in a few days or if you have white patches on the inside of your cheeks.
- Do not put up with dentures that are too big, click when you eat, or don't feel good. Dentures do take some time to get used to. But if they are still giving you trouble after the first few weeks, talk to your dentist about adjusting them. Don't try to fix them yourself.
- Replace your dentures about every 5 years.

Managing Stress

Some stress is normal and even healthy. Stress releases hormones that speed up your heart, make you breathe faster, and give you a burst of energy. This can be useful when you need to focus or act quickly. It can help you win a race, finish a big job, or get to the airport on time.

But too much stress or being under stress for too long is not good for you.

- It can make health problems like heart disease, diabetes, and asthma worse.
- It can make you moody, anxious, and depressed. You may find it hard to concentrate and may lose your temper more easily.
- It can cause headaches, back pain, and muscle tension.
- It can hurt your relationships. You may have trouble at home or at work.

You may not have these problems right away. Most people can get through short periods of stress without long-term effects. But over time, continued stress will take its toll on you.

The good news is that you can learn ways to reduce and cope with stress that will help you avoid stress-related health problems.

Ways to Reduce Stress

- **Decide what matters most and what can wait.** Maybe there are things you don't need to do at all.
- **Learn to say no.** Don't commit to things that don't matter to you.
- **Do one thing at a time.** When you try to do too many things at once, each usually takes more time than it would if you focused on it alone.
- **Get organized.** Make lists, or use an appointment book. Keep track of deadlines.
- **Don't put things off.** Use a schedule planner to plan your day or week. Just seeing on paper that there is a time to get each task done can help you get to work. Break a large project into small pieces, and set a deadline for each one.
- **Save some time for yourself.** Leave your job at the office, even if your office is a room in your home. If you give up free time to get more work done, you may pay for it with stress-related symptoms. If your employer offers a flexible work schedule, use it to fit your work style. Come in earlier so you have time for a longer lunch or a workout.
- **"Unplug" when you leave work.** Leave your work cell phone behind or turn it off. Don't check work e-mail at home.
- **Get enough sleep.** Stress can seem worse than it is when you're tired all the time. And you may not get as much done if you're tired.

How to Cope Better With Stress

For most people, there's just no way to totally avoid stress. It's part of life. But you can control how you react to stress.

Healthy Ways to De-Stress
Listen to music
Exercise
Go outdoors
Play with a pet
Laugh or cry
Spend time with someone you love
Write, draw, or paint
Pray or go to church
Take a bath or shower
Work in the yard or do home repairs
Do yoga, meditation, or muscle relaxation

Unhealthy Ways to De-Stress
Drive fast
Eat too much or too little
Bite your fingernails
Drink too much coffee
Criticize yourself
Avoid people
Yell at your spouse, children, or friends
Smoke
Drink alcohol
Get violent or aggressive

People don't always realize that they feel bad because of stress. Classic signs of stress include headache, stiff neck, or a nagging backache. You may lose your temper more often. You may feel jumpy or exhausted all the time.

Just knowing why you're feeling the way you do may help you cope with the problem. For a tool that can help you

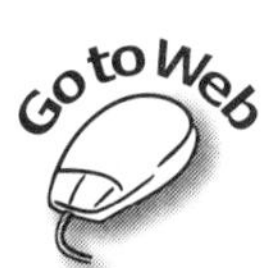

gauge your stress level now or anytime, go to the Web site on the back cover and enter **L060** in the search box.

Are You Stress-Hardy?

Some people seem to stand up to stress or bounce back from it better than others. They adjust to change more easily. They are more "stress-hardy."

How stress-hardy are you? Take a short quiz to find out. Go to the Web site on the back cover and enter **U822** in the search box.

If you would like to be more stress-hardy, here are a few things that may help:

- Know what's important to you, whether it's your family, your work, or something else. When you are under a lot of stress, it can help to remember what matters most.
- Try to have a sense of control over your life. You cannot control every detail, but look for areas where you can make a difference. Not everything is out of your hands.

More

- Try to look at change as a challenge or opportunity rather than a threat.
- Do things that let you be creative and let you be yourself. Some people can do this through their work. But sometimes activities outside of your job—hobbies, exercise, social groups, volunteer work, travel—are better chances to "do your own thing."
- Stay in touch with people who care about you. Having a strong network of family and friends can help you manage stress better.

Learn to Relax

There are many techniques you can learn to help you relax. Progressive muscle relaxation is one that seems to work well.

To learn this technique, practice it in a time and place where nothing will interrupt you. Do it once or twice a day until you can do it easily.

Progressive Muscle Relaxation

Relaxing your muscles can reduce tension and anxiety. It can help reduce stress-related health problems and often helps people sleep better.

You can buy a tape or CD that takes you through all the muscle groups, or you can do it by just tensing and relaxing each muscle group on your own.

- Choose a place where you can lie down on your back and stretch out.
- Tense each muscle group (hard, but not to the point of cramping) for 4 to 10 seconds. Then give yourself 10 to 20 seconds to release it and relax.
- At various points, check the muscle groups you've already done and relax each one a little more each time.

Muscle Groups

Remember to relax between each muscle group.

Hands: Clench them.

Wrists and forearms: Extend them and bend the hands back at the wrist.

Biceps and upper arms: Clench your hands into fists, bend your arms at the elbows, and flex your biceps (the muscles in your upper arms).

Shoulders: Shrug them. Check your arms and shoulders for tension.

Forehead: Wrinkle it into a deep frown.

Around the eyes and bridge of the nose: Close your eyes as tightly as you can. (Take out your contact lenses before you do this.)

Cheeks and jaws: Grin from ear to ear.

Around the mouth: Press your lips together tightly. (Check your face for tension.)

Back of the neck: Press the back of your head against the floor.

Front of the neck: Touch your chin to your chest. (Check your neck and head for tension.)

Chest: Take a deep breath and hold it. Then let it go.

Back: Arch your back up and away from the floor.

Belly: Suck it into a tight knot. (Check your chest and belly for tension.)

Hips and buttocks: Squeeze your buttocks together tightly.

Thighs: Clench them.

Lower legs: Point your toes toward your face, as if trying to bring your toes up to touch your shins. Then point your toes away and curl them under at the same time. (Check the area from your waist down for tension.)

When you are finished, return to alertness by counting backward from 5 to 1.

Keep Your Brain Healthy

One of the hottest topics in senior health these days is how to keep our brains working their best as we age. Studies are looking at the effects of "brain gyms" and brain-fitness training. Companies are already selling games and software that claim to give your brain a workout.

While we wait for the study results, we do know a few things:

"Use it or lose it" applies to the brain. Memory loss and decreased mental power don't have to be part of growing older. Just like exercise helps muscles stay strong, activities that challenge your brain can help it stay young.

- Take a class or read a book about a new subject that interests you.
- Take up a new hobby. Learn to knit, play an instrument, or do wood carving.
- Shake up your routines. Take a different route to places you go often. Travel if you are able.
- Stay socially engaged. Keep working if you can, or volunteer for a worthy cause. Spend time with friends and family.

What's good for your heart is good for your brain. Heart-healthy lifestyle choices also help protect your brain from aging.

- Eat a healthy diet. Get plenty of fruits and vegetables, and cut down on cholesterol, saturated fat, and salt. See page 333.
- Get regular exercise. Exercise can increase blood flow and help grow new brain cells. Pick something you enjoy: Walk the dog, work in the garden, or take dance lessons.

More

- Keep your blood pressure and cholesterol under control. If you have diabetes, keep your blood sugar in a normal range.
- Stay at a healthy weight. See page 326.
- Lower your stress level. See page 356.
- Don't smoke or drink a lot of alcohol.

If you notice sudden changes in mental sharpness, don't ignore them. Talk to your doctor. Sometimes the fix is as simple as changing a medicine you are taking or treating a vitamin deficiency.

Brain-Healthy Foods

Can the foods you eat help keep your brain sharp as you age? That question is the focus of a lot of research. Experts are most interested in foods that are high in omega-3 fats and antioxidants. Antioxidants are thought to help prevent cell damage that leads to cancer and heart disease. So they may also help prevent brain aging.

But you don't have to wait for the research. Foods with high levels of antioxidants and omega-3 fats are part of a healthy diet. They include:

- Vegetables like broccoli, spinach, and kale.
- Fruits like berries, dried plums, and red grapes.
- Oily fish like salmon, tuna, mackerel, and sardines.
- Nuts like almonds, walnuts, and pecans. (Nuts are high in calories, so watch your portion sizes.)

Remember to talk with your doctor before you change your diet if you have a chronic disease or take medicines. And remember that the best diet includes foods from all the food groups. For help planning a healthy diet, see page 333.

Sex and Aging

Sex tends to be a private matter, so you have probably heard less about sexual changes than any other part of aging. Luckily, the news is good. For most healthy adults, pleasure and interest in sex don't decrease with age.

Sex is not just for the young. People can fall into the trap of thinking that as they age, they become less sexual or less desirable. Older adults who accept this notion may cheat themselves of the joy and comfort that sex can bring.

It's true that age may cause some changes that affect your sex life. Knowing what to expect may help you adapt so you can enjoy sex as long as you choose to. It's also normal and healthy to choose not to have sex.

If you notice sexual changes that don't seem to be linked to normal aging, talk to your doctor. Some medicines and health problems can cause sexual problems that can be treated.

For Men

After 50, you may find that:

- Your sex drive has slowed down a bit.
- Your erections are not as firm. But as long as you have good blood flow, you can have erections firm enough for intercourse for your entire life. To learn more about erection problems, see page 138.
- You may be able to delay ejaculation longer than when you were young.

For Women

After menopause, you may find that:

- It can take longer to get sexually excited, and you may be less interested in sex.
- Your skin may be more sensitive and easily irritated, so you may not enjoy skin-to-skin contact as much.
- Intercourse may hurt because the vaginal walls are thinner and drier. This is called atrophic vaginitis (see page 245). A lubricant (Astroglide, Replens) or estrogen cream can help.

Not all older adults have these problems. Those who do can experiment to find ways to enjoy sex in spite of these changes.

Staying Sexual

That old saying about exercise, "use it or lose it," applies to sex too. Having sex on a regular basis is the best way to stay sexual.

To get the most out of sex:

- Remember that the brain is a sex organ. Try fantasy and imagination to increase excitement. Use candlelight and soft music, sexy movies or books, or whatever else helps you get in the mood.
- Take your time. More kissing and touching before sex (foreplay) may increase your response.

More

- Be open to new ideas. Try a new position or a different time of day. Try scented oil for a sensual massage.
- Try a lubricant if sex hurts. Use a water-based lubricant (Astroglide, Replens) or vegetable oil. Do not use petroleum jelly, such as Vaseline.
- Drink alcohol only in moderation. Having 1 or 2 drinks may help you relax and enjoy sex more. But drinking more can work against you.
- Talk to your partner about any concerns you have. Say what you would like, and find out what your partner would like. A good talk can bring you closer.

Doctors can prescribe medicines to increase sexual response. Some people find that herbs like gingko biloba help. Both prescriptions drugs and herbs can have side effects. Talk to your doctor before you try any medicines or herbs to be sure they are safe for you.

Touch and Intimacy

Whether married or single, we all need to feel loved and wanted. Two ways to fill these needs are through touch and intimacy. Both help us feel connected to others.

Even if you are not in a sexual relationship, there are ways to meet your needs for touch and intimacy.

- Get a massage. A professional massage is great, but a simple shoulder rub or neck rub from a friend feels good too.
- Give and get hugs.
- Think about getting a pet. Caring for a pet can meet your need for touch, and a pet can be good company. A dog can help you get more exercise. A cat or bird may be better if you have trouble getting around.
- Keep in touch with family. Spend time with your children, grandchildren, or brothers and sisters.
- Look up old friends. It can be easy to lose touch with people we really like.
- Make room for new friends. Join a support group, or go to a senior center.
- Give some of your time and energy to others. Volunteer for a worthy cause where you can meet like-minded people.

Safe Sex

Safe sex can help you avoid sexually transmitted diseases, also called STDs. STDs can cause a lot of problems in your body. Some of them can even kill you. And the number of people over 50 who have STDs is growing each year.

It's up to you to protect yourself and your sex partner(s) from STDs. The good news is that you can.

To learn about the symptoms of STDs and what to do if you think you have one, see page 222.

Who Gets STDs?

Anyone who has sex can get an STD. It doesn't matter how old you are, whether you're male or female, what race you are, or whether you're gay, straight, or bisexual.

You can get an STD from any kind of sexual contact, not just intercourse. STDs are spread through skin-to-skin contact between the genitals and through contact with body fluids such as semen, vaginal fluids, and blood.

How You Can Stay Safer

Only two things completely get rid of the risk of STDs and HIV infection:

1. Not having sex at all (abstinence). This means not having vaginal, anal, or oral sex.
2. Total monogamy between uninfected partners. This means you and your partner have sex only with each other, and you are absolutely sure that neither of you has a disease.

If you do not choose one of those two options, you can still greatly reduce your risk if you follow the guidelines below.

- Have safe sex every time you have sex. This means:
    - Use condoms until you are sure that neither you nor your partner has an STD or HIV. Talk to your partner before you have sex the first time. Find out if he or she is at risk for STDs. Keep in mind that a person can have HIV or an STD and not know it. Get tested for STDs together and retested 6 months later.
    - Use condoms correctly every time. Use latex condoms from the beginning to the end of sexual contact. "Natural" or lambskin condoms do not protect against HIV or other STDs.
- Agree with your partner that neither of you will have sex with anyone else.
- Do not have sex if you or your partner has symptoms of an STD, such as sores on the genitals or mouth.
- Do not have sex while you or your partner is being treated for an STD.
- If you or your partner has genital herpes, do not have sex when either of you has a blister or an open sore or feels tingling or pain in the genital area. These may be signs of an outbreak. At other times, use latex condoms. You can spread genital herpes even when no sores are present.

Preventing Falls

Every year, thousands of older adults fall and break a bone. In fact, falls are one of the main causes of injury and disability in this age group. Hip fractures are especially serious, and most of them are caused by falling.

A number of things increase your risk of falling. Your vision and hearing probably are not as sharp as they once were, so you may miss cues that would help you avoid objects that could trip you. Some health problems can affect your strength or balance. Medicines like sleeping pills or sedatives can make you dizzy or drowsy and more likely to fall.

Accidents do happen, but there are some easy things you can do to reduce your risk of falling.

Make Your Home Safer

- Remove or fix things that you could trip over, such as raised doorway thresholds, throw rugs, or loose carpet.
- Keep paths clear of electrical cords and clutter.
- Use nonskid floor wax, and wipe up spills right away.
- Keep your house well lit, especially stairways, porches, and outside walkways.
  - Put night-lights in the bedroom, bathroom, and halls.
  - Add extra light switches or use remote switches (such as switches that go on or off when you clap your hands). These make it easier to turn lights on if you have to get up during the night.
- Put sturdy handrails on stairways.
- If you live in an area that gets snow and ice in the winter, sprinkle salt or cat litter on slippery steps and sidewalks.

Many falls happen in the bathroom. To make your bathroom safer:

- Install grab handles inside and outside your shower or tub and near the toilet and sink.
- Use nonskid mats.
- Use a shower chair or bath bench.
- Try a long-handled brush or mittens with straps to help with bathing.

Be Careful

- Wear low-heeled shoes with nonskid soles.
- Do not wear socks without shoes on smooth floors.
- Store things on lower shelves so that you do not have to climb or reach high.
- Always use the handrail when you go up or down stairs.
- Do not try to carry too many things at the same time.
- Use a walker or cane with nonslip rubber tips.

Take Care of Yourself

- Get regular exercise to improve your strength, muscle tone, and balance. Walk if you can. Swimming may be a good choice if you can't walk well.
- Have your vision and hearing checked each year.
- Know the side effects of the medicines you take.
- Stand up slowly after you have been sitting or lying down.
- Limit how much alcohol you drink.

To learn what to do if you fall, see page 34.

Driving: Are You Safe?

Driving a car gives you the freedom to go where you want when you want. And years of experience behind the wheel may have made you a very safe driver. But the fact is, as we get older, our bodies change in ways that can make it harder to drive well.

- Vision gets weaker. You may not have good side vision. Your eyes may be more sensitive to glare from headlights or the sun. It becomes harder to see well at night.
- Reflexes get slower. You may not be able to brake or turn the wheel quickly in an emergency.
- Weak muscles and stiff joints can make it hard to look behind you as you back up.
- Health problems like Parkinson's, diabetes, or Alzheimer's may reduce your skills.

If you have noticed a slight decrease in your driving skills, there are things you can do that may help:

- Take a driver safety course for older drivers. AARP offers one. So do many hospitals and state motor vehicle departments.
- Limit the times and places you drive. For example, you could avoid driving at night or during rush hours. You could stay off freeways and only travel routes you know well.
- Keep your mind and your eyes on the road. If you need to use your cell phone or check a map, pull into a parking lot or onto the shoulder of the road.
- Be as safe as you can. Keep your car windows clean. Leave plenty of room between your car and the car in front of you. Use your headlights day and night. Always wear your seat belt.

At some point, you may decide (or be told) to stop driving. It may be hard to think about giving up the freedom driving gives you. But it's important to be honest about your abilities. Consider these questions:

- Do you feel nervous or scared when driving?
- Have you put a lot of dents in your car?

More

- Have loved ones expressed concern about your driving or refused to ride with you?
- Do you have a lot of close calls where you almost crash?
- Do you have trouble staying in your lane?
- Do other drivers often honk or yell at you?
- Have you gotten tickets or warnings?
- Does your mind wander while you are driving?
- Do you often get lost?

If you answered yes to any of these questions, talk to your doctor. Find out if medicines or a health condition could be causing the problems. You may need to have your driving checked by a professional.

If it has become risky for you to keep driving, try to face the facts. An accident can happen in a split second. Don't wait until you hurt yourself or someone else.

Plan Ahead

If you are still safe to drive, now is the time to start thinking about when you will stop. To plan ahead:

- Check into other ways to get around. Call a local senior center or the Area Agency on Aging to find out about buses or vans in your area. Think about family or friends who might be able to give you rides. Find out how much taxis cost.
- Total up how much driving costs you. It is probably a lot. The money you spend now on gas, car care, licensing, and insurance is money you will have in your pocket when you stop driving. It can help pay for bus fares or taxis, or you can use it for things you enjoy. If you sell your car, you will free up even more money.

Master Your Medicines

Medicines can help you feel better if you have a cold or fever. They may keep you out of the hospital and even save your life if you have a chronic disease. But sometimes medicines can hurt you.

As you age, your body becomes more sensitive to medicines. And older adults are more likely to need several medicines. One medicine may cause side effects that create problems with other medicines. Or one medicine may increase or decrease the effect of another. Even what you eat or drink can make a difference. The more medicines you take, the harder it can be to avoid problems.

You can take an active role in your health by making sure you take your medicines properly and safely. This will also help you get the best results from your medicines.

Work With Your Doctor

Your doctor can help you manage your medicines so you get the most benefit with the least risk. But your doctor can help you only if you keep him or her well informed.

- Make a list of everything you take, and keep a copy in your purse or wallet. At each doctor visit, ask your doctor to review the list.
- Remember to include herbs, vitamins, and nonprescription medicines on your list. They can have powerful effects on the body and cause problems if combined in the wrong way.
- Find out if there are any medicines or other things you should avoid. For example, people who have heart failure or kidney disease should not take ibuprofen (Advil, Motrin) or naproxen (Aleve). Grapefruit juice can cause problems with some medicines.

Call your doctor if:

- You have any side effects or problems with your medicine, or you are thinking of stopping your medicine. Do not stop taking your medicine unless your doctor tells you to.
- You have any changes in your health that might affect the way your medicine works, such as weight gain or loss or another disease.

Have a Routine

Having a daily routine is very important, especially if you take more than one medicine. Some of these tips may help:

- Make a schedule for when you take your medicines, and post it someplace where you will see it often.

More

- Make your schedule as simple as you can. Plan times to take your medicines when you are doing other things, like eating a meal or getting ready for bed.
- Take each of your medicines at the same time each day. This makes it less likely that you will miss a dose.
- Set a kitchen timer to remind you when to take your medicine.
- Try using a weekly medicine organizer. You can buy a plastic pillbox with a space to hold each day's medicine. Be sure to keep at least one pill in each original bottle so you know which one is which.

Tell your doctor if you are having problems with your routine. For example, you might be able to take one longer-acting dose of a medicine instead of two shorter-acting ones.

8 Questions You Should Ask

Anytime your doctor gives you a new prescription, ask these questions and write down the answers:

1. **What is the name of this medicine, and what does it do?**
2. **Why do I need to take it?**
3. **How much do I take, and how do I take it?** For example, do you take 1 pill at a time or 2? Do you take 1 tablespoon or 1 teaspoon?
4. **When should I take it?** If you are supposed to take it twice a day, can you take it at 8 a.m. and 8 p.m.? If you take it once a day, is it best to take it in the morning or at another time?
5. **Are there special things I should know about how to take it?** For example, should you take it with meals or just with a glass of water? Can you chew it, or should you swallow it whole?
6. **What should I do if I miss a dose?**
7. **Are there any problems I should watch for?**
8. **Is this safe with the other medicines I take?**

When you pick up your medicine at the drugstore, read the information sheet that comes with it. This will list the side effects and other important facts.

If there is anything you don't understand, ask the pharmacist to explain it. You have the right to know how your medicine works.

Medicine Safety Tips

- Store medicines in a cool, dry place. Do not store them in the kitchen or bathroom. Only keep your medicine in the refrigerator if your doctor or pharmacist tells you to.
- Check all your medicines at least once a year. Do not use a medicine if it is expired or not labeled or you don't know what it is. Do not use "left-over" prescription medicines.
- Do not throw expired medicine in the trash or the toilet. Ask your pharmacist how to get rid of it.
- Keep all medicines out of the reach of children. Keep medicines in their original child-resistant containers.
- Do not share medicines. It is never a good idea to borrow medicines or share medicines with another person.
- Before filling any new prescription, give the pharmacist your list of medicines. Ask the 8 questions on page 368. Be sure to ask about possible interactions with any other medicines you are taking. If you fill prescriptions at more than one drugstore, make sure each of them has your list.

Watch for Drug Reactions

Medicines can cause bad (adverse) reactions in some people.

- **Side effects** are unpleasant but known reactions to a medicine. They are usually mild (such as an upset stomach), but they can be serious.
- **Drug interactions** can happen when you have to take more than one medicine. And the effect of some medicines can change if you take more than one medicine. Sometimes the symptoms can be severe.
- **Drug allergies** occur when your body overreacts to something in a medicine. Most drug allergies are mild, but a severe drug allergy can be life-threatening and needs emergency care. See page 73.

A bad reaction to a medicine can cause symptoms such as:

- Hives, rash, or blisters.
- Coughing, wheezing, or trouble breathing.
- Stomach cramps, nausea, vomiting, or diarrhea.
- Headaches, dizziness, ringing in the ears, and blurred vision.
- Confusion and sleepiness.

Call your doctor if you think you are having a bad reaction to a medicine. It is important to find out what type of reaction it is.

More

Vitamins, Herbs, and Other Supplements

Dietary supplements include things like vitamins, minerals, herbal products (such as ginkgo biloba or St. John's wort), and products made from natural substances (such as glucosamine). Some people take them to prevent or treat health problems and to improve their overall health. For the most part, experts consider most supplements safe when they are used properly.

It's best to think of vitamins, herbs, and other supplements just as you do medicines. Like medicines, they can both help you and hurt you. Just because a product is natural does not mean it is harmless.

Here are a few things to keep in mind if you are using vitamins, herbs, or other supplements:

- They may have side effects or cause allergic reactions.
- They may react badly with other medicines you take. It's very important that your doctor and pharmacist know all the medicines you are taking, including supplements.
- They do not fall under federal laws and are not made the same way every time. So the products and brands may vary in how well they work and what side effects they cause.
- The long-term effects of many supplements are not known.
- Some supplements may not be safe for people who have certain health problems.

Make sure your doctor knows if you are using a dietary supplement or if you are thinking about using one. Your doctor or pharmacist can tell you whether the supplement is safe for you, based on your health and any other medicines you take. He or she can also help you know how to use the supplement safely.

Growing Older: Myths, Gifts, and Realities

Myths of Aging. 372

Gifts of Aging 374

The Biggest Challenge of Aging: Loss and Life Change 376

A Caregiver's Guide 378

Planning for the Future 382

Dying Well 387

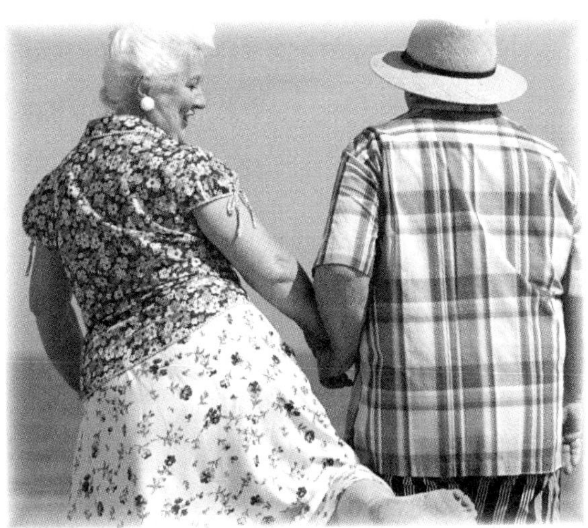

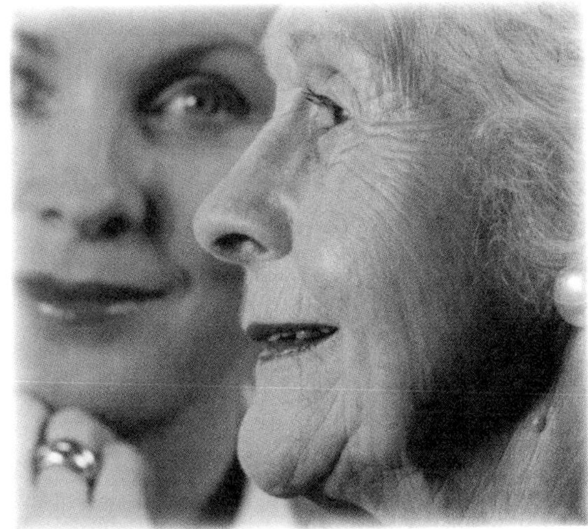

Myths of Aging

"Society teaches us to see each new crease or sag as a personal failure. We don't look in the mirror and say, 'Shucks, I wish I knew less,' so why do we wish we were younger?"
—N. R. Shabahangi

Except when thinking about antiques, fine wines, and a cheese or two, we tend to think that getting older is bad rather than good. There are plenty of myths about aging. Get the facts and avoid being "myth-interpreted."

Myth: Old people have to live in nursing homes.

Fact: Fewer than 1 in 20 older adults live in nursing homes. Most live in their own homes or with family.

Myth: Old people eventually become senile.

Fact: Many people reach very old age as mentally sharp as ever. Senility or dementia is not a normal part of aging. It's caused by health problems like Alzheimer's disease or depression. The same things that keep the rest of your body fit and healthy can keep your brain healthy too: regular exercise, healthy eating, support, and a positive attitude. "Brain fitness" ideas may also help. See page 359.

And it seems that you *can* teach an old dog new tricks. Older adults are quite good at learning new things. See page 374.

Myth: Old people don't have sex.

Fact: Many older people want, and have, an active sex life. Although there may be some changes to adapt to, both men and women can enjoy sex late in life. See page 361.

Myth: You won't live long if your parents didn't.

Fact: Good genes help, but good health habits matter more. A healthy lifestyle and a healthy environment can help you have a longer, more vital life.

Myth: Changing your health habits now won't matter.

Fact: It's never too late. If you quit smoking, your risk of heart disease and stroke will go down almost right away, no matter how long you've smoked. If you have high blood pressure or high blood sugar, eating healthier, being more active, and losing just a little weight can help get them under control.

The truth: Older people are generally healthy. We are living longer lives with less disability. This combination adds life to years as well as years to life. And it gives us the chance to enjoy the gifts of aging.

Anti-Aging Medicines

There is a lot of talk these days about possible "anti-aging" medicines. A whole industry has sprung up around products that claim to stop or slow the normal aging process. They range from vitamins and herbs to magnets and hormones.

Sounds great, doesn't it? Take a pill, potion, or shot, and turn back the clock to a younger you. As usual, when something sounds too good to be true, it probably is. So far, there is no good science to show that these products work. In fact, some (such as growth hormones and herbs like ma huang) may be dangerous.

If you are thinking about "anti-aging" medicines:

- ◆ Be aware that there is no known product that can stop the aging process.
- ◆ Be very careful about anything you put in your body. Older adults often have stronger reactions to drugs than younger people do.
- ◆ Talk to your doctor before you try any product. Even some vitamins can cause bad reactions if you take them with prescription medicines.
- ◆ Beware of claims made by people who benefit from selling these products. Instead, check with trusted public agencies like the U.S. Food and Drug Administration.

There may not be a Fountain of Youth or a pill that will make you young again. So instead of trying to stay young, how about aging as well as you can? Instead of fighting age, fight the diseases that can rob your energy and shorten your life. You can start today:

- ◆ Stay at a healthy weight.
- ◆ Eat a low-fat diet that includes lots of fruits and vegetables, whole grains, and lean protein.
- ◆ Get some exercise most days of the week.
- ◆ Stay active and involved in life, and keep a hopeful outlook.

Gifts of Aging

Benjamin Franklin was past 80 when he helped draft the U.S. Constitution. Gandhi was in his 70s when he launched India's struggle for independence. Grandma Moses started painting at 78 and kept going until she was 101. Georgia O'Keeffe, after becoming blind, learned to do pottery in her 90s.

A productive, creative, and exciting old age is not just for the superstars of art and politics, though. You, too, can make a difference, especially when you embrace the gifts that come with age: wisdom, creativity, and the chance to contribute in new ways.

Wisdom

Wisdom is simply good sense. Most of us grow wiser as we age. We learn from our experiences and come to understand what truly matters. Simply living and surviving for decades can bring us the experience and knowledge that help us make wise decisions.

Don't confuse being mentally quick with being wise. The speed of the brain may slow down with age, but our skill in using a lifetime's worth of information does not. Unless a physical problem occurs, the brain continues to adapt throughout life. The older brain constantly re-creates itself, gaining new insights and wisdom as it goes. Some researchers believe that the young mind is actually at a disadvantage: It tries to make up for a lack of information with speed.

Practice—and share—your wisdom every day. With good decisions and new learning, you can grow wiser all the time.

Creativity and Lifelong Learning

Think of life as happening in three ages:

- **The first age:** Childhood
- **The second age:** Raising a family and working
- **The third age:** Retiring from work and exploring new things

These days, most people are living about 30 years longer than their grandparents did. This 30-year "bonus" means that we may get to enjoy that third age in ways that our grandparents did not.

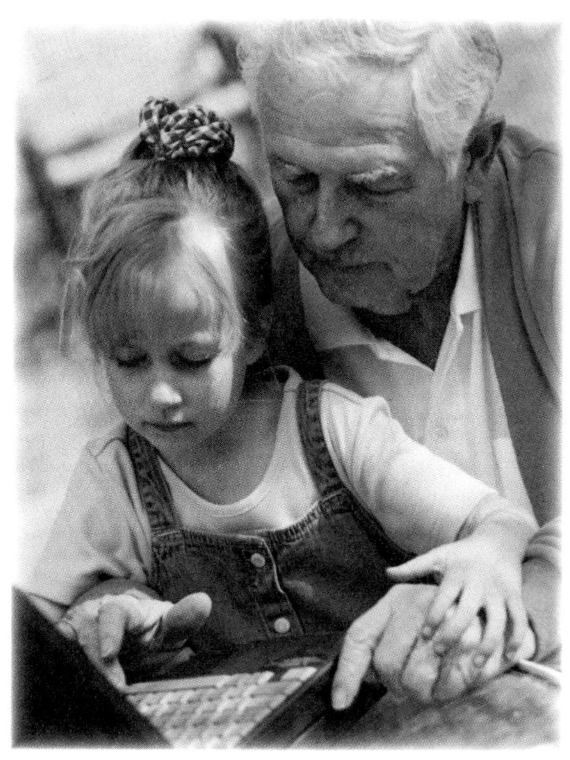

After the daily pressures of raising a family and going to work are over, some people find a source of creativity they never knew they had. The third age gives you a great chance to try things that you didn't have time for in the past. Believe in your own creativity and ability to learn, whether it's in writing a family memoir, exploring new interests through an adult learning center or Elderhostel, reconnecting with something you enjoyed in your youth, or setting off on new adventures.

Being creative is good for you too. Meeting new people, learning new things, and having new experiences helps keep you mentally sharp.

Continuing Contributions

Older adults have a lot to offer—time, talents, and energy. And never let it be said that they are a drain on the economy:

- Older adults pay taxes (just as they've done all their lives).
- Older adults volunteer.
- Older adults give money to charity.
- Older adults help friends and family, including taking care of their spouses and grandchildren.

Older adults have a chance to make their extended years better for themselves and for others. Many retirees spend at least part of their time making a difference in their communities. By using their knowledge, skills, and energy to make that difference, older volunteers see themselves as part of the larger picture. They're part of the solution. What positive difference could you make today in your family, your community, your world? You are needed.

Other contributions lie closer to the heart. Remember what you have to offer your children, your grandchildren (and great-grandchildren!), and other young people. Your listening, your play, your steady presence, your love, and your stories and life history are all much-needed gifts.

Preserving and passing along your values, your hopes, and the lessons you've learned may appeal to you as a way to give the younger generation something beyond money and property. See page 385 to learn more about Ethical Wills.

The Biggest Challenge of Aging: Loss and Life Change

Change is as much a part of our lives as breathing. We change physically—from babies to teens to adults. We change roles—from daughters and sons to mothers and fathers, from workers to retirees. Our relationships change too, as we grow and as our needs change.

Change can hurt. Any big change means a loss of some kind. And the changes seem to come faster as the years go by. More and more, you may have to let go of what used to be and embrace new things. For many people, this is life's toughest challenge.

Change and loss come in many forms: Death. Loss of a job or your home. Loss of loved ones, friends, or pets. Loss of youth, health, or physical abilities. Life is full of losses. Like everyone, you have a natural, healing process that can help you adjust to change and loss. It's called grief.

Grieving

Grief is all the feelings that come with loss. When you have a great loss, like the death of someone you love, the changes are big and the feelings will be strong. Don't try to avoid grief. It catches up with you sooner or later. Trying not to grieve may lead to mental and physical problems.

It may help you to look at some of the ways you have dealt with loss in the past. What helped you cope? Knowing that you have survived loss before can give you hope when you feel overwhelmed by grief.

Grief is also a process of adjusting to the loss. Moving through the process of grief can help you deal with your sorrow in a healthy way.

1. You will need to accept that the loss has happened. At first, you may feel so shocked and numb that you can't believe your loved one is gone. As time passes, the loss will sink in.

2. You will need to experience and accept the pain of the loss. As you start to really believe your loved one is gone, you may feel a lot of pain, both emotional and physical. Emotional pain includes sorrow, anger, guilt, loneliness, and despair. You may have real physical pain too, such as tiredness, loss of appetite, headaches, or sleep problems. This is an especially important time to keep up healthy habits.

3. You will need to adjust to changes in your life. A great loss brings other losses with it. With the loss of a spouse or partner, you lose someone close to talk to, the person who touched you every day, and the person who took on some of the daily tasks like cooking or balancing the checkbook. Each of these changes can be a loss on its own. Just knowing this may help you get through it.

4. You will need to reinvest and move on with your life. We do not get *over* losses. We get *through* them. Life will never be the same as it was before the loss. But a time will come when you will regain your balance and start to reconnect with the world.

Home Treatment

These home treatment guidelines are meant to help with a major loss like the death of a loved one. But they work for other losses too.

- Give yourself time to mourn. Don't feel like you should get back to "normal" too soon after your loss. Feel free to cut back on obligations and duties. Grieving is not easy.
- Be kind to your body. It's important to keep up healthy habits, like exercise and eating right. Be careful not to take up unhealthy habits, such as drinking too much or taking pills to numb your grief.
- Seek out people who will listen, support you, and encourage you. At first, friends may feel awkward around you. Let them know how they can help you as you grieve. Support groups can also help. Hospitals often have groups to help people with their grieving.
- Express yourself. Cry. Let yourself feel sad. Write your thoughts down in a journal, or paint or draw your grief. Many people find comfort in reading books and stories about how others have coped with grief.
- Delay major decisions if you can. Don't rush into selling your things or moving.

Remember that there is no right or wrong way to deal with a loss, but there is a healthy way. Be kind to yourself. With time, things will get better.

When to Call a Doctor

Normal grieving can last for days, weeks, months, or years. Only you know how much time you need. But if you have any of the following problems, you may need help.

Call 911 or the national suicide hotline at 1-800-784-2433 if you feel hopeless and cannot stop thinking about death or suicide.

Call a counselor or doctor if:

- You are hurting yourself, such as drinking too much, taking drugs to dull your pain, not eating well, or spending too much money.
- You feel overwhelmed by strong feelings of anger, guilt, or despair a lot of the time.
- You are spending too much time alone, and you feel isolated from other people.
- You have been grieving longer than you think is good for you, and things seem to be getting worse instead of better.

A Caregiver's Guide

Many people take care of loved ones who are sick or unable to care for themselves. Caregiving can be rewarding. It feels good to know that you are helping someone. But caregiving can also be hard, in both physical and emotional ways. Too often, caregivers end up exhausted and stressed out. This can lead to depression and other serious health problems.

Don't let this happen to you. Your own health and well-being are important. And you won't be able to take care of someone else if you are not well yourself.

To be a good caregiver, let a few key ideas guide you:

- Take care of yourself first.
- Don't be overly helpful.
- Let others help.

And take pride in being a caregiver. Caregiving is not easy, and those who do it are special people.

Take Care of Yourself

Caregivers tend to put the needs of the person who needs help first and forget about taking care of themselves. This may work for a while. But over time, it is sure to lead to problems. Staying well will mean you will have more energy and enthusiasm for giving care.

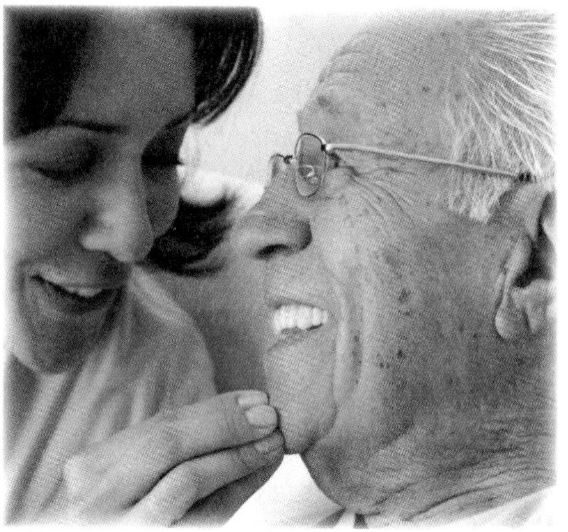

Time may be your most important resource if you are a caregiver. Don't forget to save some time for yourself every day. If you wait until you have done all of your chores, it will never happen. Make the time to do these things—just for you:

- Exercise. It will reduce stress and depression, help you sleep better, and give you more energy. Walking is a great exercise that most people can do. If you can't find time in the day for a 30-minute walk, take three 10-minute ones instead.
- Eat healthy. When you are busy, it may seem easier to eat fast food than to make healthy, low-fat meals. But healthy meals can be easy to fix, and a good diet will give you more energy. See page 333.

Plan Ahead for Caregiving

If you are taking care of someone who is ill:

- Ask the doctor how the illness is being treated, what to expect from treatment, and what will happen if the illness gets worse.
- Find out what medicines the person is taking, what side effects to expect, and if there are medicines the person needs to avoid.
- Talk about what kind of problems might come up and what other health care services might be needed (for example, home nursing, hospital, or nursing home care).
- Work with a case manager or social worker to review the person's financial status.
    - If he or she needs financial help (such as Medicaid) to pay for long-term care, find out how and when to apply.
    - Find out if your state requires you to be a legal guardian before you can manage another person's finances.
- Talk to loved ones about end-of-life issues. This may be hard, but it is the best way to be sure their wishes are met. See Planning for the Future on page 382.

- Do something you enjoy every day—reading, listening to music, painting, or doing crafts—even if you can only do it for a few minutes at a time. Get out for activities you enjoy. Ask someone you trust to stay with your loved one for an hour or two so you can do those things.
- Stay connected to friends and family. Having a strong support system is a key to good health.

Part of taking care of yourself is dealing with your emotions.

- Watch for signs of depression, and get help if you need it. See Are You Depressed? on page 146.
- Manage the stress that comes with caregiving. See page 356. Let go of guilt, and accept the fact that you can't do everything.
- Forgive yourself for mistakes. Give yourself credit for taking on a hard job and doing it as well as you can.

Don't Help Too Much

A common mistake that caregivers make is helping *too* much. One good thing you can give the person you're caring for is as much control of his or her own life as possible. Your attitude makes a big difference. Remember to:

- Expect more. If you expect the person to get dressed, take a bath, or fix simple meals, it may happen.
- Empower. Let the person make as many decisions as possible, such as what to wear, what to eat, or when to go to bed.

More

- Encourage independence. You may be able to do something better or faster, but there are real benefits to letting the person do it alone. Help the person feel good about doing things without your help.
- Modify. One very helpful thing you can do is make changes to the person's home and get the tools that will let him or her do things without help. See Devices That Can Help on this page.

Devices That Can Help

Devices that help a person do daily tasks more easily are called **assistive technology**. If you are a caregiver, finding the right tools to help others will make your job much easier.

Assistive devices can range from very simple (like a cane) to very complex (like a computer). There's a wide range of them, depending on what extra help a person needs.

- People who have problems with walking or balance can use walkers, wheelchairs, or scooters.
- People who have trouble opening or holding things can use jar openers and large-handled silverware and kitchen tools.
- People who have a hard time bending over can use long-handled shoe horns, buttonhooks, and sock pullers.
- Raised toilet seats can help people who have a hard time going from standing to sitting and then getting back up.
- People who have to take lots of medicines can use pill crushers, pill organizers, and automatic pill dispensers that come with alarms.

There are so many products that it may be hard to know which would be best. To get started:

- Talk to the experts. Ask for suggestions from the person's doctors and physical therapists. Ask other people with similar problems what has helped them.
- Learn about your choices. Look online at a site like Technology for Long-Term Care (www.techforltc.org) or ABLEDATA (www.abledata.com). These government-funded sites give information about devices but don't sell them.
- See if you can get help with the cost. Check the person's insurance policy, or find out if Medicare, Medicaid, or the Department of Veterans Affairs will help.
- Before you buy a costly device, ask to have it on a trial basis. A product only helps if the person will use it.

- Simplify. For example, if you are taking care of a person who has mild dementia, divide tasks into easy steps: First, get out the cereal box. Next, get out the milk and the bowl. Label rooms, cupboards, and drawers with pictures and words so the person can find things. For more ideas, see When a Loved One Has Alzheimer's on page 263.

Let Others Help

Some caregivers feel that they are the only person who can take care of their loved one. But if you want to be a good caregiver, you need to learn to ask for help and accept it when someone offers.

Help can come from many places and in many forms. When family or friends offer to lend a hand, be ready with specific ideas. Let them pick something they would like to do. For example, you could ask them to:

- Pick up a few items at the grocery store.
- Fix a meal or do some cleaning or yardwork.
- Stay with the person you care for so you can go out for a while.

You may also be able to find other types of support. You might:

- Hire a teenager or older adult to help for a few hours a day.
- Find a grocery store that delivers.
- Hire a home health aide or personal care assistant.
- Sign up for homemaker or chore services or "Meals on Wheels."

There are also services that can provide care on a short-term basis.

- **Respite care** provides someone who will stay with your loved one while you get out of the house for a few hours. Some respite services are free or ask only for a small donation.
- **Adult day centers** are places where a person who does not need one-on-one supervision can stay and be active during the day. They are usually open during working hours and may not be available on weekends. Day centers provide meals, personal care services, and social activities. Even using this service for a few hours a week can make a big difference.

To learn about the support services in your area:

- Call the National Eldercare Locator at 1-800-677-1116.
- Contact a local senior center or your Area Agency on Aging. Look under "senior citizen services" or "aging" in the phone book.

If you can't care for the person at home, you may have a choice of housing options.

- **Adult foster care or board-and-care homes** are private homes where older adults have 24-hour personal care, supervision, and meals. Some states require board-and-care homes to be licensed.

More

- **Nursing homes** may have different levels of care.
  - Intermediate care includes help with using the toilet, dressing, and personal care for people who do not have serious health problems.
  - Skilled nursing care is usually for people who have just come from the hospital or who need special nursing care.
  - Some nursing homes have special units for people with Alzheimer's disease or other types of dementia.

If the person is in the last stages of a disease and is expected to live less than 6 months, you may want to look into **hospice care**. See page 387 to learn more.

Do You Need Help?

Being a caregiver can be hard on your health and well-being. If any of the statements below are true, look for help.

- I feel overworked and tired most of the time.
- I don't think I'm doing a good job as a caregiver.
- I feel alone, depressed, or angry.
- I'm not getting enough rest.
- I don't have time for anything fun in my life.
- I feel like I don't have time for myself.

Remember: You need to take care of yourself too. Ask for help when—or before—you need it.

Planning for the Future

Change happens. Even if you are doing well now, it's a good idea to prepare for a time when you might not be able to care for yourself on your own. It's also wise to plan for the end of your life.

It can be hard to think and talk about these issues. But planning for the future can help you to:

- Learn your options for care and what it will take to pay for them.
- Save your loved ones the stress of making hard decisions for you.
- Make sure your wishes are respected when the time comes.

Do these things *before* you are in crisis and while you are still able to. Here are some things you can do to help shape the future you want.

- Write an advance directive. See page 383.
- Decide who will make health decisions on your behalf if a time comes when you can't make them yourself. See page 383.

- Look into long-term care insurance. See page 385.
- Get your financial and legal affairs organized. See page 386.
- Think about writing an ethical will. See page 385.
- Know what options people have when they reach the end of life. See page 387.

And don't forget to communicate! Talk with your family, your counselors, and your doctors. Your plans will do no good if no one knows about them.

Advance Directives

The best way to make sure your health care wishes are followed is to put them in writing. A written plan for your health care is called an advance care plan or advance directive. It is used only if you become so sick that you can't make choices for yourself.

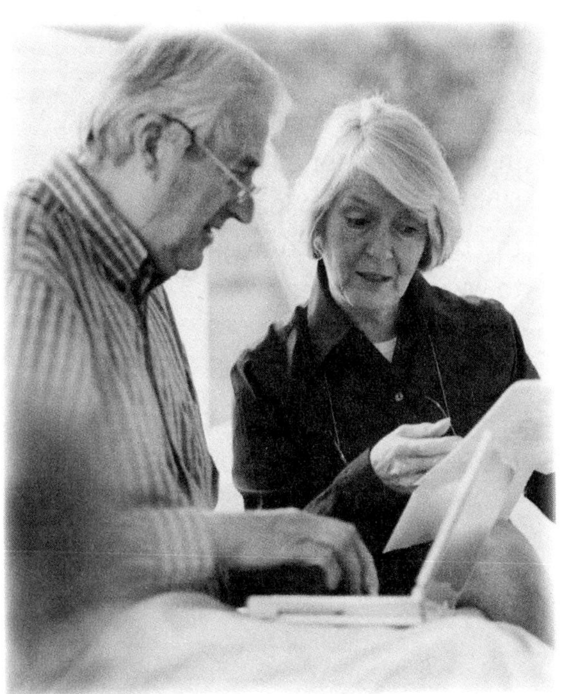

There are two main types of advance directives:

- A **living will** tells what treatment you want at the end of your life. For example, it tells when you would or would not want to be on a breathing machine or be fed through a tube.
- A **durable power of attorney for health care** lets you choose someone now who can make choices for you if a time comes when you can't make them yourself. This person is called your health care agent or health care proxy.

Do not assume that your doctor and family will know what you want if you don't have a written plan. Without one, choices about your care may be made by a doctor who doesn't know you or by the courts. In some states, hospital staff must keep you alive as long as possible if they don't know your wishes. This may or may not be what you want.

How to Write an Advance Directive

1. Get your state's forms for a living will and durable power of attorney. You can usually get them from a hospital, law office, or senior center. You also can find them online at www.caringinfo.org. Or try the *Five Wishes* document. See page 384.
2. Choose someone to be your health care agent, the person you want to speak for you if and when you can't speak for yourself. Choose someone you trust who is willing and able to take on this responsibility.

More

3. Fill out the forms. If you don't understand them, ask a lawyer or family member to help. Get them notarized or witnessed if your state requires it (many states don't).
4. Make sure your doctors, your family, and your health care agent have copies.

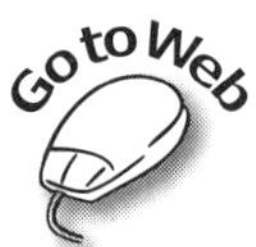

For help writing an advance directive, go to the Web site on the back cover and enter **E379** in the search box.

Deciding About Life Support Treatment

When you create an advance directive, you will need to answer questions like:

- Do you want CPR if your heart stops?
- Do you want to be given liquids or food through a vein (IV) or stomach tube if you can no longer eat or drink?
- Do you want to have a tube in your windpipe and use a breathing machine (ventilator) if you cannot breathe on your own?
- Do you want kidney dialysis if your kidneys stop working?

Think about what you would want, depending on things like how sick or hurt you were, how good your chances for recovery were, and what your life would be like if you chose treatment to keep you alive.

Five Wishes

Five Wishes is a document that helps you explain how you want to be treated if you are seriously ill and cannot speak for yourself. It is different from a typical living will because it lets you put in writing all of your needs: medical, personal, emotional, and spiritual.

Five Wishes lets your family and doctors know:

1. Which person you want to make health care decisions for you when you can't make them yourself.
2. The kind of medical treatment you want or don't want.
3. How comfortable you want to be.
4. How you want people to treat you.
5. What you want your loved ones to know.

Five Wishes also encourages you to talk about your wishes with your family and your doctors.

Five Wishes is a legal document in many, but not all, states in the United States. To learn more about the document and to get a copy, go to www.fivewishes.org.

If you have an illness that can't be cured, a time may come when you decide not to have treatment that might keep you alive. This can be a hard decision. But if you are very ill, it may be the right choice for you and your family. Sometimes, using treatment to keep a dying person alive can cause unnecessary suffering.

These are often tough choices. For help thinking through them, go to the Web site on the back cover and enter **V353** in the search box.

Long-Term Care Insurance

An important part of planning ahead is looking into long-term care insurance. In most cases, private medical insurance, Medicare, and even "Medigap" insurance will pay for only a few months of care in a hospital or nursing home. And they do not cover help with daily tasks like eating, dressing, and bathing.

Long-term care insurance pays for long-term help with daily tasks if you are not able to do them. This type of insurance is a good idea if there is a chance that you could need this type of care. Many people do, if they live into old age or have a chronic disease.

You may want to buy long-term care insurance if:

- You want to protect your assets. Long-term support and services can cost a lot and could quickly use up your savings.
- You don't want to depend on family members to care for you if you become frail or disabled.
- You want to choose where and how you receive long-term care. For example, if the insurance pays for health and personal services in your home, it could mean that you can live in your own home rather than move to a nursing home.

More

Ethical Wills: Sharing Your Values

A legal will distributes your money and your things after you die. It answers the question: "What do I want my heirs to have?" An ethical will answers the question: "What do I want my heirs to know?" It is a heartfelt way to share your values, your beliefs, and your hopes with those you love.

Your ethical will can be as simple as a personal letter or a series of notes to different people. It can be as short as one page or as long as a book. Some people may choose to record their ethical will on audio- or videotape.

Think of an ethical will as a gift to future generations. For help getting started, go to www.ethicalwill.com.

The cost of long-term care insurance can vary greatly. It depends on:

- Your age when you buy the policy. The younger you are, the lower your cost will be. On the other hand, if you buy the policy too early, you may pay for the insurance for many years before you need it.
- Your health and your medical history. It is very important to buy a policy while you are in good health. Some health problems can prevent you from getting coverage.
- What benefits you choose. You will need to decide several things, such as how long the coverage will last (a few years or your lifetime), how much the policy will pay each day, and how many days you will pay for your own care before the insurance starts paying.

When shopping for long-term care insurance, look for a policy that:

- Pays benefits without requiring a hospital stay.
- Does not raise the cost based on your age or health status.
- Pays benefits for in-home care.
- Can be renewed for your lifetime.
- Covers all levels of long-term care.
- Will cover Alzheimer's disease and any other illness that causes dementia.
- Adjusts your benefits for inflation.

Also, check the financial rating and reputation of the insurance companies. You want to choose a company that will be there and provide good service when you need it.

This is a lot to think about and decide. Talk with a trusted financial advisor or a close family member.

To learn more about your options, go to the National Clearinghouse for Long-Term Care Information at www.longtermcare.gov. Or go to the Medicare Web site at www.medicare.gov.

Estate Planning

Along with planning for future health decisions, it's a good idea to get your business and personal affairs in order.

- Write or update your will. If you don't have a will, your state's laws may decide what happens to your money and property (your "estate") when you die. Consider naming a person to oversee your estate after your death. This person is called an executor.
- Appoint someone to make financial decisions for you in case a time comes when you can't make them for yourself.
- If you are responsible for the care of your grandchildren or any other minors, choose someone to take care of them if you are gone. This person is called a guardian.

- Make sure your will and other records (life insurance policies, pension and retirement account records, real estate deeds, stocks) are in a safe place. Close family members, the executor of your estate, and your lawyer should know how to access these records in case something happens to you.

A lawyer can advise you on how best to organize your estate so your family can handle your affairs after your death. A financial planner or social worker can also help. These resources may be available in your community or through a local hospital or hospice program.

Dying Well

It's time to change the way we die.

- Most people say that they would like to die at home. But most will end up dying in a hospital or nursing home.
- Most people say that they would like to die without pain. But most have to suffer from undertreated pain during their final days.
- Most people say that they would like to end life with their family around them celebrating their lives. But far too many people are swept up in a series of aggressive medical treatments that take control out of their hands and turn their final days into a contest against death rather than an acceptance of it.

Aggressive medical treatment may keep you alive longer. But it often does so at the cost of the quality of your remaining time. When we look at dying as a medical failure rather than as a natural part of life, we make it harder to die a "good death."

How do you want to spend your final days? What are your options? These are two very important questions to talk about with your family and your doctors. One important option to think about is hospice care. You may also want to read about palliative care, sometimes called "compassionate care," on page 260.

Hospice Care

Hospice care provides medical care, emotional help, and spiritual support as you near the end of your life. It can also help your family and friends care for you and deal with their grief.

You can get hospice care when your doctor says that you have a limited time left to live. Medicare pays for hospice care when a person has 6 months or less to live if the disease runs its natural course. (If you live longer than 6 months, you can continue on hospice. If your illness gets better, you can stop receiving hospice care.)

More

You may want to choose hospice care if:

- You have decided to stop treatments that might lengthen your life.
- You want to choose where to spend the time you have left (such as in your home).
- You want family and friends to be involved in your care.

The goals of hospice are to keep you comfortable and help you get the most out of life in the time you have left.

- Hospice focuses on relieving pain and other symptoms. It does not try to cure your illness.
- It does not speed up or lengthen dying.
- Hospice includes counseling and support for you and others you care about; respite care, which gives some time off to those who take care of you; and help with things like meals and errands.
- Hospice programs can help 24 hours a day, 7 days a week, in your own home or in a hospice center. Many hospitals and nursing homes also offer hospice care.

Don't wait for your doctor or family to bring up your end-of-life care. Sometimes it's hard for a doctor to admit that a patient is nearing death. And it can be hard for your family to accept. For help working through your decisions

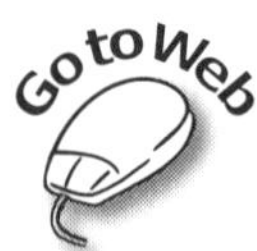

about end-of-life care, go to the Web site on the back cover and enter **D479** in the search box.

A Good Death

Everyone dies. But what is a good death? Think about what that means to you. It may mean that you want:

- To stay in control of what happens to you and know that your wishes will be followed.
- To have your pain controlled.
- To be able to choose where, and how, you die.
- To have the people you want around you when you die.
- To die with dignity.

For many, a good death is one that embraces dignity, respect, and compassion. Speak up and get the end-of-life care—and the death—that you want.

Index

A

A1c blood test 299
Abdominal aortic aneurysm, screening for 323
Abdominal injury 66
Abdominal pain 66
  after injury 66
  burning beneath breastbone 176
  diverticulitis and 129
  frequent, with bloating and gas 121, 161, 190
  gallstones and 159
  hard, swollen belly 67
  lower belly/pelvic area (men) 217
  lower belly/pelvic area (women) 245
  lower left belly 129
  lower right belly 67
  upper right belly 156, 160, 223
  with fever 67, 129
Abdominal problems, see Digestive problems
Abrasions (scrapes) 44
Abscess, see Boils 98
Abstinence, sexual 363
Abuse and violence 68
  elder abuse 69
Accidents, see Injuries
Achilles tendon
  location (illus.) 179
  tendinosis 108, 179
  torn or ruptured 50
Acid blockers and reducers 177, 244
Acid reflux 176
  sore throat and 235
Acne, adult, see Rosacea 221
Acquired immunodeficiency syndrome (AIDS) 222, 224
Actinic keratoses 232
Acupuncture, for back pain 83
Addiction, alcohol or drug 70
Advance directives 383
Aerobic exercise 343
Age spots 231
Aging
  anti-aging medicines 373
  brain fitness 359
  driving safety 365
  end-of-life care 387
  exercise and 340
  fall prevention 364
  hearing loss 171
  long-term care insurance 385
  Medicare 9
  memory loss 123
  myths about aging 372
  planning for the future 382
  positive aspects of aging 374
  sex and 361
  sleep problems 233
  vision changes 248
AIDS (acquired immunodeficiency syndrome) 222, 224
Alcohol
  alcohol problems or abuse 70
  erection problems and 139
  high blood pressure and 185
  osteoporosis and 207
  screening test for alcohol problems 71
  ulcers and 243
Allergic reaction, severe 73, 74
  to food 73
  to insect bites or stings 13, 73
  to medicines 73, 369
Allergies 73
  allergic reaction, severe 73, 74
  allergic rhinitis 73
  allergy shots (immunotherapy) for 75
  drug or medicine reactions 74, 369
  epinephrine kit (EpiPen) 13, 74
  food allergies 73
  hay fever 73
  insect stings 13
  skin tests for 75
Alopecia (hair loss) 165
Alzheimer's disease 261
  caregiving tips 263
  living with 261
  medicines for 262
  nursing home decisions 264
  see also Confusion and memory loss 122
  signs of sudden worsening 265
  warning signs 123
Amsler grid (illus.) 250
Anal problems
  see Rectal problems 180
  warts, see Genital warts 223
Anaphylaxis 13, 73, 74
Anemia 147
Anger 76
  see also Abuse and violence 68
Angina 115, 288
Angiomas, cherry 231
Angioplasty 288
Animal bites 12
Animal dander, allergies to 75
Ankle sprain 49
Antacids 177
  ulcers and 244
Anti-inflammatories, see Nonsteroidal anti-inflammatory drugs (NSAIDs)

Antibiotics
  diarrhea and 127
  for ear infections 136
  for sinusitis 228
  for urinary tract infections 92
  hearing problems and 171, 173
  nausea and vomiting and 253
Antidepressants 293, 295
Antidiarrheals 128
Antifungals 157
Antihistamines
  for allergy symptoms 73
  for itching 14, 220
Anxiety 77
Aortic aneurysm (abdominal), screening for 323
Appendicitis 67
Arrhythmia 174
Arteries, blocked, see Atherosclerosis
Arthritis 266
  back pain and 81
  dietary supplements for 268
  exercise and 268
  gout 163
  hip pain and 108
  ice and cold packs for 51
  jaw pain and 192
  joint replacement surgery for 267
  medicines for 266
  neck pain and 204
  pain management and 266
  using a cane (illus.) 270
  using a walker (illus.) 269
  weight as risk factor 326
Aspirin
  bruising and 22
  during heart attack 38
  for preventing heart attack and stroke 185, 290, 297
  hearing problems and 171, 173
  heartburn and 177
  nosebleeds and 43
  see also Nonsteroidal anti-inflammatory drugs (NSAIDs)
  ulcers and 243
Assistive devices 380
Asthma 271
  action plan for 272
  asthma attacks 272, 273, 274, 275
  avoiding triggers 274
  inhaler 274
  medicines for 273
  peak flow measurement 272, 273
Atherosclerosis 186, 208, 287
  angioplasty 288
  arteries, blocked (illus.) 287
  see also Coronary artery disease 287
Athlete's foot 158
Atrial fibrillation 175
Atrophic vaginitis 245, 361
Aura, before migraine headache 167

B

Back injuries 79
Back pain 79
  acupuncture for 83
  chiropractic treatment for 83
  exercises that make pain worse 89
  first aid for 82
  herniated disc and 80
  massage therapy for 83
  osteoporosis and 207
  pelvic tilt exercises (illus.) 82
  physical therapy for 83
  prevention 84, 86
  sciatica and 80
  spinal injury 79
  spinal stenosis and 83
  surgery for 90
  tension headaches and 167
  with fever and chills (males) 215
  with leg pain or weakness 80
  with painful urination 90
Back surgery 90
Bacterial vaginosis 246
Bad breath 164
Balance problems 130
  exercises to improve 351
  Parkinson's disease and 242
  stroke and 54
Baldness 165
Bald spots 165
Barium enema 122
Bedsores 213
Bee stings 13
Belly button
  hernia, umbilical 182
Belly pain, see Abdominal pain
Benign positional vertigo 131
Benign prostatic hyperplasia (BPH) 215, 216
Birth control, menopause and 203
Bites, animal or human 12
Bites, insect, spider, or tick 13
Black eye 22
Bladder
  control problems 92
    sudden 79
  infections 90
Bleeding
  blood thinners and 96, 175
  cuts 27
  emergencies 17
  from ears or nose after head injury 36
  gums 164
  how to stop (illus.) 17
  nosebleeds 43
  rectal 17, 66, 121, 124, 243
  see also Blood

- shock and 47
- vaginal 17, 149
  - after menopause 149
  - during or after sex 223

Blepharitis 144

Blisters 95
- burns and 23
- frostbite and 35
- how to drain (illus.) 96
- on genitals 223
- on lips or mouth 118
- painful band of (shingles) 225
- sunburn and 56

Bloating 161, 190
- after meals 244
- with frequent belly pain 121

Blood
- draining from ear 135
- in eye 143
- in sputum 96, 102, 200, 210
- in stools 17, 127, 129, 180, 190, 243
- in urine 65, 90, 193
  - in males only 215
- in vomit 17, 66, 253
- see also Bleeding
- under a nail 18

Blood clot
- in brain (stroke) 54
- in leg 96
- in lung (pulmonary embolism) 97

Blood flow problems
- atherosclerosis 186, 208, 287
- cold hands or feet 117
- foot care and 209
- high blood pressure 183
- high cholesterol 186
- intermittent claudication 209
- peripheral artery disease 208
- Raynaud's 117

Blood pressure
- high blood pressure 183
- low blood pressure and lightheadedness 131
- monitoring at home 185

Blood spots under skin 218

Blood sugar
- A1c test 299
- diabetes and 296
- monitoring 298
- too high or too low 302

Blood thinners 96, 175, 318
- bruises and 22
- nosebleeds and 43

BMI (body mass index) 330, 331

Body mechanics
- back pain and 84
- examples of (illus.) 84, 85

Boils 98

Bone density test (DEXA scan) 207

Bones, broken 49

Bone thinning (osteoporosis) 207

Botulism 155

Bowel movements
- bloody or black 121, 124, 127, 180, 190
- constipation 124
- diarrhea 127
- incomplete or irregular 121, 124, 190
- irritable bowel syndrome and 190
- leakage 124, 180
- loose and watery 127
- loss of control 79
- mucus in 190
- painful or hard to pass 124
- unexplained changes in 121

BPH (benign prostatic hyperplasia) 215, 216

Brain fitness 359

Breast cancer 100
- mammograms 100, 324

Breast exams 100, 324, 325

Breast problems 99

Breathing emergencies 19
- allergic reaction, severe 73, 74
- choking 26
- CPR 19

Breathing problems 101
- after insect sting 13
- anxiety and 77
- asthma 271
- chest and lung problems (chart) 59
- COPD (chronic obstructive pulmonary disease) 282
- emergencies 19, 26
- fast, labored, or shallow breathing 19, 47, 102
- not breathing 19
- shortness of breath 38, 96, 101, 115, 200
- sleep apnea 233
- snoring 234
- wheezing 73, 101, 200, 271
- with blurred vision 155

Broken bones 49

Bronchitis 102
- chronic 102
  - see also COPD (chronic obstructive pulmonary disease) 282

Bruises 22
- see also Pressure sores 213

Bunions 103

Bupropion (Zyban), for quitting smoking 352

Burns 23
- chemical 25
- severity (illus.) 23, 24
- sunburn 56

Bursitis 105

C

Caffeine, headaches and 168

Calamine lotion, for rashes 220

Calcium, osteoporosis and 208

Calluses 109

Cancer 276
breast 100, 324
cervical 149, 323
chemotherapy for 276
colorectal 121, 181
end-of-life care 281
endometrial (uterine) 149, 202
follow-up care 280
hair loss 279
living with 276
lung 200
ovarian 149
pain management for 278
prostate 214
radiation therapy for 276
screening tests for cancer 322, 323
side effects of treatment 278
skin 230
treatment options 276, 281
uterine (endometrial) 149, 202
weight as risk factor 326
Candidiasis (yeast infection) 245
Cane, how to use (illus.) 270
Canker sores 109
Carbon monoxide poisoning 64, 166
Cardiac rehabilitation 291, 306
Cardio exercise 343
Cardiopulmonary resuscitation (CPR) 19
Caregiving 378
depression and 379
elder abuse 69
support for 381
Carpal tunnel syndrome 110
areas of pain or numbness (illus.) 111
surgery for 112
wrist position when typing (illus.) 111
Cataracts 113
surgery for 113
Cat bites or scratches 12
Cellulitis 220
Cervical cancer 149
HPV (human papillomavirus) and 223
Pap test for 323
Chafing 219
Chantix (varenicline), for quitting smoking 352
Checkups (wellness exams) 321
Chemical burns 25
Chemotherapy for cancer 276
Cherry angiomas 231
Chest, heart, and lung problems (chart) 59
Chest-wall pain 102, 116, 210
Chest pain 114
angina 115, 288
burning beneath breastbone 176, 244
chest-wall pain 102, 116, 210
costochondritis 116
heart attack 38, 114
areas of discomfort (illus.) 38, 115
spreading to back, shoulders, neck, jaw, arms 38, 115
with productive cough and fever 102, 210
with shortness of breath, coughing up blood 96
with sweating, shortness of breath, nausea, dizziness 38, 115
Chickenpox, shingles and 225
Child abuse or neglect 68
Chiropractic treatment, for back pain 83
Chlamydia 223
Choking 26
Heimlich maneuver (illus.) 26
Cholera, shots to prevent 321
Cholesterol
high cholesterol 186
in food 186, 335
tests 187
Chondroitin 268
Chronic fatigue syndrome 147
Chronic kidney disease 308
blood pressure and 310
diabetes and 310
dialysis 313
diet for 311
emergencies 314
glomerular filtration rate (GFR) 311
kidney transplant 313
limiting fluids 310
medicines for 309
medicines that can be harmful 309
signs of worsening 314
Chronic obstructive pulmonary disease, see COPD
Cialis 139
Circulation problems, see Blood flow problems
Claudication, intermittent 209
Clots, blood 96
Cluster headaches 168
Cold, intolerance of 238
Cold hands and feet 117
Cold packs, how to make and use 51
Colds 119
sinusitis and 227
Cold sores 118
Cold temperature exposure
frostbite 35
hypothermia 41
Colonoscopy 121
Colon polyps 121
Colorado tick fever, see Tick bites 14
Colorectal cancer 121, 181
screening tests for 121
Colposcopy 324
Compassionate care, see Palliative care 260
Concussion, see Head injury 36
Condoms, safe sex and 363
Confusion 122
after head injury 36

Alzheimer's disease and 123
heat stroke and 39
hypothermia and 41
medicines as a cause of 124
memory loss and 122
shock and 47
Congestive heart failure, see Heart failure
Conjunctivitis (pinkeye) 140
Consciousness, loss of 33
Constipation 124
hemorrhoids and 180
irritable bowel syndrome and 190
with abdominal pain and fever 67
Contact lens care 142
Contusions (bruises) 22
Convulsions (seizures) 45
Cooking, low-fat 334
COPD (chronic obstructive pulmonary disease) 282
avoiding triggers 283
breathing techniques (illus.) 284
bronchitis and 102
emergencies 286
flare-ups (exacerbations) 283
medicines for 282
oxygen therapy 286
pulmonary rehabilitation 285
signs of worsening 283, 286
Corneal scratch (abrasion) 31
Corns 109
Coronary artery disease 287
angina 115, 288
angioplasty 288
arteries, blocked (illus.) 287
cardiac rehabilitation and 291
emergencies 291
exercise and 290
heart-healthy diet for 289
smoking and 290
weight as risk factor 326
Cost-saving tips
emergency rooms 6
medical tests 7
medicines 3
surgery 9
Costochondritis 116
Cough 126
bronchitis and 102
chronic cough 126, 200
COPD and 282, 286
dry cough 126
during or after exercise 101
productive cough 126, 210
smoker's cough 126
with blood pressure medicine 126
with bloody sputum 200
with chest pain 96, 102, 210
with foamy, pink mucus 307
Coumadin (warfarin), see Blood thinners
Counseling, for depression 292
CPR (cardiopulmonary resuscitation) 19
Cramps
abdominal 66
muscle 197
Cuts 27
see also Scrapes 44
stitches for 29
Cyst, ovarian 67
Cystitis (bladder infection) 90

D

Dairy (lactose) intolerance 128
DASH diet 289
Deafness, see Hearing loss 171
Death 387
grief 376
thoughts of 55
Decongestants
for allergy symptoms 73
for colds 120
for sinusitis 228
Decubitus ulcers, see Pressure sores 213
Deep vein thrombosis (DVT) 96
DEET 16
Dehydration 29
lightheadedness and 131
muscle cramps and 197
prevention 31, 339
rehydration drinks for 30
Delirium, see Confusion and memory loss 122
Dementia, see Alzheimer's disease 261
warning signs of 123
Dental care 354
Dental problems
chipped tooth 241
dry mouth 133
gingivitis 164
gums, bleeding or swollen 164
jaw pain 192
see also Mouth problems
toothache 240
tooth loss, accidental 241
Denture care 355
Dependence, alcohol or drug 70
Depression 146, 292
antidepressant medicines 293, 295
caregiving and 379
counseling 292, 295
fatigue and 146
grief 376
preventing relapse 295
seasonal affective disorder 294
St. John's wort for 293
suicide warning signs 55
symptoms of 146
thyroid problems and 238
Dermatitis, see Rashes 218
seborrheic 219

Detox, alcohol or drugs 71, 72
DEXA scan 207
Diabetes 296
  blood sugar monitoring 298
  carbohydrate and sugar 300
  emergencies 302
  exercise and 301
  eye disease (retinopathy) and 251
  foot care 209
  insulin for 296
  meal planning 300
  medicines for 296
  routine tests (chart) 299
  weight as risk factor 326
Diabetic retinopathy 251
Dialysis, kidney 313
Diarrhea 127
  bloody 127, 155
  dehydration and 30
  irritable bowel syndrome and 190
  lactose intolerance and 128
  medicines for 128
  rehydration drinks for 30, 128
Diet
  cholesterol levels and 187
  DASH (Dietary Approaches to Stop Hypertension) 289
  diabetes and 300
  food guide pyramid (MyPyramid) 338
  heart-healthy diet 289
  low-sodium 304
  portion control 327
  see also Healthy eating 333
  weight management and 326
Dietary supplements 337, 370
Dieting 329
Digestive problems
  abdominal pain 66
  constipation 124
  diarrhea 127
  digestive problems (chart) 60
  diverticular disease 129
  food poisoning 155
  gallstones 159
  gas 161
  heartburn 176
  irritable bowel syndrome 190
  stomachache (abdominal pain) 66
  ulcers 243
  vomiting 253
Digital rectal exam 215
Disc, herniated 80
  anatomy of (illus.) 80
  surgery for 90
Diverticular disease 129
Dizziness 130
  see also Fainting and unconsciousness 33
Dog bites 12
Domestic violence 68
Drinking (alcohol) 70
Driving safety 365
  after a stroke 316
Drowning, first aid for 19
Drug problems 70
  risk of HIV with needle sharing 224
  screening test for 71
Drugs, see Medicines
Dry eyes 143
Dry mouth 133
Dry skin 134
Dry vagina 246, 361
Durable power of attorney for health care 383
Dust, allergies and 74
DVT (deep vein thrombosis) 96
Dying 387

E

E. coli, see Food poisoning 155
Ear anatomy (illus.) 135
Ear infections 135
Ear problems
  dizziness 130
  drainage 135
  earache 135
  ear and hearing problems (chart) 63
  eardrum rupture 136
  earwax 137
  feeling of fullness in ear 135, 137
  hearing loss 171
  infection 135
  labyrinthitis 131
  Ménière's disease 132
  otitis media (middle ear infection) 135
  ringing or noise in ear (tinnitus) 173
  swimmer's ear 136
  vertigo 130
Earwax 137
Edema, see Swelling
Ejaculation, painful 217
Elbow pain (illus.) 107
Elder abuse 69
Emergencies
  bleeding 17
  blood sugar, too high or too low 302
  blunt abdominal injury 66
  breathing emergencies 19
  burns 23
  chemical burns 25
  chest pain 38, 114
  choking 26
  dehydration 29
  frostbite 35
  head injury 36
  heart attack 38, 114
  heat stroke 39
  hypothermia 41

seizures 45
shock 47
spinal injury 79
stroke 54
suicide 55
unconscious 33
when to use the emergency room 6
Emphysema, see COPD (chronic obstructive pulmonary disease) 282
Encephalitis 151
West Nile virus 16
End-of-life care 387
advance directives 383
End-stage renal disease, see Chronic kidney disease
Endometrial (uterine) cancer 149
Endometriosis 149
Epilepsy, seizures and 45
Epinephrine kit (EpiPen), for allergic reactions 13
Erection problems 138, 361
medicines for 139
Ergonomics
back pain and 84
examples of (illus.) 84, 85
neck pain and 205
wrist position when typing (illus.) 111
Estate planning 386
Estrogen therapy
HRT (hormone replacement therapy) 202
osteoporosis and 208
Ethical wills 385
Exercise 340
aerobic/cardio 343
arthritis and 268
back pain prevention 86
balance exercises 351
benefits of 341
cholesterol levels and 187
dehydration and 31
diabetes and 301
getting started 341, 342
heart disease and 290
heart failure and 305
heat sickness and 39
high blood pressure and 184
muscle cramps during 197
muscle strengthening 343
basic exercises (illus.) 345–349
osteoporosis and 207
safety 341, 342
stretching 349
basic exercises (illus.) 345–350
walking 344
weight management and 327
Exploitation, financial 69
Eye anatomy (illus.) 162
Eyedrops, how to insert (illus.) 142
Eyelid problems 144
see also Eye problems 140
Eye problems
black eye 22
blood in eye 143
burning and soreness 221
cataracts 113
change in size of pupils 140
chemical in eye 25
conjunctivitis (pinkeye) 140
contact lens problem 142
corneal scratch (abrasion) 32
diabetic retinopathy 299
discharge from 140, 142
dry eyes 143
eye and vision problems (chart) 62
eyedrops, how to insert (illus.) 142
glaucoma 162
infection or inflammation 140, 142
itchy, watery eyes 73, 140
object in eye 31
how to remove (illus.) 32
pain, sudden and severe 62, 162
pain in eye 143
pinkeye 140
red and irritated 140, 143
see also Eyelid problems 144
see also Vision problems
tearing, excessive 144

F

Facial pain
on one side 169
shingles and 226
with fever 227
Fainting 33, 47, 130
Falls 34
preventing 364
Fatigue 145
anemia and 147
depression and 146
irritable bowel syndrome and 190
see also Sleep problems 232
severe and frequent 147, 152
thyroid problems and 146, 238
Fats in foods 334
Fears (phobias) 77
Fecal incontinence 79, 124
Fecal occult blood test (FOBT) 122
Female health, see Women's health
Female pelvic organs (illus.) 323
Female pelvic problems 148
Fever 150
after immunizations 321
after mosquito bites 16
after tick bite 14
dehydration and 30
heat stroke and 39
with abdominal pain 67

with facial pain 227
with groin pain 182
with joint pain 270
with low back or pelvic pain (males) 215, 217
with pain in side or back 90, 193
with sore throat 235
with stiff neck, headache, vomiting 150, 151
with swelling or pain in leg or calf 197
with urinary symptoms 90
males only 217
Fever blisters (cold sores) 118
Fiber 336
constipation and 125
Fibroids, uterine 149
Fibromyalgia 152
Financial affairs and wills 386
Financial exploitation 69
Finger, see Wrist or hand problems
Fingernail, see Nail problems
Fissure, anal 181
Fitness, see Exercise 340
Flashbacks 77
Flatulence (gas) 161
Flexibility, stretching and 349
Flexible sigmoidoscopy 121
Flu (influenza) 153
antiviral medicine for 153
flu shots 154, 320
Food allergies 73
lactose intolerance 128
Food guide pyramid (MyPyramid) 338
Food poisoning 155
hepatitis A 156
Food safety 155
Foot care 209
Foot exam for diabetics 299
Foot problems
ankle sprain 49
athlete's foot 158
blisters 95
calluses and corns 109
cold feet 117
diabetes and 297
heel pain 178
ingrown toenail 189
numbness or coldness 208
plantar fasciitis 178
see also Toe problems
warts 254
Forgetfulness 122
Fractures, see Broken bones 49
Frostbite 35
see also Cold hands and feet 117
Fumes, chemical 25
Fungal infections 157
yeast infections, vaginal 245

G

Gallstones 159
surgery for (cholecystectomy) 160
Gas 161
with bloating and belly pain 161, 190
Gastroenteritis (stomach flu)
diarrhea and 127
see also Food poisoning 155
Gastroesophageal reflux disease (GERD) 177
Generic medicines 3
Genital herpes 223
Genitals
itching 223
sores 223
vaginitis 245
warts 223
GERD (gastroesophageal reflux disease) 177
Gingivitis 164
Ginkgo biloba, for memory loss 124
Glands, swollen 236
Glaucoma 162
optic nerve (illus.) 162
screening for 163
Glomerular filtration rate (GFR) 311
Glucosamine 268
Golfer's elbow 107
Gonorrhea 223
Gout 163
Grief 376
Groin
bulge or lump in 182
sudden, severe pain 182, 193
Gum disease 164
Gynecological exam 323
Gynecological problems 148, 245

H

Hair and scalp problems
alopecia 165
bald spots 165
hair loss 157, 165, 279
chemotherapy and 279
ringworm 158
thinning hair 165
Hammer toes 103
Hand-washing
colds and 120
flu and 154
food poisoning and 156
hepatitis A and 156
Hand problems, see Wrist or hand problems
Hay fever 73
HDL cholesterol 186
Head, shaking (tremor) 241
Headaches 166
after taking new medicine 64
caffeine and 168
cluster 168

during or after exercise, sex, coughing, or sneezing 166
emergency symptoms 166
encephalitis and 151
meningitis and 151
migraines 167
possible causes (chart) 64
sudden and severe 54, 64, 166
tension headaches 167
tracking your headaches 167
with facial pain 227
with fever, stiff neck, vomiting 151
with jaw pain 192
with runny nostril or red eye 168
with severe eye pain 64
with vertigo 131
with vision loss 64, 169
with weakness, numbness, vision loss, or speech problems 54, 166
Head injuries 36
prevention 37
Healthy eating 333
Hearing aids 172
Hearing problems 170
checking for 170
ear and hearing problems (chart) 63
hearing specialists 173
loss of hearing 171
Ménière's disease and 132
noise and 170, 171
prevention 170
ringing in ears (tinnitus) 173
with vertigo 130
Heart attack 38, 114
areas of discomfort (illus.) 38, 115
aspirin and 38, 290
high blood pressure and 184
prevention 287
smoking and 290
warning signs 38, 115
Heartbeat, see also Pulse rate
anxiety and 77
atrial fibrillation and 175
changes in 174
fast, with chest pain 38, 115
fast or irregular 29, 174
heart failure and 307
skipping 174
Heartburn 176
acid reflux (illus.) 176
antacids 177
gastroesophageal reflux disease (GERD) 177
hiatal hernia and 182
Heart disease, see Coronary artery disease 287
high cholesterol and 186
risk factors for 187
weight as risk factor 326
Heart failure 303
cardiac rehabilitation and 306
cough with foamy, pink mucus 307
emergencies 307
exercise and 305
heartbeat changes and 307
limiting fluids 306
low-sodium diet 304
medicines for 303
shortness of breath and 307
swelling in legs or feet 305, 307
weight gain and 305, 307
Heart palpitations 174
Heart problems (chart) 59
Heart rate, see Pulse rate
Heat exhaustion 39
Heat stroke 39
Heel pain 178
Heel spurs 178
Heimlich maneuver (illus.) 26
Helicobacter pylori (*H. pylori*), ulcers and 243
Hemodialysis 313
Hemoglobin A1c blood test 299
Hemorrhage, see Bleeding
Hemorrhoids 180
Hepatitis A 156
Hepatitis B 223
Herbal medicines 370
ginkgo biloba 124
saw palmetto 217
St. John's wort 293
Hernia 182
hiatal hernia 182
inguinal hernia (illus.) 182
surgery for 183
Herniated disc 80
anatomy of (illus.) 80
surgery for 90
Herpes, genital 223
Herpes, oral (cold sores) 118
Herpes virus
zoster (shingles) 225
Hiatal hernia 182
High blood pressure 183
DASH diet and 289
risk factors for 185
High cholesterol 186
Hip (illus.) 105
Hip fracture 34, 364
Hip pain 108
Hip replacement surgery 267
HIV (human immunodeficiency virus) 224
prevention 363
safe sex and 224
testing for 224
Hives 188
Hoarseness, see Laryngitis 196

Hormone replacement therapy (HRT) 202
Hospice care 387
  see also Palliative care 260
Hostility 76
Hot flashes 201, 202
HPV (human papillomavirus) 223
HRT (hormone replacement therapy) 202
Human bites 12
Human immunodeficiency virus, see HIV (human immunodeficiency virus)
Human papillomavirus (HPV) 223
Hydrocortisone cream, for rashes 220
Hypertension (high blood pressure) 183
Hypothermia 41
Hypothyroidism 146, 238
Hysterectomy 149

I

Ibuprofen, see Nonsteroidal anti-inflammatory drugs (NSAIDs)
Ice packs 51
Immunizations 320
  fever or rash after 321
  flu shots 154, 320
  pneumococcal vaccine 211, 320
  reactions to 321
  schedule for adults (chart) 320
  travel and 321
Immunotherapy (allergy shots) 75
Impaired glucose tolerance 298
Impotence 138
Incontinence
  fecal 79, 124
  urinary 92
Indigestion 176
Infection
  bladder or kidney 90
  breast 99
  cellulitis 220
  ear 135
  eye 140
  fungal 157
  mouth (thrush) 158
  prostate 217
  sexually transmitted 222
  sinus 227
  skin 27, 96, 98, 220
  swollen lymph nodes and 236
  tooth or gum 240
  urinary tract (bladder or kidney) 90
  vaginal 245
  wound 27, 44
Influenza (flu) 153
  antiviral medicine for 153
  flu shots 154, 320
Ingrown toenail 189
Inguinal hernia 182
Inhalers
  asthma medicines 274
  COPD medicines 282
Injuries
  abdominal 66
  back or neck 79
  belly, blow to 66
  broken bone 49
  bursitis 105
  cut 27
  dislocation 50
  fingers or toes, how to tape (illus.) 53
  head 36
  ice and cold packs for 51
  knee 194
  pulled muscle 49
  puncture wound 27
  RICE (rest, ice, compression, elevation) 50
  scrapes 44
  shock and 47
  slings for (illus.) 52
  spinal 79
  splinting (illus.) 53
  strain or sprain 49
  stress fracture 52
  tendinosis 105
Inner ear problem 131
Insect bites and stings 13
Insect repellent 16
Insomnia 232
  sleeping pills and 234
Insulin 296
Insurance
  long-term care 385
  Medicare 9
  prescriptions 3
Intertrigo (chafing) 219
Iron-deficiency anemia 147
Irritable bowel syndrome 190
Itching
  anal or rectal 181
  ear 135
  feet 158
  genitals 223
  how to relieve 134
  rashes and 218
  rectal or anal 180
  skin 134
  vaginal 223, 246
  with rash, warmth, or hives 73

J

Jaundice
  gallstones and 159
  hepatitis A and 156
  hepatitis B and 223

Jaw pain 192
  clicking or popping 192
  with signs of heart attack 38
Jock itch 158
Joint pain
  arthritis 266
  broken bones 49
  bursitis 105
  gout 163
  polymyalgia rheumatica 212
  sprains 49
  with rash or fever 270
  with swelling and redness 270
Joint replacement surgery 267

K

Kegel exercises 94
Keratoses, actinic 232
Keratoses, seborrheic 231
Kidney
  chronic kidney disease 308
  diabetic nephropathy 299
  dialysis 313
  infections 90
  kidney stones 193
  transplant 313
Knee anatomy (illus.) 195
Knee problems 194
  arthritis 266
  pain 108, 194
  see also Strains, sprains, and broken bones 49
Knee replacement surgery 267
Knocked out (unconscious) 33, 36

L

Labyrinthitis 131
Lacerations (cuts) 27
Lactose intolerance 128
Laryngitis 196
Laxatives, constipation and 125
LDL cholesterol 186
Legal affairs and wills 382, 386
Leg problems
  aching and swelling 96, 247
  blood clot in leg 96
  cramps 197
  infection (cellulitis) 220
  pain 80, 197, 208
  peripheral artery disease 208
  sciatica and leg pain 80
  shin splints 198
  sudden pain or swelling 197, 247
  unexplained tender lump 96, 247
  varicose veins 247
Levitra 139
Life support, decisions about 384
Lifting
  back pain and 85
  example of proper technique (illus.) 85
  hernias and 183
Lightheadedness 130
  see also Fainting and unconsciousness 33
Lipomas 237
Liver disease, hepatitis B and 223
Living will 383
Lockjaw (tetanus) 320
Long-term care insurance 385
Low-fat cooking 334
Low back pain 79
Lump
  in belly, groin, or behind knee 237
  in breast, armpit, or chest 99
  in groin or scrotum 182
  in leg 96, 247
  on or near anus 180
  see also Swollen lymph nodes 236
  under the skin 237
Lung problems
  blood clot in lung (pulmonary embolism) 97
  cancer 200
  chest, heart, and lung problems (chart) 59
  see also Breathing problems
Lyme disease 14
Lymph nodes, swollen 236
  location of (illus.) 237

M

Macular degeneration 250
  Amsler grid (illus.) 250
Malaria, shots to prevent 321
Male health, see Men's health
Male pelvic organs (illus.) 218
Mammograms 100, 324
Massage therapy, for back pain 83
Medical tests
  cost-saving tips 7
  screening tests (chart) 322–323
Medicare 9
Medicines
  allergic reaction to 74, 369
  anti-aging 373
  confusion as side effect 124
  cost-saving tips 3
  erection problems as side effect 139
  generics 3
  misuse or abuse of 70
  questions to ask 368
  rash after taking new medicine 218
  safe use of 124, 369
  see also Herbal medicines
  tips for taking 367
Meditation, for stress relief 357
Melanoma 230

Memory loss 122
  see also Alzheimer's disease 261
  thyroid problems and 238
Men's health
  condom use 363
  erection problems 138, 361
  exercise and fitness 340
  hernia 182
  prostate cancer 214
  prostate enlargement 215
  prostatitis 217
  sex and aging 361
  sexually transmitted diseases 222
  weight management 326
Ménière's disease 131, 132
Meningitis 151
Meniscus (knee cartilage) 195
Menopause 201
  hormone therapy and 202
  osteoporosis and 203, 207
  vaginal bleeding after 149, 201
Menstrual problems
  bleeding between periods 201
  missed or irregular periods 201
Mental health problems
  abuse and violent behavior 68
  Alzheimer's disease 123, 261
  anger and hostility 76
  anxiety 77
  confusion 122
  dementia 123, 261
  depression 146, 292
  grief 376
  insomnia 232
  memory loss 122
  panic disorder 77
  phobias 77
  seasonal affective disorder 294
  stress 356
  suicide 55
Migraine headaches 167
Milk (lactose) intolerance 128
Mineral supplements 337, 370
Minoxidil, for hair loss 165
Mold, allergies and 73
Moles, changes in (illus.) 231
Mood changes
  anger and hostility 76
  depression and 292
  drug problems and 71
  during winter 294
  menopause and 201
  stress and 356
Mosquitoes 16
  encephalitis and 151
  West Nile virus and 16
Mouth problems
  blisters on lips, mouth, or tongue 118
  canker sores 109
  cold sores 118
  dry mouth (chronic) 133
  dry mouth (dehydrated) 30
  jaw pain, clicking, or popping 192
  see also Dental problems
  sour taste in mouth 176
  sticky saliva (dehydrated) 30
  white patches inside mouth 158
Movement problems
  loss of on one side of body 54
  Parkinson's disease and 242
Multivitamins 337, 370
Muscle
  chest, pulled 116
  cramps 197
  pulled or strained 50
  relaxation techniques 358
  strengthening exercises (illus.) 345–349
  tension and stress 356
  tension with headache 167
Myocardial infarction (heart attack) 38, 114

N

Nail problems
  blood under nail 18
    how to drain (illus.) 18
  fungal infection 158
  ingrown toenail 189
Naproxen, see Nonsteroidal anti-inflammatory drugs (NSAIDs)
Nasal discharge, colored 227
Nasal spray, decongestant
  for colds 120
  for sinusitis 228
Nausea 253
  after meals 244
  see also Vomiting
  shock and 47
  with chest pain 38
  with headache 167
  with stiff neck, fever 151
Neck pain 204
  exercises for (illus.) 206
  meningitis and 151
  prevention 205
  spinal injury 79
  stiff neck with headache, fever, vomiting 151
  tension headaches and 167
  whiplash 204
  with jaw pain 192
Neglect or abuse 69
Nephropathy, diabetic 299
Nervousness, see Anxiety 77

Neuropathy, diabetic 299
Nicotine replacement products 352
Nightmares 77
Nipple, discharge from or changes in 99
Nitroglycerin 289
  erection-producing medicines and 138, 289
Noise, hearing problems and 170, 173
Nonsteroidal anti-inflammatory drugs (NSAIDs)
  hearing loss and 170
  heartburn and 177
  see also Aspirin
  ulcers and 243
Nosebleeds 43
  how to stop (illus.) 43
Nose drops, saline 228, 229
Nose problems
  nasal discharge, colored 227
  nose and throat problems (chart) 63
  nosebleeds 43
  runny or stuffy nose 73, 119, 227
  sinusitis 227
Numbness or tingling
  after head injury 36
  after injury 49
  in arm or hand 204
  in genital or rectal area 79
  in leg or foot 79, 80, 178, 194, 208
  in wrist or fingers 110
  on one side of body 54
Nursing homes 382
  Alzheimer's disease and 264
Nutrition 333
  fats in foods 334
  fiber 336
  fruits and vegetables 333
  guidelines (MyPyramid) 338
  portion control 327
  protein 337
  salt (sodium) 338
  sugar 338
  vitamin and mineral supplements 337, 370
  water 339
  weight management and 326
  whole grains 335

O

Obesity 326, 330
Object in eye 31
  how to remove (illus.) 32
Office ergonomics, see Ergonomics
Orthostatic hypotension (low blood pressure) 131
Osteoarthritis, see Arthritis 266
Osteopaths, back pain and 83
Osteoporosis 207
  back problems and 80
  menopause and 203
Otitis media (middle ear infection) 135
Ovarian cancer 149
Overweight 326, 330
Oxygen therapy, for COPD 286

P

Pain
  abdominal 66
  arthritis 266
  back 79
  back, with painful urination 90
  between belly button and breastbone 244
  breast 99
  chest 114
  chest-wall 102, 116, 210
  during ejaculation 217
  during or after sex 223
  ear 135
  elbow 106
  eye 62, 143, 162
  facial 169, 226
  flank (side), with painful urination 90
  foot or toe 103
  groin or scrotum 182
  hand or wrist 106
  heel 178
  hip or thigh 108
  in cheek, upper teeth, forehead, or behind eyes 227
  in front of lower leg 108
  jaw 192
  joints 105
  knee 108, 194
  leg 197
  lower belly/pelvic (females) 66
  lower belly/pelvic (male) 217
  neck 204
  pelvic/lower back (males) 215
  rectal or anal 124, 180
  shoulder 107
  side or groin 193
  toothache 240
  widespread, with fatigue 152
Pain management
  arthritis 266
  cancer and 278
Palliative care 260
  cancer and 281
Pancreatitis 67
Panic attacks 77
Pap test 323
Paralysis
  after head injury 36
  after injury 49
  sudden, on one side of body 54
Parasites
  diarrhea and 127
  food poisoning 155

Parkinson's disease 242
Pelvic exam, female 323
Pelvic inflammatory disease (PID) 223
Pelvic organs, female (illus.) 323
Pelvic organs, male (illus.) 218
Pelvic pain (male) 217
Pelvic problems, female 148
  cancer 149
  pain 148, 223
  sexually transmitted diseases 223
  vaginitis 245
Penis, discharge from 217, 223
Peptic ulcer 243
Periodontal disease 164
Peripheral artery disease 208
Peritoneal dialysis 313
Pertussis vaccine 320
Pet dander, allergies to 75
Phlebitis 198
Phobias 77
Physical activity, see Exercise 340
Physicals (wellness exams) 321
Physical therapy, for back pain 83
Piles (hemorrhoids) 180
Pinched nerve in neck 204
Pinkeye 140
  how to remove crusts (illus.) 141
Plantar fasciitis 178
  location of plantar fascia (illus.) 178
Plantar warts 254
Plant rashes 219
Pleurisy, chest pain and 116
Pneumococcal vaccine 211, 320
Pneumonia 210
Poisoning, carbon monoxide 64, 166
Poison ivy, oak, or sumac 219
Polymyalgia rheumatica 212
Post-traumatic stress 77
Postnasal drip 120, 227
Posture
  back pain and 84
  examples of (illus.) 84, 85
Power of attorney for health care 383
Prediabetes 298
Prehypertension 184
Presbycusis 171
Presbyopia 249
Prescriptions, see Medicines
Pressure sores 213
Preventive care, screening tests and 321
Progressive muscle relaxation 358
Prostate (illus.) 218
Prostate cancer 214
Prostate enlargement 215
  enlarged prostate (illus.) 216
Prostate exam 215
Prostatitis 217
PSA (prostate-specific antigen) test 215
Pulmonary embolism 97
Pulmonary rehabilitation 285
Pulse rate, see also Heartbeat
  exercise and 343
  fast, with anxiety 77
  fast, with chest pain 38, 114
  fast or irregular 174
  how to count (illus.) 48
  resting 48
  slowed 41
  weak and fast 47
Puncture wounds 27
Pyelonephritis (kidney infection) 90

Q

Quitting smoking 351

R

Rabies 12
Radiation therapy for cancer 276
Rashes 218
  after immunizations 321
  after taking new medicine 218, 369
  after tick bite 13, 14
  chafing 219
  expanding red rash 13, 14
  poison ivy, oak, or sumac 219
  scarlet fever 235
  see also Fungal infections 157
  shingles 225
  skin problems (chart) 61
  sore throat and 235
  sudden, with purple or red spots under skin 151
  with fever, stiff neck, headache 151
  with itching, warmth, or hives 73
  with joint pain and fever 270
Raynaud's 117
Rectal problems 180
  anal fissure 181
  bleeding 17, 121, 180, 243
  colon polyps 121
  colorectal cancer 121, 181
  constipation 124
  exam, digital rectal 215
  hemorrhoids 180
  itching 180, 181
  leakage from anus 180
  lump 180
  pain 124, 180
  warts (anal) 223
Reflux, of stomach acid 176
  coughs and 126
Rehydration drinks 30
  diarrhea and 128
Relapsing fever, see Tick bites 14
Relaxation techniques 358

Rescue breathing 19
Respiratory problems, see Breathing problems
Retinal detachment 62, 251
Retinopathy, diabetic 251, 299
Rheumatic fever 236
RICE (rest, ice, compression, elevation), for injuries 50
Ringing in ears (tinnitus) 173
Ringworm 158
Rocky Mountain spotted fever, see Tick bites 14
Rosacea 221
Rubbers, see Condoms 363
Ruby spots 231
Runny nose 73, 119

S

Sacroiliac joints 80
Sadness, persistent 146
  see also Grieving 376
Safe sex 363
Safety
  driving safety 365
  fall prevention 364
  food safety 155
  medicine, safe use of 367
Salicylic acid, for warts 255
Saliva, lack of, see Dry mouth 133
Salmonella, see Food poisoning 155
Salt (sodium) 338
Saturated fats 335
Saw palmetto, for prostate enlargement 217
Scarlet fever 61, 235
Sciatica 80
Sclerotherapy for varicose veins 247
Scrapes 44
Screening tests 321
  for alcohol and drug problems 71
  for breast cancer 100, 324
  for cervical cancer 323
  for colorectal cancer 121
  for glaucoma 163
  for hearing problems 322
  for high cholesterol 187
  for HIV (human immunodeficiency virus) 224
  for prostate cancer 215
  for thyroid problems 239
  schedule (chart) 322–323
  skin self-exam 230
Scrotum
  bulge or lump in 182
  sudden, severe pain 182
Seasonal affective disorder 294
Seborrheic dermatitis 219
Seborrheic keratoses 231
Seizures 45
Senility, see Confusion and memory loss 122
Senior health, see Aging
Sex
  aging and 361
  erection problems 138, 361
  pain during 223, 361
  safe sex 363
  vaginal bleeding during or after 223
Sexual abuse 68
Sexually transmitted diseases 222
  prevention 363
  risk for 363
  vaginitis and 246
Shaking (tremor) 241
Shingles 225
  vaccine 226, 320
Shin splints 108, 198
Shivering 41
Shock 47
Shortness of breath 101
  after insect sting 13
  asthma and 271
  bronchitis and 102
  COPD and 282, 286
  heart failure and 303, 307
  lung cancer and 200
  with chest pain 114
  with chest pain, coughing up blood 96
  with signs of heart attack 38
Shots, see Immunizations 320
Shoulder
  anatomy of (illus.) 107
  dislocation 50
  pain 107
Sinusitis 227
  antibiotics for 228
  colds and 227
  location of sinuses (illus.) 227
Sitz baths, for hemorrhoids 181
Skin cancer 230
  actinic keratoses 232
Skin problems
  actinic keratoses 232
  age spots 231
  athlete's foot 158
  bedsores 213
  blisters 95
  blood spots under skin 218
  blue, gray, or blotchy skin 19
  boil 98
  breast or nipple, changes in 99
  burns 23
  calluses 109
  cellulitis 220
  chafing 219
  chemical burns 25
  cold hands or feet 117
  cool, moist, pale, or red skin 39
  cool, pale, moist skin 47
  corns 109

cuts 27
dry skin 134
facial redness 221
frostbite 35
fungal infections 157
growths or sores 230, 231
hives 188
infected wound 27
infection (cellulitis) 220
itching 134
jaundice, with gallstones 159
jock itch 158
lip or mouth sores (cold sores) 118
lump under the skin 237
moles 230
mouth sores (canker sores) 109
pressure sores 213
puncture wounds 27
rash after tick bite 14
rashes 218
red, hot, and dry skin 39
ringworm 158
rosacea 221
scrapes 44
sebaceous gland growths 232
seborrheic dermatitis 219
seborrheic keratoses 231
self-exam for skin cancer 230
shingles 225
skin cancer 230
skin problems (chart) 61
skin tags 232
splinters 49
sunburn 56
varicose veins 247
warts 254
yellowing (jaundice) 156, 223

Sleep apnea 233
Sleeping pills 234
Sleep problems 232
Alzheimer's disease and 262
anxiety and 77
depression and 146
insomnia 232
snoring 234

Slivers (splinters) 49
Smoking
asthma and 272
chronic cough and 126
COPD and 282
coronary artery disease and 290
erection problems and 139
high blood pressure and 185
lung cancer and 200
osteoporosis and 207
quitting 351
ulcers and 243

Snakebites, splinting after 53
Sneezing 73, 119
Snoring 234
Sore throat 235
with cold symptoms 119
with fever 235

Speech problems, new or sudden 54
after head injury 36

Spiders
bites from 13
black widow (illus.) 14
brown recluse (illus.) 14

Spider veins 247
Spinal injury 79
Spinal stenosis 83
Spinning sensation, see Vertigo 130
Splinters 49
Splinting, after injury 53
Sports drinks, for dehydration 30, 31
Sports injuries
Achilles tendon problems 179
ice and cold packs for 51
knee problems 194
plantar fasciitis 178
strains, sprains, and broken bones 49
stress fractures 52

Sprains 49
St. John's wort, for depression 293
Stabbing, see Puncture wounds 27
STDs (sexually transmitted diseases) 222
Steroids, high blood pressure and 185
Stiff neck 204
Stings, insect 13
Stitches 29
Stomachache, see Abdominal pain 66
Stomach flu
diarrhea and 127
see also Food poisoning 155
vomiting and 253

Stools
bloody or black 17, 127, 180, 190
leakage 124, 180
mucus in 190
test for blood in 122

Stool softeners, for constipation 125
Strains, muscle or ligament 50
Strength training 343
Strep throat 235
rheumatic fever and 236
scarlet fever and 235

Stress
headaches and 167
sleep problems and 232
stress management 356

Stress fractures 52
Stretching 349
basic exercises (illus.) 345–350

Stroke 54
aspirin for preventing 290
atrial fibrillation and 175
caregiving tips 317
driving after 316
high blood pressure and 184
high cholesterol and 186
life after 314
rehabilitation 314
weight as risk factor 326
Styes 144
Subconjunctival hemorrhage 143
Substance abuse 70
Suicide 55
Sunburn 56
Sun exposure
actinic keratoses and 232
skin cancer and 230
Supplements
herbal 370
see also Herbal medicines
vitamin and mineral 337, 370
Sutures (stitches) 29
Swallowing
difficulty, with blurred vision 155
painful or difficult 176, 235, 243
Sweating
anxiety and 77
dehydration and 30, 31
heat sickness and 39
with signs of heart attack 38
Swelling
after bone, muscle, or joint injury 49
after insect sting 13
ice and cold packs for 51
in leg or calf with fever 197
in legs or feet, with heart failure 305, 307
lips, tongue, or face (allergic reaction) 73
lymph nodes 236
Swimmer's ear 136
Swollen lymph nodes 236
location of (illus.) 237
Syphilis 223

T

Tearing, excessive 144
Teeth, see Dental problems
Temperature, see also Fever 150
heat sickness and 39
hypothermia and 41
Temporal arteritis 169
Temporomandibular (TM) disorder 192
Tendinosis (tendinitis) 105
Achilles 108, 179
elbow (illus.) 106, 107
hip 108
ice and cold packs for 51
patellar (knee) 195
shoulder (illus.) 107
Tendon strain or tear 50
Tennis elbow 107
Tension (stress) 356
Tension headaches 167
Testicular problems
bulge or lump 182
sudden, severe pain 182
Tests, screening (chart) 322–323
Tetanus shot 320
after cut or puncture wound 27
after scrape 44
Throat problems
laryngitis 196
nose and throat problems (chart) 63
postnasal drip 120, 227
sore throat 119, 235
sour taste in throat 176
strep throat 235
swallowing problems 176, 235, 243
Thrombophlebitis 96
Throwing up 253
Thrush 158
Thyroid problems
fatigue and 146
hair loss and 165
hypothyroidism 238
TIA (transient ischemic attack) 54
Tick bites 13
how to remove a tick (illus.) 15
Lyme disease and 14
Tinnitus 173
TM (temporomandibular) disorder 192
Tobacco use, quitting 351
Toenails, how to cut (illus.) 189
Toe problems
bunion 103
calluses and corns 109
hammer toe 103
ingrown toenail (illus.) 189
joint pain 163
nail, blood under 18
nail, fungal infection 158
pain and swelling 103, 163
Tonsils, coating on 235
Toothache 240
sinusitis and 227
Tooth injury or loss 241
Trans fats 335
Transient ischemic attack (TIA) 54
Tremor 241
Trichomoniasis 223
Trigeminal neuralgia 169
Triglycerides 186
Type 1 or type 2 diabetes, see Diabetes 296
Typhoid, shots to prevent 321

U

Ulcers 243
  location of (illus.) 244
Unconsciousness 33
  head injury and 36
  shock and 47
Underweight 326, 330
  nutrition tips 340
Upper respiratory infections
  colds 119
  flu (influenza) 153
  sinusitis 227
Urinary problems
  blood in urine 193
  burning with urination 91, 223
  dribbling (males) 216
  frequent urination 91
    in males only 216, 217
  incontinence 92
    Kegel exercises for 94
  kidney stones 193
  loss of bladder control (incontinence) 92
  not able to urinate 90
  painful urination 91, 223
    in males only 217
  see also Urine
  trouble starting or stopping urine stream (males) 216
  urinary problems (chart) 65
  urinary tract infections 90
  weak urine stream (males) 216, 217
Urinary tract (illus.) 91
Urine
  blood in 65, 90, 193
  blood in (males) 215
  cloudy 91
  dark yellow urine 30
  leakage 92
  pus in 90
  pus in (males) 215
  reduced amounts 30
  unusual odor 91
Urticaria (hives) 188
Uterine (endometrial) cancer 149, 202
Uterine fibroids 149
UTI (urinary tract infection) 90

V

Vaccinations, see Immunizations 320
Vaginal bleeding, after menopause 149
Vaginal discharge 223, 245, 246
Vaginal dryness 245, 361
  lubricants for 203, 361
  menopause and 201, 202
Vaginal itching 223, 246
Vaginitis 245
  types of (chart) 246
  yeast infections 245
Varicella, see Shingles 225
Varicose veins 247
Vein, inflamed (phlebitis) 198
Venereal diseases (VD), see Sexually transmitted diseases 222
Vertigo 130
Viagra 139
Violent behavior or abuse 68
  see also Anger 76
Vision problems
  adapting to reduced vision 251
  after blow to eye 22
  after chemical exposure or fumes 25
  after head injury 36
  blank or dark spots 249, 250, 251
  blind spots 162
  blurred vision 54, 162, 250
  blurred vision with trouble swallowing or breathing 155
  cataracts 113
  cloudy or foggy vision 113
  diabetic retinopathy 251
  double vision 113
  driving safety and 365
  eye and vision problems (chart) 62
  floaters or flashes of light 62, 249, 251
  glare 113
  glaucoma 162
  loss of focus 249, 250
  macular degeneration 250
  normal changes with aging 248, 249
  retinal detachment 62, 251
  screening test for glaucoma 163
  see also Eye problems
  vision loss, sudden 54, 62, 162, 249, 251
Vitamin D, osteoporosis and 208
Vitamin supplements 337, 370
Voice, loss of (laryngitis) 196
Vomiting 253
  after head injury 36
  after meals 244
  bloody 17, 176, 253
  dehydration and 29, 30
  with abdominal pain and fever 67
  with dizziness or vertigo 131
  with groin pain and fever 182
  with painful urination 90
  with pain in groin, side, or back 193
  with stiff neck, headache, fever 151

W

Waist size (circumference) 330
Walker, how to use (illus.) 269
Walking 344
Warfarin (Coumadin), see Blood thinners
Warts 254
  genital warts 223
Water, daily intake 339

Water, untreated, and diarrhea 127
Weakness 145
  anemia and 147
  bone (osteoporosis) 207
  heart failure and 303
  in arm or hand 204
  in leg or foot 79, 80
  shock and 47
  sudden, on one side of body 54
    after head injury 36
Weight gain
  heart failure and 305, 307
  see also Weight management
  thyroid problems and 238
  unexplained 145
Weightlifting 343
Weight loss
  excessive 330
  unexplained 121, 145, 176, 190, 243
Weight loss, see also Weight management
Weight management 326
  body mass index (BMI) 330, 331
  diets and 329
  exercise and 327, 341
  gaining if you are underweight 330
  healthy eating and 326
  healthy weight ranges 331
  high blood pressure and 184
  portion control 327
  waist size (circumference) 330, 332
Wellness exams 321
West Nile virus 16
Wheezing 19, 101
  after insect sting 13
  allergic reaction 73
  asthma and 271
  bronchitis and 102
  COPD and 286
  lung cancer and 200
Whiplash 204
Whooping cough (pertussis) vaccine 320
Wills 386
  ethical 385
Withdrawal
  from alcohol or drugs 70, 71
  from antidepressants 294
  from nicotine 352
Women's health
  breast exams 324, 325
  breast problems 99
  cancer, pelvic and gynecological 149
  endometriosis 149
  exercise and fitness 340
  fibroids, uterine 149
  hormone therapy 202
  hysterectomy 149
  mammograms 324
  menopause 201
  osteoporosis 207
  Pap test 323, 324
  pelvic infections 223, 245
  pelvic pain 148, 149
  sex and aging 361
  sexually transmitted diseases 222, 223–224
  vaginal bleeding 148
  vaginal dryness 201, 245
  vaginitis 245
  weight management 326
  yeast infections 245
Worrying, see Anxiety 77
Wrist or hand problems
  carpal tunnel syndrome 110
  cold intolerance 117
  pain 106
  shaking (tremor) in hands 241
  weak grip 110
  wrist sprain 50

X

Xerostomia, see Dry mouth 133

Y

Yeast infections
  mouth (thrush) 158
  vaginal 245
Yellow fever, shots to prevent 321
Yoga, for stress relief 357

Z

Zyban (bupropion), for quitting smoking 352